Progress in Clinical Science Series

Progress in the Treatment of Fluency Disorders

Edited by

Lena Rustin
Speech Therapy Services
Finsbury Health Centre, London

Harry Purser
School of Speech Pathology
Leicester Polytechnic

David Rowley
School of Speech Pathology
Leicester Polytechnic

Taylor & Francis
London New York Philadelphia
1987

UK   Taylor & Francis Ltd, 4 John St., London WC1N 2ET

USA   Taylor & Francis Inc., 242 Cherry St., Philadelphia, PA 19106–1906

British Library Cataloguing in Publication Data

Progress in the treatment of fluency disorders.

  (Progress in clinical science series)
  Includes indexes.
  1. Stuttering.   2. Speech therapy.   I. Rustin, Lena.
II. Purser, Harry.   III. Rowley,   David.   IV. Series
[DNLM: 1. Stuttering—therapy.   WM 475 P964]
RC424.P95   1987   616.85′ 54   87–7074
ISBN 0–85066–664–3
ISBN 0–85066–683–X (soft)

Typeset by Chapterhouse, The Cloisters, Halsall Lane, Formby
Printed in Great Britain by Taylor & Francis (Printers) Ltd.
Basingstoke, Hants.

Progress in the Treatment of Fluency Disorders

PROGRESS IN CLINICAL SCIENCE SERIES

Clinical Information Technology
by David Rowley and Harry Purser

Progress in the Treatment of Fluency Disorders
Edited by Lena Rustin, Harry Purser and David Rowley

Counselling Individuals: The Rational Emotive Approach
by Windy Dryden

Disorders of Communication: The Science of Intervention
Edited by Margaret Leahy

Linguistics in Clinical Practice
Edited by Kim Grundy

Contents

Contributing Authors   vii
Foreword   xi
Preface   xiii
Acknowledgments   xv

Introduction: A Tutorial on Stuttering
Gavin Andrews   xvii

I   THE NEUROPSYCHOLOGY OF STUTTERING   1

1 **Neuropsychological Models of Speech Dysfluency**
   David B. Rosenfield and Harvey B. Nudelman   3

2 **Hemispheric Processing and Stuttering**
   Walter H. Moore, Jr and Einer Boberg   19

3 **An Approach to the Study of Motor Speech
   Mechanisms in Stuttering**
   C. Woodruff Starkweather, Joy M. Armson and
   Barbara J. Amster   43

**II   THE ASSESSMENT AND TREATMENT OF
       STUTTERING**   59

4 **Linguistic Profiling of Stuttering Behaviour**
   Susan Edwards and William Hardcastle   61

5 **Assessment and Diagnosis of Childhood Dysfluency**
   Edward G. Conture and Anthony J. Caruso   84

6 The Treatment of Stuttering: Recent History and
   Contemporary Issues
   Hugo H. Gregory   105

7 The Cooper Personalized Fluency Control Therapy
   Program
   Eugene B. Cooper   124

8 Personal Construct Theory and the Treatment of
   Adolescent Dysfluency
   Willie Botterill and Frances Cook   147

9 The Treatment of Childhood Dysfluency Through
   Active Parental Involvement
   Lena Rustin   166

10 Paradoxical Therapy in the Treatment of Stuttering
   Armin Kuhr   181

11 Self-help for Stutterers — Experience in Britain
   Bryan Hunt   198

12 Informing Stutterers About Treatment
   Gavin Andrews, Megan Neilson and Mary Cassar   213

   III   THE EFFECTS OF TREATMENT FOR
         STUTTERING   233

13 The Effectiveness of Treatment for Stuttering
   Kenneth O. St. Louis and Janice B. Westbrook   235

14 The Psychology of Treatment Evaluation
   Harry Purser   258

References   274
Index   305

Contributing Authors

Barbara Amster
Assistant Professor
Department of Pediatrics
Medical College of Pennsylvania
USA

Joy Armson
Doctoral Candidate
Department of Speech Pathology
Temple University
Pennsylvania
USA

Gavin Andrews
Professor of Psychiatry
Department of Psychiatry
St. Vincents Hospital
Sydney
Australia

Einer Boberg
Professor of Speech Pathology
University of Alberta
Canada

Willie Botterill
Senior Speech Therapist
Bloomsbury, Hampstead &
    Islington DHAs
London
UK

Anthony Caruso
Research Associate
Speech Motor Control Laboratories
Waisman Center
University of Wisconsin
Wisconsin
USA

Mary Cassar
Speech Pathologist
St. Vincents Hospital
Sydney
Australia

Edward Conture
Professor of Speech Pathology
Department of Speech Pathology
Syracuse University
Syracuse
New York
USA

Frances Cook
Chief Speech Therapist
Bloomsbury, Hampstead &
  Islington DHAs
London
UK

Eugene Cooper
Professor of Speech Pathology
University of Alabama
Texas
USA

Susan Edwards
Lecturer in Linguistics
Department of Linguistics
University of Reading
Reading
UK

Hugo Gregory
Professor of Speech Pathology
Northwestern University
Illinois
USA

William Hardcastle
Senior Lecturer in Linguistics
Department of Linguistics
University of Reading
Reading
UK

Dr Brian Hunt
Association of Stutterers
Hendon
London
UK

Armin Kuhr
Senior Lecturer in Clinical Psychology
Hannover Medical School
West Germany

Walter H. Moore
Professor of Neuropsychology
California State University
Long Beach
USA

Megan Neilson
Scientific Officer
St. Vincents Hospital
Sydney
Australia

Harvey Nudelman
Professor
Department of Neurology
Baylor College of Medicine
Texas
USA

Harry Purser
Senior Lecturer in Clinical Psychology
Leicester Polytechnic
Leicester
UK

David Rosenfield
Director — Stuttering Centre
Baylor College of Medicine
Texas
USA

David Rowley
Senior Lecturer in Experimental
  Psychology
Leicester Polytechnic
Leicester
UK

Lena Rustin
Director — Speech Therapy Services
Bloomsbury, Hampstead &
  Islington DHAs
London
UK

Kenneth St. Louis
Professor of Speech Pathology and
  Audiology
West Virginia University
West Virginia
USA

Woodruff Starkweather
Professor and Director
Program in Speech Language and
  Hearing Sciences
Temple University
Pennsylvania
USA

Janice Westbrook
Fluency Specialist
Dallas Independent School District
Texas
USA

Foreword

This book is one of a series whose primary aim is to inform the professional practice of speech and language clinicians and their colleagues in the caring professions. The starting point for this series was a systematic review of those topics in human communication which are essential to the development of effective treatment programmes and the development of effective clinicians.

Whilst we have seen considerable advances in the scientific understanding of communication disorders in recent years much that is relevant to the practising clinician is either published in specialist scientific journals or exchanged on the conference floor. Bringing this theoretical and practical material together in book form seemed the first priority for a series of this kind. *Progress in Clinical Science* therefore aims to emphasise the scientific basis of modern clinical practice.

In addition we saw a need for texts capable of addressing broader issues in clinical practice. We wanted to provide a new resource for clinicians who wished to further their own social, interpersonal and scientific skills through further study. Topics here range from discussion of specific models of clinical intervention to the skills required for the scientific evaluation of the treatment enterprise.

Research into both the process and outcome of therapy programmes has revealed that individual therapist characteristics play a crucial role in the success or failure of treatment over a wide range of treatment approaches and client groups. Every therapist needs an injection of new stimulation in order to continue the process of evolution that characterises effective clinical practice. We need to be self-critical and we need to introduce systems of peer review in order to ensure that the work we do on behalf of our clients is of the highest possible standard. This series emphasises the need for efficacy research and the responsibility each individual clinician carries for the evaluation of their own clinical skills.

We are grateful for the help and support we have received from colleagues in many professional groups during the development of *Progress in Clinical Science*. It is our hope that the books in this series will cut across traditional disciplinary boundaries. The problems of theory construction, skill acquisition and treatment evaluation are common to every caring profession. We hope that *Progress in Clinical Science* will bring a fresh incentive for interdisciplinary collaboration at every level of professional development.

Harry Purser and Dave Rowley
Series Editors
Leicester Polytechnic, UK.

Preface

Progress in the Treatment of Fluency Disorders was conceived during the summer of 1985 as a consequence of a conference jointly sponsored by the Speech Foundation of America and the UK College of Speech Therapists. The *Oxford Dysfluency Conference* had the distinction of being the first international symposium dedicated to the problem of speech dysfluency to be held in the United Kingdom.

The aims of the Oxford conference were twofold: first, to provide an opportunity for fluency specialists from the UK, USA and Europe to meet and discuss contemporary issues relating to both the nature and treatment of stuttering; second, to disseminate clinical treatment skills through a number of practical workshops led by acknowledged international experts in the therapy process. The event stimulated an enormous amount of interest amongst therapists and research workers and attracted delegates from all over the globe. By the end of the conference it was evident that there was both the will and the demand for a new volume of readings which captured the spirit of the event. This book is the result.

The conference programme was specifically commissioned to reflect new developments in theory and practice as well as highlighting established positions on the treatment of speech dysfluency. When we sat down to plan this volume we decided to emphasise two main themes. The first concerns the neuro-psychological and neuromotor dimensions of fluent speech. In the search for working models of stuttering we are inevitably drawn to the complex contemporary research literature on brain–behaviour relationships. We were conscious of the keen interest that many clinicians have in this area and therefore resolved to dedicate a section of this volume to a systematic review of the field. The second theme is of course the treatment of stuttering. Here our intention has been to provide a blend of new ideas as well as some of the very best examples of tried and tested treatment approaches. The material selected for inclusion ranges from innovative perspectives on the assessment and treatment of stuttering, through specific therapy programmes, to detailed accounts of the treatment process from the client's viewpoint. We hope that the ideas contained here will provide a further stimulus to the development of effective treatment for stuttering.

In the course of bringing together the material for this book we have commissioned a number of specific reviews of particular topics as well as chapters based on material presented at the Oxford Conference. We are indebted to all our colleagues who worked with such patience and determination to provide the profession with what we hope will become a valued resource for both practising clinicians and their students in training.

Lena Rustin, Harry Purser, David Rowley

Acknowledgments

We wish to thank Jane Fraser and the Speech Foundation of America, the College of Speech Therapists and the University of Oxford for their help and support during the initial stages of this project. We also wish to thank Chris Code for his advice in the editorial process and Sentinel Software, Mekom and Andy Shimell for technical support.

Introduction: A Tutorial on Stuttering

Gavin Andrews

Overview

Stuttering is a disorder in the rhythm of speech in which individuals know precisely what they wish to say, but at the time are unable to say it because of involuntary repetition, prolongation or cessation of sound. It is quite distinct from the non-fluencies of normal speakers for these consist of whole word repetitions, phrase repetitions and interjections, with virtually no repetitions or prolongations of single sounds. Ordinary or idiopathic stuttering is a disorder that begins in childhood, usually between the onset of speech and the age of school entry, and almost always before puberty. Most stutterers begin by repeating syllables, and these repetitions, together with prolongations are necessary and sufficient for the disorder to be diagnosed. In some children, particularly as the stutter becomes more severe, speech becomes more disrupted because of tense pauses, breathing irregularities and other facial and body movements associated with the act of speaking. In severe stutterers even the speech between stutters is abnormally dysrhythmic.

Just under 5 per cent of all children will experience a period of stuttering that lasts three months or more, but because of cases of late onset and early remission, the prevalence seldom rises above 1 per cent. Four out of five children who experience a period of stuttering will no longer be stuttering by the age of 16. Three times as many boys as girls stutter and the sex ratio increases with age, for the girls recover more quickly than boys.

Stuttering can be caused by brain disturbances in both children and adults and hence there is an increased prevalence associated with perinatal brain damage, cerebral palsy, epilepsy, head injury and other neurological conditions. In adults a typical repetitive stutter can follow a severe psychological trauma but this syndrome is usually self-limited unless perpetuated by the prospect of compensation or other primary gain.

Idiopathic stutterers come from families in which there is an increased risk of family members themselves having been troubled by stuttering. The risk of stuttering among these first degree relatives varies by sex of relative and sex of stutterer so that for men who have stuttered, 9 per cent of their daughters and 22 per cent of their sons will stutter; while for the fewer women who ever stuttered the risk are higher, as 17 per cent of their daughters and 36 per cent of their sons will be affected. The risk of stuttering in a monozygotic co-twin of a stutterer is 75 per cent. These data are consistent with inheritance being a major determinant in most cases, although severity of stuttering itself does not appear to be under genetic control. As discordant monozygotic twins exist environmental factors clearly do play some part, but despite considerable research, brain damage acquired at birth or subsequently is the only factor to have been demonstrated.

When children who stutter are compared with children who do not stutter they are found to score half a standard deviation lower on tests of intelligence. They show half a year school grade disadvantage and are over represented in classes for educationally subnormal children. Stutterers are more likely to be delayed in speech development, to perform less well on tests of language proficiency, and to show articulation defects independent of and in addition to their stutter. Many comparisons of neurological functioning have been performed. There are no established differences in laterality as measured by handedness, dichotic word test, or intracarotid sodium amytal, although there is increased right hemisphere alpha suppression during speech related tasks. Stutterers perform less well on tests of central auditory function, and are slower in auditory and visual voice reaction times and in auditory–motor pursuit tracking tasks.

Stuttering is not an emotional disorder and stutterers and their parents are just as, and no more neurotic than nonstutterers. Stutterers seen in the clinic are often able and intelligent, for they are precisely the people who are referred for treatment because of their handicap to verbal communication. This selection bias means that research findings on groups of stutterers obtained primarily from clinic sources may well not reveal the actual state of affairs among stutterers as a whole.

Much is often made of the variability of stuttering, but this is more apparent than real, for a severe stutterer will be severely afflicted whenever measured in an ordinary speaking situation and a mild stutterer will likewise always be mild. Thus there are no systematic variations in frequency of stutter that are common to all stutterers across time or across ordinary speaking situations although individuals will know of factors which cause variation in their own severity. Severity, for most stutterers, does vary systematically in some unusual or laboratory conditions. Stuttering is more frequent when reading to an audience of increasing size or when saying the initial words of sentences or words of greater complexity or uncertainty. It can be temporarily eliminated in seven conditions: *chorus reading, lipped speech, prolonged speech, rhythmic speech, shadowing, singing,* and *when speaking very slowly.* The prolonged speech technique is the basis for many current treatment programmes.

Stuttering can be progressively eliminated by response contingent stimulation. It can be immediately reduced in six conditions: *speaking alone, speaking with rhythmic movement, delayed auditory feedback, masking, change in pitch,* and *whispering*. Lastly, there are three conditions which progressively reduce stuttering: *adaptation, speech muscle EMG feedback,* and *taking haloperidol*. Many of these changes are dramatic, some are used as the basis of therapy, but most seem to work because they simplify the information that has to be integrated if speech is to be accurately controlled. Thus these conditions are also effective in aiding normal speakers to eliminate their normal nonfluencies.

Treatment and the Nature of Stuttering

Some years ago we used the meta–analytic technique to compare the efficiency of all treatment techniques on which empirical data was available. Five treatments appeared promising: *prolonged speech, precision fluency shaping, rhythmic speech, airflow therapies,* and *attempts to modify attitudes*. More recent data have convinced us that only the prolonged speech and precision fluency shaping techniques have the capacity to produce long term fluency in a majority of stutterers.

What then is stuttering? We have hypothesised that due to an inherited or acquired deficit in their central cortical capacity for speech, stutterers have a diminished ability to deal with the relationship between motor activity and the associated sensory activity produced during speech. As a consequence the stutterer, in order to speak fluently, must either spend additional time occupied with this relationship or must utilize additional capacity at the expense of other mental functions. This view would suggest that whether one will become a stutterer depends on a trade off between one's neurological capacity for speech and the level of communication demand.

Thus stuttering should have a peak frequency of onset at a time when an explosive growth in language ability outstrips a still immature speech motor apparatus and the peak age for spontaneous recovery should occur when the motor ability catches up with the language demand. The peak ages for onset and remission are consistent with these ideas. As said before, one explanation for the effect of the fluency inducing conditions is that they simplify the speech motor control task. No one has yet shown that persons with the more severe forms of dysfluency have the most reduced central capacity for sensory motor integration and it is not clear what determines the frequency of the primary symptoms of stuttering. The secondary symptoms of stuttering are different and are probably learned as instrumentally acquired adjustive responses.

The data on which this tutorial is based are contained in two review papers: *Andrews, Guitar and Howie (1980)* and *Andrews, Craig, Feyer, Hoddinot, Howie and Neilson (1983)*.

I THE NEUROPSYCHOLOGY OF STUTTERING

Ever since the early pioneering work of the nineteenth century neurologists there has been a special place accorded to speech and language functions in the exploration of brain–behaviour relationships. The classic work of Broca and Wernicke in their studies of aphasiology has stimulated subsequent generations of research workers to address the general issue of the neural mechanisms underlying speech and language.

From those early anatomical studies of the human brain a number of new 'neurosciences' have gradually evolved. Perhaps the most clinically relevant perspective is offered by the fusion of neurology and neurophysiology with the methods of experimental psychology: *neuropsychology*. In neuropsychology the focus of study is the working relationship between neural structures and overt perceptual, motor, cognitive and emotional behaviour. This branch of the neurosciences has been developed by many eminent research workers and clinicians whose work underpins our understanding of the clinical brain disorders. Modern clinical neuropsychology is a complex and wide ranging field of endeavour which offers exciting new insights to the practicing therapist.

The problem of stuttering has received its fair share of attention from neuropsychologists during the past fifty years. Indeed it has come to the point where the literature on the topic is quite overwhelming. Further, many clinicians, trained in a different tradition, find this area difficult to penetrate. Yet equally there is a feeling amongst many therapists that it will be a neuropsychological model that ultimately provides the key to unlock the puzzle of stuttering.

In the following section we present three papers specially commissioned for this volume that aim to shed light on the state of our current knowledge of the neuropsychology of stuttering. David Rosenfield and Harvey Nudelman open this section with a discussion of the fundamental logic of neuropsychological explanations. They go on to outline an interactionist model of stuttering which places neuropsychological models of speech fluency in perspective. In the second paper in this section Walter Moore and Einer Boberg have undertaken the most comprehensive review of the

1

literature on hemispheric processing and stuttering that has been produced to date. In this extended paper they critically review the main experimental studies that have attempted to elucidate the relationship between stuttering and individual differences in hemispheric processing. Their conclusions offer intriguing new insights into both the nature and treatment of stuttering. In the final paper Woodruff Starkweather and his colleagues focus on the neuromotor literature on stuttering. They conclude that whilst stuttering may be a phenomenon of the motor speech system it is *not* the consequence of any specific motor disorder. Here too there are clear implications for the clinical treatment of the problem.

1 Neuropsychological Models Of Speech Dysfluency

David B. Rosenfield and Harvey B. Nudelman

Introduction — the Evolution of Models

Stuttering is a part of the human genome. As a global, pan-cultural motor disturbance of speech it has afflicted human beings for thousands of years. All languages have words that describe stuttering. Twentieth Century BC hieroglyphics, representing the word 'nit-nit', suggested stuttering. Mesopotamian clay tablets dating from centuries before the birth of Christ comment on stuttering, as do the Old Testament and the Koran. Isaiah noted: 'And the tongues of stammerers shall be ready to speak plainly (Isaiah 28:11)' (Rieber and Wollock, 1977; Rosenfield, 1984).

Hippocrates (460–377 BC) used the term 'trauloi' to refer inclusively to stuttering, cluttering, dysarthria, and other articulatory disturbances. Aristotle (384–322 BC) employed 'ischnophonia' specifically to stuttering, contending that the speech disturbance resulted from conflict between various body humors. Galen (131–200 AD), viewing human beings as individual microcosms of the universe, believed that people stuttered for individually different reasons depending upon their respective components of heat, dryness, moisture, and cold. 'Phlegmatic' individuals stuttered for reasons different from those of 'choleric' individuals. Galen's theories regarding the humoral system formed the basis for Medieval and Renaissance medicine, but this approach promoted little understanding of the motor dynamics of speech output (Reiber and Wollock, 1977; Rosenfield, 1984).

The history of stuttering offers a window on how the scientific community has developed models of illness. When human beings were viewed as being microcosms of the universe the alleged components of that universe (heat, dryness, moisture, and cold) were thought to be out of balance and therefore predisposing the individual to disease. In this setting there was no nosology for organ dysfunction, nor for symptoms. Brain disease (or liver disease, heart disease, etc.) was not viewed as relating to trauma, degenerative changes, vascular disease, infection, and the like; rather, it was viewed in terms of alleged components of the universe. It was not until the dissolution of laws against autopsies that a more cohesive approach to function and dysfunction of the human body came into being. Even in that setting it was some time before people realized what part of the body related to what function. For example, it was not until the 18th century that the larynx was thought to have more importance in sound production than the hyoid bone (Rosenfield, 1984).

Why should speech–language pathologists and their colleagues be concerned with the above? Simply put, the milieu of our society and the undercurrents of our thinking strongly influence the questions we pose as well as altering how we interpret our data. If we view speech output as something 'automatically done', but performed with error in the stutterer, then our questions and experimental paradigms will differ from those put forth when we view speech as a well-sequenced, well-timed motor output, subserved by various neurophysiologic mechanisms underlying efficient speech–motor control.

Theories of stuttering have certainly evolved over the years. No longer do we hear about Mercurialis' sixteenth century recommendation of rubbing lotion on the heads of moisture–deficient stutterers! Theories of stuttering have paralleled progress made in other realms of medicine and science. As time has gone by they have incorporated new ideas of altered self-concept (Johnson, 1955; Sheehan, 1970b), cerebral hemisphere abnormalities (Adams, 1982; Jones, 1966; Orton, 1928; Rosenfield, 1980, 1984; Travis, 1931), and disturbance of laryngeal motor control (Adams, 1978; Freeman, 1979; Rosenfield, 1980; Starkweather, 1982; Wyke, 1971). The historical continuum of theories of stuttering have slowly progressed from philosophical permutations to models of neurophysiologic abnormalities of voice function.

Orton (1928) and Travis (1931) first proposed that the frequent stumbling dysfluencies noted in children learning to speak arose from a poorly established cerebral dominance for language which in turn resulted in abnormally programmed speech output. Individuals who continued to stutter did so as a result of a continuing incomplete lateralization of cerebral dominance for language. Stuttering was not so much a reflection of an individual's psychological milieu but rather reflected this underlying cerebral disturbance. The past several decades have witnessed considerable altercations regarding these matters. Is language in the brain of stutterers programmed such that they are destined to stutter? If so, where and what might be that abnormality? Is something actually 'broken'? What would be the therapeutic implications were we in a position to answer these questions?

The search for a 'nidus' cause for stuttering has seen the application of newly discovered techniques for analyzing cerebral laterality for speech production to the problem. In this setting there have been expanded paradigms of handedness questionnaires, dichotic listening, application of barbiturate injection to assess laterality (Wada testing), as well as other techniques (Andrews *et al*, 1983; Bloodstein, 1981; Geschwind and Behan, 1982; Rosenfield, 1980). The search for something abnormal in the stutterer's nervous system became further sponsored by the recognition that previously fluent individuals could become dysfluent following brain damage. Studies of acquired stuttering, palilalia, cluttering, and spasmodic dysphonia opened these horizons regarding cerebral control of disturbed speech–motor output. Yet despite multiple review articles and putative models no singular cause for stuttering has been proposed (Andrews *et al*, 1983; Kent, 1983; Rosenfield, 1984; Starkweather, 1982). Further, despite the myriad of pages in the stuttering literature and the increased number of speech clinicians, stutterers have neither disappeared nor even decreased in prevalence (Porfert and Rosenfield, 1978).

Neuropsychological Models and the Explanation of Stuttering

One frequently hears questions regarding the 'neuropsychological models' of stuttering. All models pertaining to stuttering must, on some level, be neurologic. Speech is a motor output subtended by a central nervous system coordinating respiratory, articulatory, and laryngeal movements taking place against a background of continuous auditory and proprioceptive feedback. Stutterers, like anyone else, do not speak with their mouths; they speak with their brains. If the brain does not exist, there is no programming for the speech–motor system.

Stutterers, for whatever reason, have abnormal speech–motor output. Any model that purports to explain this phenomenon, regardless of its orientation, must address how it is that the brain produces these dysfluencies. Too frequently researchers have investigated stuttering by applying a paradigm employing some recent technological measure that tests whether a group of stutterers differs from a group of non-stutterers. It is in this setting that we have witnessed a growing number of studies employing dichotic listening, voice onset time, and laryngeal reaction time, as well as others. Some investigators detect minimal group differences but others have not. Controversies exist over the results and their interpretation (Andrews *et al*, 1983; Freeman, 1982; Rosenfield, 1984).

As we will see later this type of approach is not very rewarding in elucidating the cause of stuttering. To be sure, the pursuit of observations is, if nothing else, an appropriate step towards syndrome delineation. However, we must build models that permit asking probing questions with heuristic merit. There seems to be, as highlighted by Kent (1983), a popular approach in the behavioral sciences where if there are a number of studies yielding results on both sides of an issue, the majority report, pro or con, often rules the decision. Many review articles tend to add up the number of positive and negative studies on a particular topic, and if over half the studies favour a given proposition, that view wins support. What is necessary is the establishment of a unified theory or model of the process under examination which must, by definition, include *all* the established facts.

Interpretation of observation is seldom theory–free. Researchers often obtain and contaminate observations through methodologies embedded with theoretical expectations and constraints (Andrews *et al.* 1983; Kent, 1983). Let us consider some relevant examples. Suppose an individual comes home and finds that his house is burning. If he places his hands over his chest, complains about transient chest pain and then proceeds in his usual state of health his neighbours might comment that his chest pain is psychological. Were that individual to fall over dead people might query whether the stress of watching his house burn caused heart attack and death, relating the input (stress) to the output (death) through coronary artery spasm, causing decreased blood flow to the heart and subsequent cardiac malfunction.

Were one to have too strong a 'psychological' bias in the genesis of the chest pain one might assume that the individual did not have coronary artery spasm. Yet, the emotional stress of watching his house burn might have triggered athero-sclerosis–compromised blood vessels into spasm, resulting in chest pain. Merely because that person's output (pain without death) differed from the second example (pain followed by death) does not mean that the two examples do not share a common mechanism. This is analogous to a person stuttering more when under scrutiny in a classroom than when alone. One cannot say that stress is the sole culprit. What are the *mechanisms* causing dysfluency, and what are the mechanisms promoting increased dysfluency when stressed in class?

Let us pose another example. An individual may type without error at 60 words per minute. If someone is standing near that individual, watching him type, the typist might be more predisposed to error and his rate may decrease. Certainly one can argue that stress makes that typist produce more errors. But, *why* does the motor system of the typist produce more errors in this situation? The degree of anxiety that the typist experiences, although it may be mild, is somehow sufficient to alter coordination and timing mechanisms/relationships between the brain and finger dexterity. Similarly, why might a professional athlete make errors if he or she is distracted at the time of execution of the athletic motor skill?

What the above situations share is a component we term *affect–sensitivity*. Affect–sensitivity refers to the fact that stress alters motor output, a phenomenon which we see every day. Although seldom explicitly stated this line of thinking has gradually become more prominent in our view of stuttering. We no longer say stutterers become dysfluent simply because they are nervous. Stutterers have an affect–sensitive problem, and may well stutter more in situations of stress. What is needed is a milieu of thinking that promotes investigation of the dynamics of the stutterer's output, with testable models and hypotheses that can explain why stutterers are more dysfluent in some situations than in others.

It is in this setting that we now find the field of speech science juxtaposed to the field of neuroscience. The crossover between the two is difficult. Individuals of either 'camp' may find themselves facing unfamiliar vocabulary and requiring particular skills with which they are not familiar. This thrust has been accompanied by a strong interest in the physiology of normal speech production.

Normal Speech Production

As noted above, speech production must be controlled, on some level, by the central nervous system. Speech–motor production requires coordination between respiratory activity, laryngeal activity, and supralaryngeal articulators. The vocal folds, part of a neuro–motor system consisting of the brain, brainstem, nerves, striated muscles, and articulatory joints, are set into action by muscular movements and modified by particular reflexes. This whole system is controlled by the brain. The brain monitors its output through sensory feedback (proprioception) and through auditory feedback. The role of auditory feedback becomes apparent when one witnesses the dysfluent output of fluent speakers in a delayed auditory feedback setting, as well as recognizing that normal speakers develop abnormal speech ('deaf speech') following hearing loss. The brain is constantly analyzing and processing its output (speech) as well as its input (proprioception and hearing) (Abbs and Rosenfield, 1986; Jurgens and Ploog, 1981; Rosenfield, 1984).

Mammalian vocalization involves coordination between respiration, laryngeal activity, and supralaryngeal articulatory movements. Lower motor neurons controlling respiratory movements reside in the anterior portion of the cervical, thoracic, and upper-lumbar spinal cord. Motor neurons controlling laryngeal closure reside in the nucleus ambiguous, situated in the lower part of the brainstem. The neurons directly responsible for supralaryngeal musculature are the trigeminal motor nucleus, facial nucleus, rostral portion of the nucleus ambiguous, hypoglossal nucleus, and the anterior horn cells of the rostral portion of the cervical spinal cord. This wide array of spinal tissue extends from the pons to the lower portion of the spinal cord (Abbs and Rosenfield, 1986; Jurgens and Ploog, 1981).

Sectioning an animal's brainstem above the trigeminal motor nucleus makes the animal mute. Thus, the neural network below this nucleus (i.e., below the pons) is not sufficient on its own to produce sound. Input from higher cerebral levels is required for vocalization. Transecting the brainstem in the upper portion of the midbrain, above the inferior colliculus (one of the midbrain structures), does not abolish vocalization. Multiple studies have investigated whether the lower part of the midbrain, or only a specific portion of it, actually 'controls' vocalization. In this setting scientists have stimulated different parts of the hemispheres and brainstem in an attempt to see whether sounds specific to the species being tested can be elicited. They have also analyzed whether ablation of selective brain structures prohibits these species–specific vocalizations. These stimulation and ablation studies have resulted in considerable information regarding speech output (Abbs and Rosenfield, 1986; Jurgens and Ploog, 1981).

Control of mammalian vocalization appears to be organized hierarchically. The lowest level is represented by the phonatory motor neurons, primary sensory neurons, and reticular spinal interneurons. Anatomically this consists of widely scattered neurons extending from the rostral pons (trigeminal nucleus) down to the upper-lumbar spinal cord (respiratory motor neurons). This level, by itself, does not initiate vocalization. Vocalization requires facilitatory input from the next level, the caudal periaqueductal gray and laterally adjacent tegmentum, both of which are in the midbrain. The periaqueductal region probably couples particular motivational states to corresponding vocal expressions by coordinating the diverse internal and external stimuli which normally induce an animal to generate a sound. The periaqueductal region, in turn, receives input partly through fairly direct sensory projections (spino–thalamic tract, superior and inferior colliculus, anterior cingulate cortex) and partially from motivational control areas (hypothalamus, midline thalamus, amygdala and septum) within the limbic system (Jurgens and Ploog, 1981).

Our limbic system, much entwined with our emotional milieu, is tied into the production of speech. One's emotional milieu can influence speech output: stress alters limbic system activity and the limbic system has major input into speech–motor output. Thus, an individual's speech may change in a particular emotional setting. One's voice becomes 'shaky' when one is stressed because emotional stress induces motor tremor. One can also have other speech–motor abnormalities, such as stuttering, that are affect-sensitive. Stress affects the limbic system and the limbic system affects speech output. If a stutterer has an unstable speech–motor system, causing him to stutter, stress can easily make him worse (Rosenfield, 1984).

Acquired Stuttering

Querying the role of the brain in stuttering, investigators have asked whether fluent speakers (having allegedly normal brains) can become dysfluent if they develop brain damage. If so perhaps areas of brain dysfunction might be found that explain acquired dysfluency and yield information applicable to stutterers. Rosenfield (1972) reported a patient who became a stutterer, in the absence of aphasia, following left hemisphere insult. Many cases of brain damage rendering fluent individuals dysfluent have subsequently been reported. Individuals can become nonaphasic stutterers following damage to the right and/or the left side of their brain. Patients with unilateral damage have a much better prognosis for recovery of fluency than do those with bilateral compromise (Ardila and Lopez, 1986; Fleet and Heilman, 1985; Helm-Estabrooks *et al.* 1986; Helm, Butler and Benson, 1978; Rosenbek *et al.* 1978; Rosenfield, Miller and Feltovich, 1981).

The underlying assumption in research pertaining to acquired stuttering is that if fluent individuals can become stutterers following brain damage, then perhaps developmental stutterers have damage in similar areas of their brain causing their stuttering behaviors. However, the acquired stutterers can have lesions in various areas in the left side and/or the right side of the brain, either anteriorly or posteriorly. There is no data that developmental stutterers have lesions in these areas. Also, the acquired stutterers, although dysfluent, do not have all the characteristics of developmental stutterers, the former being frequently resistant to fluency-evoking manoeuvres and having their dysfluencies scattered throughout the sentence rather than at the beginning of sentences and phrases.

Most papers on acquired stuttering contend that brain damage somehow alters the normal underlying cerebral laterality for language, causing speech dysfluency. Others focus attention on palilalia and cluttering (Daly, 1985; Horner and Massey, 1983; Sussman, 1982), trying to ascertain what portions of the brain are not working appropriately. Again, brain compromise causing acquired stuttering can be so scattered, ranging from basal ganglia to subcortical white matter to cortex, in either or both hemispheres, that no singular cause for acquired dysfluency has been found.

Specific attention to the integrated sensorimotor dynamics of speech production is seldom sufficiently addressed in acquired stuttering. Instead, attention has mainly focused upon employing newer techniques for getting a 'handle' on laterality. It is in this setting that the literature on acquired stuttering has helped sustain an interest in looking for *the* experimental paradigm that would enable language laterality function to be tested more definitively, such that differentiation between individual stutterers and individual non-stutterers can be achieved.

Cerebral Laterality

Cerebral dominance refers to the predominant lateralization of a particular neuropsychological function on one side of the nervous system or the other. A more narrow definition, suitable for our discussion, refers to the capacity of a region on one side of the brain for processing and storing certain types of information that is greater than that in the corresponding region on the opposite side. Left hemisphere dominance for language implies that regions on the left are more specialized for the acquisition and processing of language than regions on the right (Geschwind and Galaburda, 1985c).

The two hemispheres of the brain are connected through interhemispheric pathways. The hemispheres also receive information from, as well as send information to, the brainstem. Most of the programming and processing of language is done in the hemispheres. Almost all right-handed individuals have the majority of their language in their left hemisphere. A left hemisphere lesion will, in 99 per cent of right-handed individuals, result in aphasia. Right hemisphere disease, with very few exceptions, seldom produces aphasia in right-handed individuals. Individuals who are not right-handed probably have language in both hemispheres, with a substantial component being in the left (Benson and Geschwind, 1985; Goodglass and Quadfasel, 1954).

It is not known *how* language comes to reside primarily in one hemisphere but we know language is usually well lateralized by the age of eight years (Geschwind and Galaburda, 1985c). Although morphology does not necessarily infer function, there are significant anatomical differences between the two hemispheres, especially in the areas subserving language function.

As mentioned earlier Orton (1928) and Travis (1931) popularized the thesis of 'incomplete' cerebral dominance as the cause of stuttering, theorizing that stuttering resulted from incomplete lateralization of language. Since handedness reflects language lateralization many investigators focused attention on handedness and stuttering. A wide disparity of results soon emerged. Estimates of left-handedness among groups of stutterers have ranged between 2 and 21 per cent with ambidexterity reported as high as 61 per cent. The reason for these discrepancies probably relates to the various definitions of stuttering, ambidexterity and handedness that have been employed in different studies (Bloodstein, 1981; Rosenfield, 1980).

Initially the discrepancy of data pertaining to handedness among stutterers made the Orton–Travis thesis unpopular. The thesis then lay fairly dormant until Jones (1966), a neurosurgeon, reported that he had occasion to operate upon four stutterers who have developed, *subsequent* to their stutter, cerebral disease necessitating surgical intervention. Jones was aware that language might reside in both hemispheres of stutterers and was concerned that the contemplated surgery would result in aphasia were he to operate upon the dominant hemisphere (e.g. Would a stutterer undergoing left brain surgery become aphasic if classical areas of speech were surgically compromised? Could the same happen if he operated on the right?). He needed to ascertain preoperatively the status of language function in each hemisphere. Thus, he performed a Wada test.

The Wada test (Wada and Rasmussen, 1960) consists of intracarotid administration of a short-acting barbiturate. Each carotid artery supplies the ipsilateral cerebral hemisphere, although sometimes there is crossover of blood flow. The barbiturate transiently anesthetizes the ipsilateral hemisphere. Patients are transiently hemiplegic on the side contralateral to the injection, and become aphasic if the language-dominant hemisphere is exposed to the barbiturate.

Jones observed that all four stutterers became aphasic following injection of the barbiturate into both the right and the left carotid artery. This implicated input from both hemispheres into major areas of the stutterers' language output. Subsequently, each patient required surgery in one hemisphere as a result of the underlying brain lesion. All four patients ceased stuttering following surgery. A repeat Wada test elicited aphasia only following injection on the non-operated side. Barbiturate injections in the carotid artery ipsilateral to the operated-upon hemisphere no longer produced aphasia. The patients no longer had bilateral speech representation and they no longer stuttered.

Jones' paper is intriguing but prompts several criticisms. All but one of his four patients were left-handed, implying bilateral language representation. All had a strong family history of left-handedness, further implying bilateral language representation. He did not state how the absence/presence of stuttering was evaluated, nor did he have long-term follow-up postoperatively.

Other investigators, pursuing Wada tests in stutterers, have had varying results. In sum 11 stutterers have undergone bilateral Wada testing with bilateral speech representation being noted in five. The conclusion is that some stutterers may have abnormal laterality whereas others do not, suggesting non-homogeneity among stutterers (Rosenfield, 1984).

The Wada test is not without risk because it involves intra-arterial puncture and catheterization. However, other tests for the analysis of cerebral dominance are virtually risk-free. One of these is the dichotic listening paradigm. The major hallmark of dichotic listening experiments is systematic manipulation of the acoustic parameters of auditory stimuli. Although the cochlea of each nerve is neurally attached to both hemispheres, a group of listeners will consistently report hearing the target stimulus in only one ear when different auditory stimuli are simultaneously presented to both ears. Kimura (1967) demonstrated that verbal signals, such as words or digits, are more accurately reported from the right ear (i.e., left hemisphere) than from the left ear (i.e., right hemisphere) after simultaneous dichotic presentation. The reverse is true for melodies (Bryden and Murray, 1985; Kimura, 1964).

Dichotic listening paradigms involve many variables ranging from types of sound heard to the order in which the subject reports the left and right ear sound to the examiner. The majority of these studies show that right-handed individuals process verbal data with the left hemisphere and process non-verbal data with the right. However, these findings primarily hold for groups, not individuals. Indeed, Blumstein, Goodglass and Tarter (1975), testing a group of subjects in a dichotic paradigm and then testing them again at a later time, observed that 85 per cent of normal right-handed males have a right ear advantage in a dichotic listening paradigm and that any such test sample contains 15 per cent misclassified subjects. As many as 30 per cent changed ear dominance when retested.

Multiple studies have addressed dichotic listening among stutterers. Results have varied in part due to different types of stimuli employed, and also possible population differences (e.g., Were the stutterers from a clinic? Were they all males? All adults? What was their handedness?). Many but not all of these studies have found evidence of cerebral laterality differences between groups of stutterers and groups of non-stutterers. These differences, when found, have not been great. Most of the studies, regardless of whether they noted differences between a group of stutterers versus a group of non-stutterers, frequently identified at least a subgroup of stutterers who were substantially different from non-stutterers, prompting the thesis of non-homogeneity and begging further investigation (Andrews *et al.* 1983; Bloodstein, 1981; Rosenfield, 1984). It is in this setting that studies of pursuit auditory tracking, contingent negative variation, central auditory processing, and laryngeal function have been performed (Andrews *et al.* 1983; Moore, Craven and Faber, 1982; Starkweather, 1982; Sussman and MacNeilage, 1975; Zimmermann, 1980; Zimmermann and Hanley, 1983).

Handedness studies, in a continuing attempt to clarify further the issue of cerebral dominance for language in stutterers, have recently surfaced again. When one employs strict definitions of strong handedness preference, such as only using one particular hand for multiple tasks (i.e., opening the lid of a box, writing, throwing, cutting, etc.) and never using the other, one finds differences between stutterers and non-stutterers (Geschwind and Behan, 1982; Schachter, McIntyre and Rosenfield, 1986). There appears to be a higher prevalence of strong left-handed preference among stutterers than among non-stutterers, but there is also a higher prevalence of strong right-handed preference. It therefore does not appear that handedness is a distinguishing property for stutterers.

One could fill hundreds of pages reviewing articles that have investigated cerebral laterality and other neurologic disturbances in stutterers. Again it appears that there is no clear-cut delineation between the stutterers and the non-stutterers. To be sure, some studies note group differences between stutterers and non-stutterers; however, no study has found significant differences between *all* stutterers and *all* non-stutterers within the groups. In other words the major differences that have been found are *average* group differences. There is no study that finds a laterality marker separating any individual stutterer from any individual non-stutterer. One finds similar results in analyzing laryngeal paradigms, such as voice onset time, voice termination times, laryngeal electromyographic recordings, laryngeal reaction times, and cineradiographic recordings. Further, studies of central and peripheral auditory function have fared likewise. Many studies identify a subgroup of stutterers who appear different from non-stutterers and conclude that stutterers are a non-homogeneous group requiring further investigation (Andrews *et al.* 1983; Bloodstein, 1981).

In summary, research during the past several decades has underscored the implicit desire to delineate a role for the brain in stuttering. After all it is the brain that controls laryngeal reaction time, voice onset time, auditory function, language laterality, etc. However, these paradigms have consistently failed to provide a measure whereby stutterers can be separated from non-stutterers. Yet stutterers do have one thing in common, separating them from non-stutterers: stuttering. Acquired stutterers, clutterers, and palilalics also all share the common denominator of dysfluency.

Motor Dynamics

Perhaps it is not too surprising that most experiments have failed to delineate significant stutterer non-stutterer differences. After all stutterers do not stutter on all sounds, nor on all words. Further, sounds that are difficult for a stutterer to produce on one occasion are sometimes produced fluently on others. Also, fluent speakers have occasional dysfluencies (Bloodstein, 1981). Since stutterers are sometimes fluent and fluent speakers sometimes stutter, perhaps we should not expect to find any single measure, or even a cluster of measures, that separate the stutterer from his fluent counterpart. Perhaps in order to understand better the disturbed motor output of stuttering we need to ask different questions, in a different milieu.

Let us hypothetically assume that all stutterers are left-handed and that all non-stutterers are right-handed. Further, assume that all stutterers have language in both cerebral hemispheres whereas all non-stutterers have language solely in their left hemisphere. Investigators might then argue that stuttering results from competing/disrupting speech output messages between the two hemispheres, both having language. They might argue that language scattered throughout the brain causes programming errors, resulting in dysfluency.

Now, let us query the opposite. Suppose that all non-stutterers have language in both hemispheres and that all stutterers have language in only one hemisphere. Investigators might now argue that stuttering results from not having enough language distributed throughout the brain. Language in only one hemisphere would be deemed insufficient to produce appropriate coordination of the speech–motor system, resulting in stuttering.

The thrust of these hypothetical situations is poignant: why should too much or too little language in any part of the brain make anyone stutter? If stutterers have 'too much' language scattered throughout the brain, why should that make them stutter? Why should this not make them more intelligent? Or, with language scattered throughout the brain, why is the processing of their world not altered such that they become schizophrenic? And even if stutterers have language in only one hemisphere, why should that make them stutter?

We are faced with an interesting dilemma. In truth some individuals have language lateralized to the left side of their brain and are fluent; some individuals have language lateralized to the left side of their brain and are dysfluent; some individuals have language insufficiently lateralized to either hemisphere (i.e., bilateral representation) and are fluent; some individuals with language localization similar to any of these situations are dysfluent (Milner, Branch and Rasmussen, 1966; Rosenfield, 1984). On an individual basis, one can find stutterers and non-stutterers who are strongly left-handed, strongly right-handed, or have mixed handedness. A theory of disturbed language laterality producing stuttering behaviors has considerable difficulty unless it can explain *why* an individual stutters and not just whether there is a difference in a measure of language laterality function between groups of stutterers and groups of non-stutterers. Considering that we do not know whether it is 'good' or 'bad' to have language bilaterally disseminated or more uni-hemispherically orientated we should query whether we are asking appropriate questions.

As noted above many investigations of stuttering frequently emanate from technological advances that permit quantification of neurological parameters that might underlie speech output. Although these studies implicitly incorporate paradigms of motor control they insufficiently address what the motor system is actually doing. Speech scientists, increasingly aware of motor control theory, are now incorporating concepts such as quantitative dynamics of feedback loops into their models of the speech–motor system. Speech production requires fine coordination between laryngeal, articulatory, and respiratory systems. The central nervous system monitors proprioceptive feedback from the laryngeal, articulatory, and respiratory systems while simultaneously measuring speech output through the auditory system. The actual speech output is compared to the intended speech output and corrective adjustments are made.

Neurophysiology suggests that this coordination is achieved through the employment of negative feedback control systems. This type of feedback control is referred to as being negative because there is a comparison between the actual output and the desired output. Negative feedback control has been observed from crayfish to mammals and has been used to analyze behaviors ranging from spinal reflexes and pupil diameter to control of blood sugar levels in the body.

Systems that use negative feedback (closed loop systems), such as the central nervous system, are capable of much finer control than those that do not (open loop systems), due to their ability to monitor performance and make adjustments in output. There is a price paid for this increased performance: the possibility of the system becoming unstable. This is due to the fact that the adjustments that are made may tend to degrade the performance rather than improve it (Anand, 1974; Milsum, 1966). Viewing speech production as a complex control system, an idea initially advanced by Fairbanks (1954), suggests that stuttering can be modelled as an instability in this complex system. A simple example of what is meant here by an 'instability' is appropriate.

Most of us are familiar with the ringing of a public address system in an assembly hall. This is caused by positive feedback from the loudspeaker to the microphone. If the effect of this positive feedback is large enough the system (microphone/amplifier/speaker/sound/microphone) becomes unstable and produces a ringing sound. Whether or not this occurs depends upon the properties of the individual components of the system: the sensitivity of the microphone, the gain (volume) setting of the amplifier, the sensitivity of the speaker, and how close the speaker is to the microphone. As can be seen there are many ranges of component settings for which this system will become unstable. In one instance the microphone might be very sensitive while the amplifier gain is low; in another the microphone may be very insensitive but the amplifier gain is high. Both conditions can produce instability and, consequently, were one to investigate the cause of the ringing sound, one could be misled by investigating only the amplifier gain. The ringing can be understood only in terms of the overall properties of the system. This is an often overlooked property of complex systems: the system can be unstable while all of its components are still functioning.

This type of approach (Systems Analysis) permits evaluating motor output without necessarily addressing what, if any, part of the brain is 'broken'. Tens of thousands of synapses participate in the brain's execution of any motor movement, synapses that involve input, output, and the interplay between the two. Thus there are numerous possibilities for breakdown and error. Stutterers need not have one particular focus of their central nervous system 'broken'.

One can posit that stutterers have a brain such that they are likely to develop problems in speech output. Their speech–motor control systems are closer to the instability threshold than those of fluent speakers. Andrews *et al.* (1983), referencing Neilson, hypothesise that stutterers lack an adequate central capacity to deal with the relationship between motor activity and the associated sensory activity produced during speech. Kent (1983) argues that stuttering reflects a reduced capability to generate fine temporal programs that are necessary for appropriate integration of auditory input and language output.

These recent approaches reflect speech scientists entering the area of motor dynamics. Let us ask ourselves how to model and quantify what is actually transpiring. How does one access the input in the sensorimotor integration necessary for speech production? How does one analyse the output? The field of control theory offers methods that help resolve these issues.

If we are to understand the causes of instability in the speech–motor control system then we need to determine the relationship between its input and output. The complete description of these dynamic relationships requires a differential equation. This can be better understood by the following example:

> Suppose one throws a ball into the air ten times, each time the ball having a different trajectory. One can describe the dynamics of this experiment by using an algebraic expression to describe each trajectory as a function of time. The description of the dynamics requires separate expressions for each toss. However, there is a more efficient way of describing this experiment employing the use of differential equations derived from Newton's Law that describes the position of the ball as a function of time. Here the solution of the differential equation describes all the trajectories and each trajectory is determined by the application of the initial conditions, (i.e., the position, speed, and angle of the ball at the time of release).

Systems analysis offers empirical methods for determining the equivalent of the differential equation for a linear system. A system can be linear only if any sine wave input into that system results in a corresponding sine wave output having the same frequency as the original input, although the amplitude and phase might differ. A full description of the mathematics in this model is beyond the scope of this chapter, but readers will find a detailed account in Nudelman *et al.* (1987). The important point we wish to emphasize here is that mathematical approaches exist for measuring movement. Nudelman *et al.* (1987) have developed these measures by asking subjects to engage in a vocal tracking paradigm in which the subject hums (output), attempting to match the changing frequency of a computer-generated tone (input). They measured the frequency changes of both sets of sound waves and analysed whether the frequency changes (modulations) produced by the subject gave the same amplitude as the modulations heard (i.e., they measured *gain*). They also investigated whether the modulations are in *phase* with one another. The authors demonstrated that the complex non-linear system underlying speech–motor production (composed of respiratory, laryngeal, and articulatory motor systems) can be modelled by a linear term when the subject is tracking. That is, the production of speech can be described by equations involving mathematical measures of input and output. Using the concept of *phase margin* as defined by control theory they found that the speech–motor system of stutterers is closer to the threshold of instability than it is in fluent speakers.

These authors contend that instabilities in the speech–motor control system (i.e., dysfluencies) can best be understood by viewing speech as having two nested loops (each one of these nested loops consists of multiple subsystems of inputs and outputs). One loop is an inner phonatory control loop for producing sound; the second is a linguistic control loop, choosing and analysing the sounds that are to be produced. What part(s) of the brain is actually doing this is not known. It may involve several areas with different areas participating in different ways at different times.

In assessing the overall speech–motor control system the authors address how the input and output are processed, and by so doing they address the dynamic relationships within the motor system. From their measures of the dynamics of the inner loop they hypothesize that during speech stutterers are more prone to instability than are fluent speakers. Their measurements also indicate that stutterers are less likely to be unstable at lower frequencies of speech–motor movements, thus explaining why 'slow speech' helps promote fluency. Using their data they compute how much time speakers have at different sound output frequencies before the speech system becomes unstable, producing the breakdown (i.e., dysfluency). Their predicted values are in keeping with those measured by Fairbanks (1955) for fluent speakers in delayed auditory feedback studies.

Conclusion

The past several decades have witnessed a continuum of experiments in speech–motor output that have begun to overlap with other areas in neurosciences. An increasing number of experiments pertaining to laterality of language have failed to differentiate individual stutterers from individual fluent speakers. The only differences that have been found, and then not consistently, have been those between groups. Often these differences have not been great in absolute terms. It is in this setting that researchers find themselves increasingly addressing the actual dynamics of speech output, and thereby overlapping with motor control researchers.

The stuttered dysfluency is *not* the major problem that the stutterer has. Indeed, one can stop the dysfluency by simply telling the stutterer to stop talking. Stuttering, unlike a convulsion, is not totally involuntary. One cannot make a patient having a major motor seizure stop seizing by simply asking him to cease convulsing. The seizure is beyond the patient's control. But, one can tell a stutterer, in the midst of a dysfluent utterance, to stop talking and the sound will stop.

The stuttered dysfluency is a *response* to the major problem at hand: the break-down of coordinated speech–motor output. This breakdown causes errors in output sometimes resulting in absence of sound production, sometimes resulting in abnormal sound production. Regardless, the stutterer must reckon with the breakdown. He may struggle, back up, and start again, or engage in varying and different strategies to 'get the word out'.

Some stutterers may well have disturbances in cerebral laterality, laryngeal motor control, or in their processing of signals. These disturbances can occur singularly, in combination, some of the time, or all of the time. Stutterers are probably not homogeneous, a fact not only underlined by the findings from different research methodologies, but highlighted by different responses among stutterers to different therapies. We must remember the microphone–speaker analogy. There are multiple possibilities for the ringing sound and these correspond to the heterogeneity among stutterers.

Application of motor control theory to speech production offers systematic mathematical descriptions of the speech–motor control system such that one can develop descriptive models of altered speech function. It is in this setting that Nudelman *et al.* (1987) contend that fluency-evoking manoeuvres for stutterers have efficacy because they lower the frequency of the stutterer's speech movements (pitch changes) to the range where gain and phase parameters promote less momentous instabilities. (Fundamental frequency during speech varies with time. These variations of fundamental frequency can be described as a sum of sine wave modulations at different frequencies. The frequency content describes how much of the pitch changes occur at each of these modulation frequencies). Speech therapy programs produce fluency when therapy is directed toward speech motor system dynamics in this less unstable range. This explains the efficacy of many well-established therapy techniques (i.e., slowed speech, air flow, etc.). A stutterer will have lasting conversational and social effectiveness when he is fluent in the frequency–content range of normal speech. Fluency in a lower frequency–content range, a range which most speech therapists address, will not produce the effective communication he desires. Investigation of speech motor dynamics and the establishment of therapies based on these findings will hopefully lead to increasingly effective treatment for dysfluent individuals.

Acknowledgment

The authors thank the Kitty M. Perkins Foundation, the M. R. Bauer Foundation, and the Ariel-Benjamin-Jeremiah Lowin Foundation for their support.

2 Hemispheric Processing and Stuttering

Walter H. Moore, Jr. and Einer Boberg

Introduction

This chapter reviews cerebral hemispheric processing research as it relates to stuttering. It describes methods for investigating hemispheric processing and central nervous system (CNS) involvement in the problem of stuttering. Findings from investigations relevant to stuttering will be summarised. In particular we aim to explore the relationships between right hemispheric processing and stuttering, and present tentative conclusions, hypotheses, and some suggestions for future research.

During the last decade we have seen a major resurgence of interest in neurophysiological components of stuttering. With modern investigative techniques researchers have explored whether stutterers differ from normal speakers on various dimensions of CNS function. Although the existence of such differences was first suggested by Orton (1927) and Travis (1931) recent technological advances have encouraged modern researchers to study CNS function and dysfunction in ways that were not available to those innovative pioneers. We are persuaded that data accumulated through recent investigations constitute compelling evidence of CNS involvement in stuttering, and that this evidence will play a critical role in our understanding of the etiology and management of stuttering. Therefore, we have undertaken to review the literature and relate our findings to our understanding of the disorder of stuttering.

The literature on CNS function and hemispheric processing is replete with controversy. As Gazzaniga (1970) aptly commented:

> The field of brain research is so enormous, so complicated, and so prolific that it is almost impossible to introduce any subject in a scholarly fashion by pointing to the antecedent studies which clearly spell out the nature of the next logical question for inquiry. One quickly gains the impression that for every issue are two opposite views with authoritative investigators on each side. Moreover, as in almost no other field of scientific investigation, what

19

looks good today will look weak tomorrow. Indeed, because of this more than one scientist has confessed a certain feeling of futility in reporting his research (p. vii).

Since the literature in neuropsychology is vast, complex and controversial we have not attempted an exhaustive review of all the issues. Instead, we will consider a number of representative studies in some detail, and attempt to integrate hemispheric processing research with physiological studies on stuttering, and normal speech. Our first aim is to outline the various experimental procedures used in modern neuropsychology to build models of brain function. In particular we draw attention to the limitations inherent in each procedure.

Methods for the Investigation of Hemispheric Processing

Several methods have been used over the years to investigate hemispheric asymmetries in normal and stuttering subjects. It is important to recognize that the procedure used will influence the investigator's interpretation of the results obtained. For example, dichotic procedures have been employed by many investigators, yet this procedure has poor temporal and spatial resolution. That is, very little can be said about the morphological structures of the brain involved in processing the stimuli, and little can be said about the changes in processing that occur over time when dichotic procedures are used. Test retest reliability with dichotic procedures is also poor. On the other hand, EEG procedures have very high temporal resolution, and can be used to study hemispheric processing over time using a variety of stimuli that are not limited to short durational information (such as nonsense syllables). Yet, the fact that scalp electrodes are used in EEG methods means that results reflect activity of many small zones of cortical and non-cortical structures beneath the electrodes. Consequently, a small, discrete area cannot be said to be responsible for the observed electrical activity.

These differences in methods must be taken into consideration when results from a variety of different studies, all using different methods, are being considered. Indeed, the same interpretations and conclusions cannot always be reached across investigations that have employed different procedures. Here we will look only at the major methods that have been used in stuttering research, and the limitations that each possesses.

Dichotic listening

With this procedure two auditory stimuli of equal intensity and onset times are delivered to the left and right ears simultaneously. Following presentation of single pairs, or several sets of pairs (typically nonsense syllables), listeners are asked to indicate, by recall or recognition, what they heard. The number of responses associated with left and right ear presentations is recorded and an 'ear preference score' is determined (see Kimura, 1961a; 1961b). If reports from one ear are more frequent or correct than from the other ear, then it is concluded that the hemisphere opposite the higher scoring ear is more efficient at processing the stimuli (Gruber and Segalowitz, 1977). This interpretation is thought to reflect the more numerous and direct neural connections between the hemisphere and the higher scoring contralateral ear.

There are several major limitations to this procedure. Due in part to the relative ease in aligning syllable pairs the majority of studies employ consonant-vowel syllables beginning with stop-plosives to explore hemispheric processing for language. Such stimuli provide a limited view of hemispheric linguistic processing, and do not reflect the semantic and syntactic components of language. Additionally, contextual and attentional variables must be carefully considered. For example, Spellacy and Blumstein (1970) found that the context in which vowels were imbedded affected ear-preference scores. Vowels embedded in a series of English words were associated with a right-ear advantage (REA), whereas those embedded in a series of melodies and sound effects resulted in a left-ear advantage (LEA). Further, Haggard and Parkinson (1971) found that when subjects were instructed to attend to the emotional tone of a sentence an LEA was produced. However, when asked to attend to linguistic or acoustic cues an REA was shown. These two studies point to the importance of both linguistic and psychological variables in the interpretation of results from dichotic listening studies.

Tachistoscopic visual methods

In this procedure visual stimuli are presented to the left and/or right visual half fields. Typically a vertical array of information is presented to the visual half fields, either monocularly or binocularly, for brief (< 100 msec) durations. The pathways from the left half field project to the right hemisphere, and those from the right half field to the left hemisphere. Similar to dichotic studies, a visual half field preference score is determined from the number of responses associated with left and right visual half field presentations. If reports from one half field are more frequent or correct than those reported from the other field, then it is concluded that the hemisphere associated with the higher scoring field is more efficient at processing the stimuli. Often a right visual half field preference is found for verbal information with a left visual half field preference for nonverbal information (McKeever and Huling, 1971; Moore, 1976).

In order to control for eye movements stimuli can only be presented for short durations, and, as a further consequence, only short stimulus arrays can be used. Not only must temporal durations be carefully controlled, but luminous conditions and center fixation must be too. Such variables as the imagery value (Paivio, 1978) of the stimuli presented must be considered when interpreting results from tachistoscopic studies. Day (1979) for example reported that high visual imagery nouns and adjectives could be processed by both hemispheres, while low visual imagery nouns and adjectives were processed by the left hemisphere alone. In the same study Day reported that all verbs, regardless of their imagery value, were processed by the left hemisphere. These results underscore the need to examine methods and procedures in some detail when comparing results across studies.

EEG procedures

Electrophysiological responses measured at the scalp may provide us with an understanding of what is going on in the hemispheres during information processing (Valsiner, 1983). Unlike behavioral input–output procedures (e.g., dichotic and tachistoscopic testing) electrophysiological measures allow us to ask more direct questions about hemispheric information processing by observing electrophysiological correlates of hemispheric activation over time. In the hemispheric alpha (8–13 Hz) asymmetry procedure *decreases* in alpha amplitude are associated with *increased brain activity* in specific brain areas. Asymmetries in alpha power have been reported between the left and right hemispheres relative to stimulus, task, and/or subject variables. Averaged evoked response (AER) techniques allow the investigator to measure a temporally stable and reliable waveform, which is generated by mechanisms within the cortex, in response to external and internal stimuli (Molfese, 1980). Various components of the AER have been found to reflect stimulus properties as well as cognitive states and activities.

Hemispheric alpha asymmetries

A number of independent investigators (Galin and Ornstein, 1972; Haynes and Moore, 1981a, 1981b; McKee, Humphrey and McAdam, 1973; Moore and Haynes, 1980a, 1980b; Morgan, MacDonald and MacDonald, 1971; Robbins and McAdam, 1974) have shown increased suppression of alpha brain wave (8–13 Hz) amplitude over the hemisphere which is primarily involved in processing specific kinds of information under specific task conditions. This differential suppression of alpha activity over the hemispheres has been the basis of claims of functional asymmetry. The alpha suppression points to the hemisphere that is allegedly processing the stimuli, or is at least involved in developing strategies for processing the stimuli.

The interpretation of EEG data related to hemispheric processing differs from that used to evaluate results with a focus on cerebral dominance. Proponents of the hemispheric processing model look for differences in the relative participation of the hemispheres during stimulus and task conditions, and do not infer absolute hemispheric mechanisms for the processing of broad classes of stimuli (i.e., 'verbal' and 'nonverbal' stimuli). For example, Faber-Clark and Moore (1983) have reported greater left hemisphere alpha suppression during linguistic tasks requiring recall, and greater right hemispheric alpha suppression during recognition tasks. Additionally, Warren, Peltz and Haueter (1976) reported that initial processing of high imagery arousal words, of both negative and positive arousal value, resulted in relatively greater left hemisphere alpha suppression than a neutral word list, which produced the opposite effects.

While the EEG procedure has high temporal resolution (moment-to-moment changes in the EEG can be studied) the results actually reflect the activity of many small zones of cortical and noncortical surface beneath the electrodes and, consequently, spatial resolution is reduced. Nor does the EEG signal provide much information concerning specific stimulus characteristics.

Scalp recorded averaged evoked responses

This neuroelectrical method uses surface electrodes to measure electrical potential (relative voltage) referenced to a ground. Recordings are time-locked to stimulus presentations and cortical electrical activity is averaged over trials. With averaging, consistent voltage changes are detectable because the background random activity is cancelled when averaged (Gruber and Segalowitz, 1977; Seitz *et al.* 1980).

An advantage to the averaged evoked response (AER) method is that it allows for observation of a specific cortical response, which may be pertinent to localization of hemispheric function (See Molfese [1983] for a review of AERs and language). It can also be used to study the relative activation latencies of different cortical areas (Brown, Marsh and Smith, 1973, 1976; Molfese, 1980; Molfese, Freeman and Palermo, 1975; Thatcher, 1977).

Using AER procedures Molfese (1980, 1978a, 1978b) has shown that both hemispheres are involved in the processing of voice and tone onset time at different epochs during stimulus presentation. According to Molfese (1978a)

> . . . one point appears remarkably clear: Prior notions of hemispheric differences which insist that only the LH [left hemisphere] is involved in the processing of language related materials must be seriously questioned, if not rejected.

A clear strength of the AER method which Molfese used lies in its high temporal resolution; this allowed him to observe the participation of the two hemispheres at different times during processing.

Cortical blood flow (CBF)

Blood flow through the various tissues of the body changes as a direct result of metabolism and activity in the tissue (Lassen *et al.* 1978). Consequently if one hemisphere, or region of a hemisphere, is more or less active than another, then we expect to see differences in regional cerebral circulation.

Perhaps the greatest advantage of this procedure resides in its capacity to detect areas of the brain that are activated (inferred from greater cortical blood flow) during information processing, both between and within hemispheres. Yet, temporal resolution is poor. According to Wood (1980) the EEG procedures have much greater temporal resolution than do CBF techniques, which require a minimum of two to three minutes of repetitive behavioral activation prior to blood flow measurement, and sampling must continue for a further fifteen to thirty minutes for adequate measures to be obtained. Using the CBF procedure Gur and Reivich (1980) were able to corroborate and extend the findings of the existence of individual differences in hemispheric activation. The authors concluded:

> . . . if one tries to determine whether a particular task is subserved by one or the other hemisphere, the results may be obscured if factors such as sex, handedness, and the extent to which the task is open to individual differences in hemispheric activation are ignored. Furthermore, an approach that ignores these variants will be unable to account for the large variation that is known to exist in cognitive organization (p. 89).

Temporary anesthetization of the cerebral hemispheres: the Wada technique

This procedure was developed by Wada (1949) and requires a general anesthetic to be injected into the left and/or right carotid artery. The drug travels up the artery and circulates in the target hemisphere producing a temporary anesthesia which lasts for 2 or 3 minutes. With the hemisphere temporarily inactivated any task which requires the processing strategies of that hemisphere will be impaired. Thus, when the left hemisphere is anesthetized speech tasks are generally impaired in right handed subjects. Anesthetization of the right hemisphere on the other hand is known to impair musical performance (Bogen and Gordon, 1971).

Temporal resolution in this procedure is poor, and spatial resolution is low. At best, one can say that one or the other hemisphere may be involved in a particular task if impaired performance is obtained following injection of the hemisphere. This is obviously a procedure which carries risks to the individual and it is not used with normal subjects because of risks to the integrity of their brains. Consequently the procedure is restricted to the investigation of the brain damaged population, and our evaluations of relevant work based on this technique must acknowledge that we are drawing inferences based on findings derived from atypical brains.

Sequential finger tapping

According to Mateer (1983) the left hemisphere is specialized for control of certain kinds of complex, sequenced motor performance requiring changes in upper limb position and orientation (See Stuss and Benson [1984] for a review of neuropsychological studies of the frontal lobes). Studies that have investigated the interaction between speaking and manual activity have demonstrated that speech interferes with a variety of manual tasks performed with the right hand (Lomas, 1980; Lomas and Kimura, 1976). Recently Lomas stated:

> It appears . . . that the lateralized interference effects of concurrent cognitive and manual activity are observed only when there is competition between verbal systems and a system for the control of posture transitions in the absence of visual guidance. It is no longer reasonable to attribute this effect simply to the processing of two tasks within one hemisphere, the effect is far more specific (p. 148).

Generally, the sequential finger tapping task requires the subject to sequentially finger tap telegraph keys with the right and/or left hands, independently, while speaking or conducting another task with the free hand. Depression of task performance is thought to reflect interference and utilization of brain mechanisms in the hemisphere needed to maintain sequential finger tapping, but which are also common to speaking. Thus, lateralization of brain mechanisms is inferred from depressed performance on sequential finger tapping.

Temporal and spatial resolution for this procedure is poor. Similar to other behavioral procedures only gross statements about lateralization of function can be made, and any interaction of the hemispheres cannot be observed. Clearly, this is a very indirect method since we must make the assumption that there is a direct link between hand skills and brain control for language.

Hemispheric Processing Investigations with Stutterers

Few researchers have established a systematic research program for the study of hemispheric processing in stutterers. Most have contributed a single study with no subsequent follow-up. More often than not behavioral input–output procedures have been employed (e.g., dichotic listening procedures), to infer underlying hemispheric mechanisms with little attention to subject, stimulus and task variables. This failure to compare subject, stimulus and task variables across investigations often leads to an impression of inconsistent and fragmentary findings.

Dichotic listening procedures

Dichotic listening procedures have long been used in brain research and have generated the largest number of studies in the area of stuttering. This has in part been due to the limited equipment needs and the development of computerized dichotic tapes which several laboratories and researchers have been willing to share with others. Perhaps one of the greatest difficulties with these studies is that relative efficiency (a preference score) has been used to infer an absolute psychological mechanism in the hemispheres of stutterers (e.g., 'reversed cerebral dominance' or 'left cerebral dominance') based upon observations with nonsense syllable stimuli.

In the stuttering literature those investigations that have used meaningful linguistic stimuli (that is, words) have consistently reported a significantly larger proportion of stutterers, compared to normals, with a left ear preference (Curry and Gregory, 1969; Perrin and Eisenson, 1970; Quinn, 1972, Sommers *et al.* 1975; Davenport, 1979). Investigations using nonsense syllables, on the other hand, have reported findings consistent with research involving normal populations (Cerf and Prins, 1974; Sussman and MacNielage, 1975; Dorman and Porter, 1975; Brady and Berson, 1975; Pinsky and McAdam, 1980; Rosenfield and Goodglass, 1980; Liebetrau and Daly, 1981; Cimorell-Strong, Gilbert and Frick, 1983; Blood, 1985).

However, in many of these investigations using nonsense syllables a larger number of stutterers were shown to have either a left ear preference, or no ear preference under dichotic stimulation with nonsense syllables (Brady and Berson, 1975; Strong, 1978; Rosenfield and Goodglass, 1980; Liebetrau and Daly, 1981; Cimorell-Strong *et al.* 1983; Blood, 1985). The only study to systematically observe stutterers' ear preference scores for both words and nonsense syllables was reported by Perrin and Eisenson (1970). They found a left ear preference for words, but no ear preference for nonsense syllables in a group of stutterers under dichotic listening conditions.

A finding in both the Rosenfield and Goodglass (1980) and Pinsky and McAdam (1980) studies with nonsense syllables was the stutterers' inferior performance in reporting CV nonsense syllables. Rosenfield and Goodglass (1980) suggested that this reflected a 'phoneme perception deficiency'. This is an interesting observation when one considers that the right hemisphere may be less capable of processing nonsense syllables than the left (Zaidel, 1979). Interpretation of dichotic studies with stutterers using nonsense syllables is difficult at best. Indeed, the processing of meaningful linguistic stimuli is vastly different from nonsense syllables and continues to be a confusing area in this literature.

Tachistoscopic procedures

Results from visual tachistoscopic procedures with stutterers have been reported in three independent investigations (Moore, 1976; Plakosh, 1978; Hand and Haynes, 1983). These studies used meaningful linguistic stimuli, and all three of these studies found left visual half field advantages (LFA) in their stuttering subjects, implying right hemispheric activation. In contrast a right visual half field advantage (RFA) was found in their nonstutterers.

These three investigations are of importance for several reasons. Most importantly they demonstrate that differences in processing are not restricted to the auditory modality in stutterers. This suggests a more pervasive and central mechanism associated with the hemispheric processing of stutterers, and that they are more dependent upon the right hemisphere for processing of both auditory and visual linguistic stimuli.

An investigation by Wilkins, Webster and Morgan (1984) studied reaction times of stutterers to stimuli presented to either the left or right visual half fields using letter and figure recognition tasks. They found longer left visual field (right hemisphere) reaction times prior to therapy. Following therapy, left visual field reaction times showed the greatest reduction from pretreatment scores. The authors suggested that these findings may relate to right hemisphere interference in stuttering. Importantly, these results demonstrate changes in the stutterers' processing of visually presented stimuli associated with clinical manipulation of stuttering and they provide support for the role of right hemispheric interference in stuttering.

The Wada technique

Temporary anesthetization of the cerebral hemispheres with intracarotid injection of sodium amytal has been employed in relatively few studies investigating stutterers. The 1966 investigation by R.K. Jones using this procedure rekindled interest in hemispheric processing in stutterers. Jones (1966) reported bilateral speech control in four stutterers prior to surgery. Following surgery the procedure showed speech was no longer controlled bilaterally, and all four of his stutterers were then reported to have normal speech.

The results of this investigation must be weighed relative to several variables that may have confounded the outcome. Three of the four subjects were left-handed, all had neurological lesions, and all had undergone a neurological surgical procedure. Subsequent studies by Andrews *et al.* (1972) and Luessenhop *et al.* (1973) failed to replicate the earlier observations of bilateral control while avoiding some of the confounding variables in the Jones study.

Investigations using this procedure are difficult to interpret for several reasons: the number of subjects used has been small; handedness has varied between studies; neurological integrity was heterogeneous; onset of stuttering was not always controlled; age of subjects varied; memory tasks differed; and the nature of the linguistic task differed. Furthermore, the procedure deals with motor speech tasks following unilateral general anesthesia and this has little temporal or spatial resolution. For these reasons, any categorical statement concerning the contribution of cerebral processing to stuttering through the use of this procedure is difficult to make.

Electrophysiological methods

Using meaningful words embedded in phrases to evoke AER potentials Ponsford, Brown, Marsh and Travis (1975) computed correlations between the averaged responses to the words in two conditions using electrodes placed over Wernicke's and Broca's areas, and over homologous points in the right hemisphere. Results revealed correlation coefficients amongst normal speakers were lower in the left hemisphere, particularly over Broca's area. However, stutterers showed a reversal of this trend, with lower correlations in the right hemisphere, and greater variance among subjects. Similarly, Zimmerman and Knott (1974), using the contingent negative variation (CNV) method with nonverbal and meaningful linguistic stimuli, concluded that stutterers, when processing verbal stimuli, show more variable interhemispheric relationships, and do not show a consistently larger shift in the left hemisphere than in the right.

Using nonverbal stimuli and simultaneous button pushing with both thumbs in one condition, and the utterance of the same fluently spoken word in another condition, Pinsky and McAdam (1980) concluded that their results, using the CNV method, provided insufficient evidence to support hemispheric asymmetry differences between stutterers and nonstutterers.

Methodological differences in the above studies may be responsible for the different results. When verbal stimuli are used and when stutterers are required to utter words, whether fluent or dysfluent (Zimmerman and Knott, 1974), differences in hemispheric activation using AER procedures have been recorded. This underscores the importance of comparing the methods used in investigations of hemispheric processing with stutterers and other groups.

Moore and his associates (Moore, 1986a; Moore, 1984a; Moore, Craven and Faber, 1982; Moore and Haynes, 1980a; Moore and Lang, 1977; Moore and Lorendo, 1980), using the EEG hemispheric alpha asymmetry procedure, have consistently reported greater alpha suppression in the right posterior temporal–parietal area in male stutterers using meaningful linguistic stimuli (high and low imagery words and connected verbal discourse) under conditions of recall and recognition. Recently, Boberg, Yeudall, Schopflocher and Bo-Lassen (1983) have found greater alpha suppression in the right posterior frontal brain areas of stutterers prior to clinical management. Following clinical management which increased fluency these investigators reported a shift in hemispheric alpha suppression to the left posterior frontal area. This observation suggests that gains in fluency that are obtained with clinical management produce a change in the processing strategies employed by the stutterer to establish and maintain fluent speech, as reflected in a shift from right to left hemispheric alpha suppression. In support of this finding, Moore (1984a) reported right hemispheric alpha suppression during baseline with a gradual and consistent suppression of left hemispheric alpha as stuttering decreased using biofeedback (EMG) in a single subject experimental design.

In a more recent publication (Moore, 1986a) a negative relationship between measures of stuttering and hemispheric alpha ratios obtained during recall tasks has been observed. These data indicate that as the frequency of stuttering increases, right hemispheric alpha decreases during active tasks requiring verbal recall. More severe stutterers tend to have greater right hemisphere activation during recall tasks. These data would suggest that hemispheric activation in stutterers is not a dichotomous variable, but rather a continuous one, with greater stuttering related to greater degrees of right hemispheric activation during recall tasks.

Sequential finger tapping

Webster (1985a; 1985b) has compared male stutterers and fluent speakers on sequential finger tapping and index finger tapping with one hand while carrying out concurrent pace tasks with the other hand under conditions of visual guidance and no visual guidance. For right hand sequential tapping, left hand concurrent task performance produced more interference among stutterers than fluent speakers. Webster (1985a) has interpreted these data as ' . . . being consistent with a neuropsychological model of stuttering that includes enhanced left hemisphere vulnerability to interference by concurrent right hemisphere activity' (p. 2). In a third study Webster (1985b) found that stutterers achieved fewer correct sequences and made more errors than fluent speakers without visual guidance.

Two investigations have been reported using nonsequential finger tapping. Sussman (1982) reported that finger tapping and concurrent reading revealed a lateralized left hemisphere interference effect only for his right handed subjects. Sussman's left and right handed stutterers revealed highly symmetric interference effects, which is suggestive of bilateral language representation. Interestingly, stutterers demonstrated left hemisphere representation for visuo–spatial processing in the Sussman study. It was not clear from the procedures, however, if visual guidance was used in this investigation.

Results reported by Brutten and Trotter (1985) using nonsequential finger tapping, visual guidance (a light was illuminated when the subjects tapped a button imbedded in a sloped box), no fluent control group, and a sample of children ranging in age from 6.5 to 17.9 years are difficult to interpret. The authors reported that interference was significantly present in both the speech and vocalic conditions, and that their results were not consistent with a laterality model. Rather they suggested that their findings of increased interference with increased attentional demands were consistent with a 'capacity framework'. The use of visual guidance in the Brutten and Trotter study may have influenced their results and interpretations. Their findings must be considered relative to Lomas' (1980) study which indicated ' . . . that the lateralized interference effects of concurrent cognitive and manual activity are observed only when there is competition between verbal systems, and a system for the control of posture transitions in the absence of visual guidance' (p. 148). The failure to include an age matched control group does not allow us to compare the performance of normal subjects for the procedures used in this investigation; nor does it allow us to evaluate the authors' interpretations of their findings.

Cerebral blood flow

Wood *et al.* (1980), using a noninvasive measurement of blood flow with two stutterers, reported greater flow in Broca's area in the right hemisphere during stuttering. However, when the subjects were fluent greater blood flow was found in the left anterior hemisphere. This study demonstrates an important relationship between stuttering and hemispheric activation. Stutterers did not simply have greater right hemispheric activation, but rather there was greater right hemispheric activation during periods of greater stuttering. This finding has also been reported by us using EEG procedures, and underscores the need to report stuttering severity data along with measures of hemispheric activation relative to stimulus, task and subject variables.

Neuropsychological test batteries

Additional evidence of CNS differences in stutterers has come from investigations that have used neuropsychological test batteries. Daly and his colleagues (Daly, Kimbarrow and Smith, 1977; Smith and Daly, 1980) have tested stutterers on the Michigan Neuropsychological Test Battery (Smith, 1975). They carefully selected 54 'functional' stutterers without concomitant disorders such as hearing loss, cleft palate, learning disabilities, mental retardation or articulation problems. They were surprised when 35% of these carefully screened subjects showed three or more positive neurological signs of cerebral dysfunction. Those stutterers with three or more positive signs were classified as 'organic' cases and this study suggested there was a high probability of cerebral and neurological dysfunction in and among certain members of the entire stuttering population. In a later study Liebetrau and Daly (1981) used performance on a neuropsychological test battery to classify stuttering as 'organic' (three or more positive signs) or 'functional' (one or less signs) cases.

Boberg and Yeudall (1984) also used a neuropsychological test battery to investigate possible CNS differences between two controlled stutterers who had made substantial gains in therapy, and maintained those gains for more than five years, and two stutterers who made minimal gains in therapy, and were unable to maintain the minimal gains achieved. The battery revealed substantial differences between the two successful and two unsuccessful stutterers. The subjects also performed verbal and visuo–spatial tasks while the experimenters measured proportional alpha power through an EEG spectral analysis. The two unsuccessful subjects showed substantially more areas of abnormal cerebral function than did the two successful subjects. It was suggested that relative gains in therapy might be related to CNS function as reflected in EEG differences and subtest results.

Summary of Findings

Looking over these findings there appears to be compelling evidence from many studies, using a wide variety of investigative techniques, that there are differences in CNS functioning amongst stutterers. Data from well controlled dichotic, EEG, blood flow, tachistoscopic, sequential finger tapping and Wada technique studies show that stutterers typically do not use primarily left hemispheric strategies to process language as do normal speakers. Rather, most stutterers use primarily right hemispheric, or greater bilateral strategies in processing language. Additionally, there is evidence of cerebral dysfunction amongst stutterers based on the results of standard neuropsychological test batteries. Finally, there is some experimental evidence that following successful clinical management stutterers demonstrate a shift from right to left hemispheric processing strategies for language (Boberg *et al.* 1983; Moore, 1984a).

A careful perusal of the methodologies and procedures employed in studies designed to explore the relationship between hemispheric activation and stuttering reveals some consistent trends. When the nature of stimuli, severity of stuttering, memory task, and processing strategies of the left and right hemisphere are considered, there is evidence that greater right hemispheric processing occurs in more severe stutterers when meaningful linguistic stimuli are used under verbal recall conditions. As with normals there is variance in the data, but tests of statistical significance have consistently revealed stutterers and normals to be drawn from different neuropsychological populations. Studies that do not control severity, task, and the nature of the linguistic stimuli used should report sub-groups of the population that show greater or lesser degrees of right hemispheric activation. Hemispheric activation is a continuous (not dichotomous) phenomenon and can only be understood in terms of those independent variables which affect it at any given moment. To suggest that all stutterers, under all conditions, use only right hemispheric processing strategies would be to deny the body of research indicating variables known to effect hemispheric activation (see below).

Effects of Right Hemispheric Processing

Relatively few investigators have studied the effects of right hemispheric language processing in stutterers. Yet, right hemispheric processing for language was first observed in stutterers over 15 years ago (Curry and Gregory, 1969), hinted at over 40 years ago (Douglass, 1943; Knott and Tjossen, 1943) and demonstrated repeatedly since. It might, therefore, be instructive first to examine evidence from other areas to understand what happens when right hemispheric strategies are predominantly used for language processing.

Dennis and her associates (Kohn and Dennis, 1974; Dennis and Kohn, 1975; Dennis and Whitaker, 1976; Dennis 1980a, 1980b) investigated linguistic and visuospatial abilities in patients who had undergone unilateral surgical decortications during infancy in order to control convulsive seizures. Although left hemisphere decortication during infancy did not produce severe aphasia, or any obvious language deficits, such patients did exhibit difficulty in using complex language; in particular the ability to respond appropriately to structural or syntactic aspects of heard utterances. There was also a delayed acquisition of word relationships. Similarly the investigators found that patients with right hemisphere decortications in infancy performed normally on simple tests of visuospatial function, but were significantly impaired on complex tasks such as maze problems and map-reading tests. In summarizing this work Kolb and Whishaw (1980) state that each hemisphere can assume some of the opposite hemisphere's function if that opposite hemisphere is removed or damaged early in infancy. Many tasks and stimuli can be processed by the resources of both hemispheres. According to Friedman and Polson (1981):

> ... the difficulties involved in obtaining reliable, replicable data in this field may similarly reflect the fact that tasks can usually be performed with a number of different resource compositions, each of which draws in varying amounts the supplies of the two hemispheres. Tasks that allow an assortment of resource compositions will tend to be easily influenced by parameter manipulations and may thus produce the most variable results across different populations of subjects (p. 1053).

However, neither hemisphere appears totally capable of mediating all of the missing opposite's functions. Milner (1975) and Teuber (1975) have emphasized that there is an intellectual 'price to pay' when one hemisphere has to assume the functions of a damaged or absent hemisphere. Kolb and Whishaw conclude that although the developing brain gives evidence of considerable plasticity, there is convincing evidence against full equipotentiality of the hemispheres: both appear functionally specialized at birth or shortly thereafter, but both may use different processing strategies to perform the same task, or comprehend the same stimuli.

This last point, equipotentiality of the hemispheres for language, has produced considerable controversy. Because of the striking difference in how early and late lesions affect language it has been proposed that the two hemispheres are equally able to mediate language at birth and in early childhood and only become specialized or 'lateralized' during development. Lenneberg (1967) proposed that lateralization of function develops rapidly between the ages of two to five, and then proceeds more slowly until puberty, by which time it is complete. Other investigators (Dennis and Whitaker, 1976; Molfese, 1977; Entus, 1977) have demonstrated language asymmetry is present at birth or shortly thereafter. Using the sodium amytal test Rasmussen and Milner (1975) have reported that only direct damage to the left hemisphere before the age of five results in a shift in hemispheric processing strategies. However, other investigators (Moore, 1984b; Kinsbourne, 1971; Pettit and Noll, 1979; Johnson, Sommers and Weidner, 1977; Moore and Weidner, 1974) using a variety of methods have demonstrated greater right hemispheric activation in left brain damaged aphasic subjects during the course of language recovery. These studies support the notion that right hemispheric processing strategies can be used to process some aspects of language in adult brain damaged subjects.

Rasmussen and Milner (1975) have found that the locus of the original damage is a critical factor in determining whether language will shift to the right hemisphere. For example, they report that damage confined to Broca's area may shift those speech functions to the right hemisphere while the undamaged Wernicke's area will retain the functions usually associated with it. Such a patient would then appear to have bilateral speech, as can be shown in sodium amytal testing. On a related point there is evidence (Teuber, 1975) that although language processing may be assumed by the right hemisphere when the left is damaged, the left hemisphere does not appear to process visuo-spatial material when the right hemisphere is damaged.

It is also conceivable that other factors play an important role in determining which hemisphere's strategies will be used to process language. One fascinating observation is that the congenitally deaf use different processing patterns when compared to hearing individuals (Neville, 1977). Deaf children who use sign language showed right hemisphere processing of language whereas nonsigning deaf children did not show hemispheric asymmetry. This finding may reflect the greater role of visuo-spatial strategies in language processing of the children who were taught to sign; a further indication that the predominant mode of hemispheric activation may be related to environmental factors, including training.

Another instance of the effects of environment on hemispheric processing comes from the case of Genie, an individual deliberately isolated from normal social and experiential stimuli until she was discovered, at approximately 14 years of age (Fromkin *et al.* 1974). When she was rescued Genie did not speak at all, possibly because she had been abused by her father for any attempt to make sounds. Also her mother was not allowed to talk to her during feeding. Genie was first treated in the Rehabilitation Center of the Los Angeles Children's Hospital and then placed in a foster home. When there was clear evidence that she had begun to learn language several tests were administered. The results of the dichotic listening tests are of special interest as they showed a strong left ear preference, hence right hemispheric processing, for both verbal and nonverbal sounds (Genie is right-handed).

The results from dichotic testing imply that Genie is using right hemispheric strategies to process both verbal and non-verbal stimuli. This observation may reflect the fact that Genie's stimulation during those years of isolation came mainly from visual input; this finding provides further support for the effects of environmental variables on an individual's predominant mode of information processing.

Thus there is a growing body of evidence which suggests that the right hemisphere can be used to process language and speech. This has been demonstrated when the left hemisphere is absent or damaged, either through lesions or surgery. It may also occur through environmental factors, including auditory deprivation and specific training in the use of a visual communication system, as in the case of deaf children. While many investigations have reported the left hemisphere to be specialized for processing verbal material, and the right hemisphere specialized for nonverbal material, an absolute dichotomy (i.e., left–linguistic, right–nonlinguistic) cannot be supported from the literature.

Recent studies have shown that the stimuli to be processed may be less important than the mode of information processing used. Willis and her associates (1979) have supported the notion that hemispheric processing is related to both task processing demands and to the stimulus–perceptual aspects of the material to be processed. Moore and Haynes (1980a) found studies that reported no differences between the sexes in processing, studies which found females to have equal hemispheric participation, and studies showing males using more left hemispheric processing. Their analysis indicated that these apparently disparate findings could be directly related to the effects of using different tasks and methods of stimulus presentation. Their findings are in agreement with a statement by Gruber and Segalowitz (1977):

> . . . as is becoming increasingly clear in recent years, although the stimulus may be a well-specified linguistic one, the brain response may be greatly dependent on psychological functions. How the brain responds is a function of phychological set, context, motivation, and so forth — factors that are not easily specified at the neurobiological or linguistic level (p. 11).

These investigations suggest that 'hemispheric dominance' or 'lateralization' should be viewed in relation to the information processing strategies available to the left and right hemispheres, and not simply in terms of the stimuli to be processed. The nature of right hemispheric processing is qualitatively distinct from left hemispheric processing. The right hemisphere has been characterized as a holistic, parallel, nonsegmental, and time-independent processor contrasted with the left, which has been seen as analytic, linear, sequential, and time-dependent (Moscovitch, 1977; Gordon, 1979). According to Zaidel (1979) the right hemisphere may comprehend spoken words by performing an acoustic pattern match with stored exemplars, rather than performing a phonetic analysis, as does the left hemisphere. The lexicons of the left and right hemispheres reflect their differences in cognitive modes of processing. The lexicon of the right hemisphere, compared to the left, has been described as ' . . . connotative, associative, and imagined rather than precise, denotative and phonological' (Bradshaw, 1980, p. 178).

While the right hemisphere can process some linguistic information it appears less efficient at processing syntactic information; and it is 'literal' in its processing strategies. The research literature has shown that the right hemisphere can process high imagery nouns and adjectives (Day, 1977, 1979); is less capable of processing the phonological components of language (Zaidel, 1979); can process sounds of longer duration (usually greater than 100 milleseconds [Tallal and Newcomb, 1978]); can process semantic–pragmatic structuredness (Heeschen and Jurgens, 1978); can process active sentences (Dennis, 1980a, 1980b); and can perform recognition tasks (Faber-Clark and Moore, 1983). It is quite apparent, therefore, that numerous variables interact to influence the activation of left and right hemispheric processing strategies. It is also evident that both the left and/or right hemisphere can process the same linguistic information under certain conditions.

Relationship of Right Hemispheric Processing to Stuttering

In the studies reviewed above we have argued that there is consistent evidence that stutterers appear to process speech/language mainly in the right hemisphere. We also considered evidence that some individuals such as hemi-decorticates, who are required to use right hemispheric strategies for language and visuospatial functions, typically show some deficits and decreased efficiency in speech and language. We are now ready to consider whether there is evidence of reduced efficiency or discoordination in the speech of stutterers, and whether such effects are linked to right hemispheric processing strategies.

We turn first to an examination of the symptoms and characteristics of stuttering. However, we must first clarify that in this chapter, when we use the term 'stuttering' we are referring to 'core' or 'primary' stuttering. The wide array of struggle be-haviors, ancillary body movements and associated features of stuttering (Wingate, 1964) that characterize much of stuttering are generally regarded as learned byproducts of the 'core' aspects of stuttering, and will not be considered further in this review.

Numerous studies and investigators have described the symptoms or character-istics of stuttering. Bloodstein (1981), for example, notes that we can identify certain features of speech including sound or syllable repetitions, broken words, prolonged sounds, and signs of unusual effort or tension that are more closely related to what most listeners judge to be stuttering. He goes on to state that during stuttering there is abnormal functioning of the whole speech system, including the larynx, and that a notable aspect of the abnormal functioning is excessive muscular tension. Even in the fluent speech of stutterers, careful examination will reveal ' . . . slowness or limitation of movement, lateness of response, or incoordination of the vocal apparatus'. Andrews *et al.* (1983) reached similar conclusions in their recent review of stuttering research findings.

Several researchers have investigated specific aspects of this abnormal functioning of the speech system. Adams and Runyan (1981) and Adams (1981, 1984a, 1985) have studied the physiology and aerodynamics of stuttering, specifically voice onset (VOT) and voice initiation time (VIT). Adams reports that both VOT and VIT are slower in young stutterers compared to control subjects. He suggests that difficulty in quickly initiating voicing is one of the immediate causes of stutterers' repetitions and prolong-ations of articulatory gestures. He further considered that these apparent difficulties might be attributed to some central disturbance that would reduce the speed with which the stutterers organized and started transmitting neural signs to the periphery for voice production. In his latest review Adams (1985) points out that the timing relationships between laryngeal events, reaction times and phonetic durations appear to be the most sensitive and reliable discriminators between stutterers' 'tenuous fluency' and normal fluency.

Freeman (1984) has used electromyographic studies to provide information about a different level of speech production, namely patterns of muscle contraction and relax-ation. Her findings suggest that the stutterer, while speaking, experiences many moments of disruption of normal coordination or physiological blocks. Depending on such factors as the nature, duration and timing of the disruptions, these effects may or may not result in perceptible stuttering. From the perspective of EMG research the stutterings that listeners identify are ' . . . only a sampling of the pathophysiological behaviours underlying the disorder and constitute only a fraction of the speech co-ordination breakdowns (blocks) experienced by stutterers' (p. 111).

Conture (1984) has used fiberscopic and electroglottographic techniques to study laryngeal movements in stutterers. He reports abnormal movements during sound/syllable repetitions in adult stutterers and, in children, excessive or inappro-priate vocal fold adduction, especially at the transitions between sounds. He observed that young stutterers may have a tendency to 'tighten' or adduct their vocal folds when they move from consonant to vowel or vowel to consonant, regardless of the voicing characteristics of the consonant.

Zimmerman (1980a, 1980b) has focused on parameters such as velocity, displacement and duration of movement, and the coordination or timing between articulator events in stutterers. The objective of this research has been to relate these events to underlying neurophysiological processes. His studies revealed differences in the movement patterns in perceptually fluent utterances of stutterers and nonstutterers. Those findings led to speculations about possible associations between dysfluent events and aberrant activation of brainstem pathways that physiologically link the articulators. It was suggested that incoordination may occur when either turning or triggering inputs are aberrant. The tension noted in some stutterers prior to speech, the aberrant position of articulators, and the fact that most stuttering occurs on initial gestures, are indicators that the period before speech movements occur may be a time when aberrant neurological inputs are transmitted.

In summary, there appears to be considerable evidence that stutterers, both in their fluent and stuttered utterances, demonstrate distinctively aberrant behaviors. There is agreement that stutterers display an abnormal number of sound and syllable repetitions, broken words, prolonged sounds and unusual tensions. Numerous experimental investigations using a variety of techniques have shown stutterers to have abnormal laryngeal patterns during speech, some of which are perceptible, and some of which are revealed only by sensitive instrumentation. Finally, there are aberrant movement patterns on the speech musculature in stutterers. Additionally, evidence of stuttering in alaryngeal speakers (Freeman and Rosenfield, 1982; Rosenfield and Freeman, 1983; Tuck, 1979) suggests that these patterns are not likely to originate at the laryngeal level. In short, the accumulated evidence supports the hypothesis that the elusive dysfunction should be located in the CNS.

We believe that there is a strong suggestion of a link between right hemispheric processing strategies in stutterers and the aberrant behaviors displayed by stutterers in the peripheral speech mechanism. We have seen that right hemispheric processing of language is correlated with deficits, and we suggest that those deficits are related to the strategies available to the right hemisphere for information processing. In other words, if stutterers process language with right hemisphere strategies it is predictable that some type of deficit will be manifested in the timing and coordination of the peripheral speech mechanism. For example, discoordinations at the laryngeal level and aberrant movements of the articulators appear to be consequences of speech that is processed with right hemisphere strategies. Stuss and Benson (1984) in a review of the functions of the frontal lobes noted that temporal ordering of events is hemisphere specific. Benton (1968) reported that patients with left frontal damage are impaired in verbal fluency, but right damaged patients had more difficulty on constructional tasks and the copying of designs. Additionally, Milner (1982) has reported that left frontal lobe patients were impaired on all voluntarily controlled ordering of actions, but that right frontal lobe patients were deficient only if the task was nonverbal. The research data indicate that the asymmetric functions of the frontal lobes, relative to the hemispheric processing data with stutterers, may have important implications for the peripheral aberrant timing behaviors by stutterers.

The Missing Pieces of the Puzzle

There are at least three major gaps in this picture that attempts to relate stuttering to hemispheric processing. The first is that although there is an indication of a deficit or asymmetry, there is no clear evidence to indicate where the deficit or difference may reside in the CNS. Although there is evidence of different cortical processing strategies, right hemispheric rather than left hemispheric, it cannot be assumed that the difference originates at the cortical level. If there is, in fact, asymmetry at the brainstem level this might indeed trigger or lead to the different processing pattern at the cortical level. On the other hand, the difference may reside in the midbrain at the thalamic level (Yeudall, 1985), or at all three levels.

Support for the possible influence of subcortical structures is found in the work begun by Ojemann, Fedio and Van Buren (1968) and Fedio and Van Buren (1975). According to this work the left and right pulvinars (thalamic nuclei) function differentially to alert and activate the cerebral cortex for incoming stimuli. Generally, the left pulvinar provides a specific alerting response to the left cortex for verbal/auditory stimuli, and the right pulvinar to the right cortex for visual stimuli. Thus, subcortical structures have specific functions associated with information processing and hemispheric activation. Much innovative and precise research will be needed before this part of the picture is made clearer.

Secondly, there is no clear explanation or evidence as to why stutterers process speech/language in the right hemisphere. It could be related to differing myelinization rates in the CNS. There is evidence, for example, that the right hemisphere matures earlier in infants than the left hemisphere (Kolb and Whishaw, 1980). It is conceivable, therefore, that the environmental stimulation for speech development is out of phase with the timetable of biological maturation. If this were the case then the individual might begin to use right hemispheric strategies because the left hemisphere has not yet matured sufficiently to undertake this task, due to slower myelinization in the left hemisphere. If such an explanation were valid it might lead to an hypothesis of an interaction between environmental stress and a deficient or immature neurophysiological mechanism.

Another possibility is that some stress or trauma (environmental, chemical or biological) could have rendered the left hemisphere less capable of language processing, or slowed the rate of development of the left hemisphere. Such injury would have to be rather subtle as we know of no neurological evidence of lesions which might account for right hemispheric processing in stutterers. However, it is conceivable that a difference could exist apart from an observable lesion, and still bias the development of the two hemispheres in favor of the right hemisphere. In fact, Kidd (1984) has shown that stuttering among the relatives of stutterers occurs in a pattern indicating vertical transmission of a susceptibility to stutter with sex-modified expression. Kidd has also indicated that ' . . . simple genetic models can be rejected easily, but several that allow environmental interaction and sex differences are consistent with (the) data.' These latter observations appear to link a genetic factor to stuttering; this factor may be related to hemispheric asymmetries and the utilization of hemispheric processing strategies.

The third area where research evidence is still scanty is the actual relationship between hemispheric processing and language development. Although a considerable effort in the field of neuropsychology has been directed at this problem, the relationships, sequences and correlations with neurological development are still poorly understood. And in the area of stuttering, and other disorders of speech and language, few researchers have systematically investigated the relationship between hemispheric processing and speech/language disorders.

In conclusion, we offer two possible hypotheses which might account for the onset of stuttering. These are, naturally, speculative and are offered only to stimulate further research in these provocative areas.

The segmentation dysfunction hypothesis

This was first advanced by Moore and Haynes (1980a). According to these authors:

> Stuttering may emerge when both hemispheric processing of incoming information and motor programming of segmental linguistic units is in the right hemisphere (a non-segmental processor). These processing differences may be related to an inability, under certain circumstances, to handle the segmentation aspects of language. This may suggest the importance of linguistic segmentation as it relates to motor programming in some stutterers. Indeed, Carroll and Tanenhaus (1978) have suggested that segmentation is functionally related to the 'coherent processing' of language. As such, stuttering may be the result of a linguistic 'segmentation dysfunction' (p. 243).

Support for this hypothesis is found in those investigations (reviewed above) that have found greater anterior and posterior activation in the right hemisphere of stutterers during linguistic tasks. Additionally, the work which has shown that the temporal ordering of events is hemisphere specific, with left frontal damage impairing verbal fluency (Stuss and Benson, 1984), adds further support to a segmentation dysfunction hypothesis. Webster's (1985a, 1985b) data and interpretation using finger tapping tasks with stutterers and nonstutterers, which indicated enhanced left hemisphere vulnerability to interference by concurrent right hemisphere activity, also support the segmentation dysfunction hypothesis of stuttering.

By examining the language variables associated with increased stuttering we gain insights into the predominant mode of information processing used, and its effects on linguistic segmentation. It has been shown that stuttering increases in the same words of initial segments of long sentences compared to short sentences (Tornick and Blood-stein, 1976), on low frequency words compared to high frequency words (Schlesinger, Melham and Levy, 1966; Ronson, 1976; Palen and Peterson, 1982), from base structure sentences to transformations (Soderberg, 1967a; Bloodstein and Gantwerk, 1967; Hannah and Gardner, 1968; Ronson, 1976; Palen and Peterson, 1982), at clause bound-aries compared to internal positions of clauses (Wall, Starkweather and Cairns, 1981), with an increase in the number of relative clauses (Wells, 1979), and when voicing adjustments are required (Adams and Reis, 1971; 1974; Wall, Starkweather and Harris, 1981). Stutterers' recall of verbal information compared to normals has been shown to be reduced (Daly, 1981b; Moore *et al.* 1982). Homzie and Lindsay's (1984) review of the language variables associated with stuttering and stutterers has shown that language deficits are both a contributing factor and a continuing component in stuttering.

When the non-segmental processing strategies of the right hemisphere are con-sidered, the linguistic variables associated with increased stuttering gain further importance. Due to the resources available to the right hemisphere (Friedman and Polson, 1981) it is less capable of analyzing the constituent parts of a sentence in the same manner as the left hemisphere. Therefore, it is less capable of interpreting passive and negative sentences as contrasted with active sentences (Dennis, 1980a, 1980b; Dennis and Whitaker, 1976; Zaidel, 1979). Additionally, the right hemisphere is not as efficient as the left in the recall of verbal information (Faber-Clark and Moore, 1983; Zaidel, 1979), but is capable of verbal recognition using high visual imagery stimuli (Day, 1977, 1979; Faber-Clark and Moore, 1983). Perecman and Keller (1981) and Molfese (1978a; 1978b) have shown that processing of voice in normal subjects can be carried out by the right hemisphere, but place of articulation requires the resources of the left hemisphere. In a more recent study Molfese (1984) has indicated that the right hemisphere must rely on a number of different areas, activated at the same time, to make phonemic discriminations.

The language variables associated with increased stuttering appear to be those which the right hemisphere is less capable of processing and thus provide support for an hypothesis of increased dependency on right hemispheric non-segmental processing being associated with stuttering. In a recent investigation Moore (1986a) has shown that stuttering severity and hemispheric activation during verbal recall tasks are related; the greater the stuttering frequency the greater the right hemispheric activation. Segmentation dysfunction may be related to the longer time duration required by the right hemisphere in information processing (Kent, 1984; Thatcher, 1980) which reveals itself under certain tasks and conditions requiring greater left hemispheric participation in more severe stutterers.

This hypothesis does not speculate as to the cause of greater right hemispheric processing in stutterers. The greater incidence of right hemispheric processing may be related to morphological differences in stutterers or it may be related to environmental/learning factors. Future researchers will need to devise innovative research methods in an effort to unravel the physiological and experiential aspects of hemispheric processing and stuttering.

The subcortical interference hypothesis

This would suggest that right hemispheric activation is initiated by subcortical structures, and not solely cortical mechanisms. Research findings have implicated the ventrolateral thalamus as an anatomic correlate for perceptual and mnemonic operations in man. Investigations conducted by Ojemann and his associates (Ojemann, Fedio and Van Buren, 1968; Ojemann, 1975; Fedio and Van Buren, 1975) have demonstrated that the left and right pulvinars evoke specific alerting responses which serve to direct attention to information in the external environment. Fedio and Van Buren report that stimulation of the left pulvinar induces transient dysphasia and a retrograde loss in recent memory for verbal material. Stimulation of the right pulvinar failed to disrupt verbal behaviour, but interfered with discrimination and recognition of complex visual patterns. These authors concluded that their findings suggested an asymmetry in the functional organization of linguistic and nonverbal processes at the level of the lateral thalamus.

Brown (1975) has provided data indicating that the pulvinar mediates between anterior and posterior 'speech zones' (Penfield and Roberts, 1959) and is involved in hemispheric activation. According to Brown:

> ... there appears to be a simultaneous realization out of a common deep structure into the final perceptual and motoric forms of the language act. In the microgeny of action and perception, temporal relationships, both within a given stratum and from one stratum to the next, are maintained through cortico–cortical or cortical–subcortical pathways (p. 26).

Inferentially, anything which would interfere with the function of the left pulvinar during verbal tasks would interfere with the activation of the left hemisphere, and its temporal functions relative to language. While there is a paucity of research to support the effects of left pulvinar dysfunction on language disorders (*q.v.*, Brown, 1972, 1975) there is some information linking stuttering to brainstem dysfunction (Hall and Jerger, 1984; Toscher and Rupp, 1978; Liebetrau and Daly, 1981; Rosenfield and Jerger, 1984). Our present knowledge of the relationships between the thalamus and stuttering are in the preliminary stage, but do suggest that a thalamic–cortical mechanism may be associated with the greater incidence of right hemispheric activation during linguistic processing in stutterers. Research in this area will need to explore the relationship between verbal and nonverbal stimulation on both cortical and subcortical activation in stutterers to support a three dimensional mechanism underlying right hemispheric activation in stutterers.

Acknowledgments

This project was supported by a Study Leave granted to Einer Boberg from the University of Alberta, Edmonton. Support for Walter H. Moore, Jr. was provided by a Class A Sabbatical Leave and a grant for scholarly and creative activity awarded by California State University, Long Beach.

3 An Approach to the Study of Motor Speech Mechanisms in Stuttering

C. Woodruff Starkweather, Joy M. Armson and Barbara J. Amster

Introduction: The Motor Perspective of Stuttering

People who stutter often present an appearance, acoustically and visually, that suggests nervousness (Woods and Williams, 1976). Perhaps for this reason, several theories of stuttering are based on the idea that the disorder is caused by anxiety of one sort or another (Brutten and Shoemaker, 1967). Stutterers are often anxious, of course, as well they should be, since they are never quite sure where, when, or to what extent they will surprise their listeners with speech that is out of step with the rhythm and tempo of normal discourse. Nor is it entirely clear to what extent high levels of emotion, positive or negative, interfere with the smooth and effortless production of speech that characterizes fluency, either at a linguistic or a motoric level, in children or in adults. Because of these uncertainties, we wish to set aside momentarily the question of the role played by emotion, either as a primary cause of the disorder or as a proximal precipitator of dysfluency, and look at stuttering from a motoric perspective. We will return to the role that emotion may play in stuttering, as viewed from the motoric perspective, in the last section of this paper. It does seem evident that, whatever its cause, stuttering manifests itself as a disorder of speech motor control.

We will first look briefly at a few studies from which a perspective on stuttering as a disorder of speech motor control can be derived. We will then describe some motoric interpretations of information that has heretofore been interpreted non-motorically. In the second section, we will discuss in somewhat more detail, despite the space limitations of this chapter, the more general motor control literature as it relates to stuttering. Finally, we will present what we believe are the clinical implications of our position.

43

Stuttering as a disturbance of motor function

Freeman and Ushijima (1978) inserted hooked wire electrodes into the bellies of muscles located within the larynges of four stutterers in order to monitor the level of electrical activity during their speech. They found that movements associated with words on which stuttering occurred were accompanied by abnormally high levels of muscle activity and activity in muscles antagonistic to the movement in question. Shapiro (1980) later replicated this experiment with additional subjects and also included insertions of the electrodes into some of the muscles associated with oral articulation. Shapiro's findings were similar to Freeman and Ushijima's; muscles that one would presume not to be active at a given moment for the smooth and rapid movement of the speech mechanism are too active and active at the wrong times in the stuttered words of stutterers. There was also a lesser tendency for words judged by listeners as nonstuttered to show the same pattern of overactive and temporally uncoordinated muscle activity.

Another, somewhat curious, study showed a similar pattern in a nonspeech muscle group. Barrett and Stoeckel (1979) made careful measurements, via replayed videotape, of the eyelid movements of stutterers and nonstutterers when they were asked to wink. They found a significant tendency for the stutterers to move the contralateral (nonwinking) eye more than the nonstutterers.

Finally, Delaney (1979) observed the muscle activity of the stapedius, which is known to be active during speech production but the function of which is uncertain, to be significantly more active *prior* to speech attempts in adult stutterers than in matched adults who did not stutter.

Taken together these studies suggest that stutterers do not inhibit, to the same extent as their nonstuttering counterparts, the activity levels of muscles that are related to the muscles involved in a specific movement. In the case of Freeman and Ushijima's (1978) and Shapiro's (1980) observations, the functional relationship was one of agonist–antagonist, while in the Barrett and Stoeckel (1979) observations, the relationship was one of ipsilateral–contralateral, and in the Delaney (1979) study, there is no known functional relationship between the stapedius and the vocal mechanism, but instead a relationship of concomitant variation. It is of course of some importance that two of these studies concerned muscle systems that were not part of the speech production mechanism. Is it possible that the entire motor system in stutterers is abnormally active? If so, and if this condition is related to the etiology of stuttering (which we do not know), why is the disorder restricted to the speech mechanism? It might be noted that observations have been made on relatively small muscle systems. Is it possible that small muscle systems, including the speech mechanism, are abnormally active in stutterers but not large muscle systems? There are questions that can only be answered by further investigation.

The many studies showing that stutterers are slower in reaction to an external stimulus than their nonstuttering peers (Starkweather, Hirschman, and Tannenbaum, 1976; Cross and Luper, 1979; Adams and Hayden, 1976; and many others) may also be conservatively interpreted as evidence that the vocal mechanisms of stutterers are slowed in their movements by the presence of extraneous activity in muscles related to, but not required for, the reaction time task.

Explanations of apparently contrary data

How can the notion of overly active and improperly timed muscle activity square with other observations of stuttering? One of the most well known facts about stuttering, and one that seems to fly in the face of motoric perspectives on the disorder, is the tendency of stuttering to occur at certain linguistic locations at the beginnings of sentences, on longer sentences, on long and infrequently used words, and on stressed words and syllables (Sodenberg, 1966, 1967a; Jayaram, 1984; Wingate, 1976).

The motoric explanation is that these linguistic locations are all places where the speech mechanism must move either more quickly, more precisely, or both. Longer sentences are spoken more quickly than shorter ones in the speech of adults (Huggins, 1978; Lehiste, 1972; Malecot, Johnston and Kizziar, 1972) and children (Amster, 1984). Longer words are spoken with shorter segment durations, and therefore presumably more quickly, than shorter words (Umeda, 1975; Klatt, 1976). Words that occur less frequently in the language are spoken more slowly (Klatt, 1976), but may be presumed to have greater demands for precision of articulation in order to increase intelligibility. Stressed words and syllables are produced with clearer intelligibility as signalled by a narrower range of acceptable articulations and full vowel colour (Hunnicutt, 1985), and this increased intelligibility is presumably produced through the execution of more precise movements. Finally, words placed at the beginnings of sentences, which is a predictable location of stuttering, require both a rapid rate of movement (Umeda, 1975) *and* precision to achieve high levels of intelligibility because of the smaller amount of context. So the fact that stuttering can be predicted from knowledge of linguistic location does not necessarily imply that language formulation, or indeed some more general emotional state, is responsible for the location. There are also motoric explanations for the phenomenon.

Another area of information about stuttering that requires explanation is the well known tendency of stuttering to be more probable of occurrence in certain social situations. Typically, the situations a stutterer finds difficult are not necessarily the same as the ones another stutterer would find difficult, and this individuality of 'difficult' situations is often taken as evidence that stuttering is a learned behaviour. Although much of what a stutterer does when trying to talk must be learned behaviour, it is noteworthy that: (a) there are certain situations that are frequently reported as difficult, and (b) the situations are never arbitrary but rather related to the use of speech. Situations that are often labelled as difficult are: talking on the telephone, responding to a request for repetition, saying one's name, or when excellence in speech is desirable, i.e., a job interview or a public speech. These commonly reported difficult situations are all ones in which more precise articulatory movements are required either because of a raised load of information, e.g., saying specific words, the acoustical imperfections of telephone transmission, or because the speaker is striving for a higher level of performance.

The second point, that difficult situations are never arbitrary, suggests that something other than learning causes situational variability. If stutterers found situations difficult because they were associated with stuttering that had occurred in the past, then there would occasionally be stutterers whose difficult situations were entirely arbitrary, for example, talking to men wirh red hair, or talking on sunny days, or at midday, or when wearing a certain type of clothing. The situations stutterers report as difficult are never as arbitrary as one would expect if they were learned by the usual conditioning processes, but are instead related to the use of speech and language. In other words, they are situations in which the pragmatics of communication is altered. With a change in language pragmatics typically goes a difference in the rate of speech or the precision of articulation, such as with authority figures, talking on the telephone, ordering in a restaurant, giving a set speech, etc. Consequently, it seems likely that there is a motoric difference in the kinds of situations that stutterers report as difficult.

The fact that stutterers speak fluently under certain circumstances, e.g., singing, rhythmically paced speech, choral speech, speaking in a dialect not one's own, DAF, whispering, etc., has also been cited as evidence that stuttering is a psychobehavioural disorder with the argument that these conditions are distracting or relaxing. An equally tenable explanation, however, is that these conditions are ones in which speech is different — either slower or lacking a need for precision of articulation. Although some research has shown that reduced rate alone is not sufficient to explain at least choral speech (Adams and Ramig, 1980) or metronomically paced speech (Fransella, 1967), neither of these studies has shown that the other important aspect of speech motor control, precision of movement, is not affected in these conditions. And in fact, one would expect that when the timing of syllables is assisted either by another speaker or by a metronomic device, the necessity for precision of movement is reduced.

The fact that many stutterers say that their stuttering is worse when they are anxious or excited may also be explained motorically. Zimmermann (1980c) has argued that the smoothness and speed with which a movement is made by the speech mechanism is determined by, among other things, the level of background tonus in the muscles. This level of muscle tension is influenced by a number of factors, one of which is the emotional state of the speaker. Anyone who plays tennis (or any other fast game) will recognize the extent to which even so subtle an emotional variable as self-confidence can influence the smoothness and precision of motor acts.

Many stutterers, particularly young ones, also report that the severity of their stuttering varies from day to day or week to week in a cyclical pattern. In the young stutterer this results in the typical episodic variation, while in the older stutterer it is seen as fluctuations of severity. This phenomenon too may be related to fluctuations in the level of background tonus. It seems almost as though the stutterer whose speech has been very poor for the past few days can not anticipate any stuttering more severe than the level he has most recently been experiencing. Consequently, on the next instance of stuttering, he is likely to find his stuttering not as bad as he expected. As a result, he feels somewhat better, which reduces his background tonus, which in turn makes him a little less likely to stutter the next time. This continues to happen, so he begins to stutter less and less and will continue to improve until he reaches a level of severity that is the best speech he ever gets. At this point, his expectations shift upward. His recent experience tells him that he should expect to speak well, and it becomes more and more likely that he will stutter more severely than he expects to. Consequently, he will usually have negative deconfirmation of his expectations, which makes his emotional level sink, his background tonus increase, and he begins to stutter more severely, on a downward course that does not end until he reaches the lowest point once again.

Although the arguments just presented suggest that stuttering is functionally related to motoric variables, we think it would be speculative to suggest that the disorder of stuttering is caused outright by some motoric deficit. Perhaps more likely, the motor system of some children is vulnerable to environmental pressures or demands, and these children are more likely to develop stuttering as a result of the interaction between environmental and genetically predetermined motoric factors. Motor coordination is learned at an early age, and so it is with stuttering. A child may develop the habit of approaching speech with struggle and avoidance because he or she has learned that speech production is difficult or not usually up to the expectations and demands of the environment.

Consequently, although we think stuttering can be properly conceived as a motoric dysfunction of the speech mechanism, we are not trying to suggest that it is a problem *caused* by a motor disorder. That remains a possibility, but there is not enough evidence from which to draw such a conclusion.

Another point which we feel has not been made; chronic stuttering itself may alter the properties of the speech mechanism. Because stuttering is accompanied by (or *is*) extraneous muscle tension, the chronic occurrence of stuttering episodes may produce long-term changes in the muscles of speech. Specifically, it should make the speech muscles stronger, thicker, and heavier. It seems reasonable to consider that the flexion of speech muscles against the extra resistance provided by antagonistic muscle sets that are abnormally tense would be likely to result in an increase in the mass of muscle tissue. Such changes would be expected to influence the mechanical properties of the speech mechanism. These mechanical changes may, in turn, make it more difficult to produce smooth, rapid, and precise movements of the articulators. A vicious cycle of this sort would go a long way to explain the fact, apparent from clinical accounts, that the longer a child has been stuttering, the longer it takes for him to recover to normal fluency (Starkweather and Gottwald, 1985). We are attempting to test this prediction.

Review of Speech Motor Control Literature and Application to Stuttering

The matter of how the brain orchestrates the production of speech has been studied from several different perspectives. Lashley (1951), in his classic paper *The Problem of Serial Order in Behaviour*, set the stage for one approach by proposing that just before production complex motor activity such as speech is represented in the brain as a string of serially ordered elements. In other words, preparation for speaking requires that an array of elements representing components of the intended final product be assembled as a plan of action in the brain. The plan is implemented as speech when the elements are 'read out' by the motor system. According to this conception, discrete elements serving as input to a motor system are fundamental units of motor control, with each control unit containing specific movement instructions or commands. This idea of a neural plan of action consisting of an ordered sequence of elements, each of which corresponds to a unit of movement commands, has been widely used by scientists as an explanatory model of speech production. They proposed that the elements of a neural action plan for speech are coded as linguistic units, the phoneme being a popular choice of the earlier models.

Models postulating that concatenable strings of elements, such as phonemes, serve as input to the speech production system must deal, however, with the fact that the output of this system, both acoustic and kinetic, is not itself segmentable into discrete, concatenable elements. Speech is produced continuously within breath group units as a stream of multiple, asynchronous articulatory movements. Moreover, movements for adjacent phonemes often overlap one another in coarticulation, as for example, when lip rounding for /u/ in 'two' is produced at the same time that the tongue tip is brought into contact with the alveolar ridge for production of /t/. In addition, the movements for a given phoneme are not constant from production to production but vary with the context of adjacent phonemes. To explain features such as coarticulation and variability, theorists have proposed a variety of schemes for coding input command units, each scheme, however, retaining the idea that the control element is identical with a linguistic unit. For example, to explain phoneme production variability, Wicklegren (1969) proposed that representations of all possible allophones are stored in the brain and may be retrieved for arrangement in a neural plan of action. To deal with the phenomenon of coarticulation, Henke (1966) suggested that commands are issued in units the size of distinctive features, while Kozhevnikov and Chistovich (1965) suggested that they were issued in units the size of syllables, since movement overlap is greater within rather than across syllable boundaries. These are only a few of the many theories that have tried to reconcile the concept of discrete, context–invariant units of motor control with the nonsegmental, context–sensitive nature of speech output.

It should be evident that theorists responsible for developing models of this sort are primarily interested in explaining speech from one particular perspective: that is, as a means by which language is given expression. Such explanations posit abstract mental processes which conceptualize or describe underlying neural activity in convenient but purely hypothetical ways.

Taking another approach to the study of how speech is produced, certain researchers have argued for the value of making minimal *a priori* assumptions about neural processes and instead using knowledge about physical and physiological characteristics of the motor speech system to guide inferences. This approach requires careful analyses of movement parameters such as displacement, velocity, and acceleration, and/or muscle activity in various speech tasks and under conditions of experimental manipulation. In taking this perspective, these researchers are primarily interested in speech as a motor skill rather than as a symbolic mode of expression and regard the study of the speech motor system to be similar in principle to the study of other motor systems; e.g., hand, limbs, etc. As a result, these investigators have been able to make use of concepts and experimental paradigms from the general field of motor control to guide their research endeavours. For example, Kelso and his colleagues (1982) have been intrigued with the finding that stable temporal patterns can be identified in such activities as locomotion or handwriting. What this means is that a constant phase relationship among movements is maintained despite changes in overall conditions (such as the speed of task execution). Thus, for example, when speed (but not amplitude) of handwriting is varied, velocity records show that while the overall duration taken to write a given word changes markedly across speeds, the timing relationships of a given movement relative to total execution time is preserved (Viviani and Terzuolo, 1980). According to Kelso and others (see, for example, Kelso and Tuller, 1984) this kind of temporal stability reveals a major feature about nervous system organization for action, namely that the movements necessary to produce the basic properties of an act may be constrained to occur in some fixed temporal pattern. In this organizational framework, fundamental units of production in speech are identical with, or defined by, units of temporal stability. Evidence for one such unit of temporal stability in speech has been reported by Tuller, Kelso, and Harris (1982); they found phasing constancy among movements employed in the production of a consonant and two flanking vowels, though this finding has been questioned subsequently on statistical grounds (Munhall, 1985).

Another group of investigators who have strongly advocated objective study of the peripheral mechanism as the route to better understanding of speech motor control are Abbs and his colleagues at the University of Wisconsin's Speech Motor Control Laboratories. Much of their efforts have been directed toward exploring afferent (i.e., sensory) contributions to mechanisms of speech production. For this purpose, they have relied extensively on use of the 'external disturbance' or 'perturbation' paradigm as a research method. In this paradigm, brief unanticipated disturbances of a structure (e.g., lip or jaw) are applied either prior to or during its movement for production of a speech sound. An example of one such task is as follows: subjects were asked to sustain production of a vowel until they heard a tone at which time they were to produce a /b/ as rapidly as possible; for a small percentage of /b/ productions, brief downward perturbations were introduced to the lower lip either prior to or during initiation of bilabial closure (see Gracco and Abbs, 1985).

For all perturbation tasks employed (see Abbs, Gracco and Cole, 1984), subjects universally were observed to make automatic adjustment so that the intended speech sound was produced with no perceptible distortion despite the briefly induced movement disturbance. Compensatory adjustments have been found to occur in both the perturbed structure (e.g., lower lip in the task described above) as well as in coactive unperturbed structures (e.g., upper lip). A general conclusion of Abbs and his fellow workers is that through its ability to make use of afferent input in flexible ways, the speech motor system is able to be highly resistant to external perturbation in achieving intended perceptual goals.

All in all, despite its more than 30-year history, the study of how speech is produced has yielded relatively little in the way of concrete, fundamental information about neuromuscular mechanisms. There is, however, reason for optimism. With increased knowledge of physiological characteristics of the peripheral mechanism, development of quantitative models which are tested through simulation techniques, and advances in technology for the study of nervous system function at all levels, future speech scientists should eventually have a sophisticated understanding of motor function in speech.

In the meantime, what can be gleaned from the existing body of literature for application to the study of stuttering? For one thing, the approach of studying physio-logical characteristics of the speech system under varying experimental conditions should be as valuable for the study of stuttering speakers as it is presumed to be for the study of normal speakers. An example of this type of research and its role in generating models of motor function/dysfunction in stuttering may help to illustrate this point. Zimmermann (1980a,c) used high speed cineradiography to obtain movement signals as stutterers produced fluent and stuttered speech and during the production of fluent speech by nonstutterers. He determined values for displacement and velocity of lip and jaw movement and made various measures of temporal and spatial patterns. Some of his findings were as follows: during fluent productions, stutterers as a group showed consistently lower peak velocities, smaller displacements, and longer transition times for both lip and jaw movement than did the normal speakers (though these differences were not statistically tested); during stuttering, stutterers assumed articulatory postures which were different from those exhibited for fluent production of the same sound; termination of stuttering was coincident with articulatory repositioning.

Based on these findings Zimmermann (1980b) proposed a preliminary model of stuttering. He suggested that speech structures normally operate within a certain range of movement parameters and interact within a range of spatial and temporal values. If these values are exceeded, afferent input to brainstem reflex centers alters the gain of the reflexes they control. This alteration in reflex gain then throws the motor system out of balance, and the result is either oscillation or static positioning of speech structures; i.e., stuttering behaviours. In subsequent research, Zimmermann and Hanley (1983) tested the hypotheses that low values of movement excursion and velocity as well as long transition times between movements are associated with fluency in stutterers by using an adaptation paradigm and tracking the changes in movement parameters over adaptation trials. The results, however, did not support his hypothesis; stutterers, like nonstutterers, increased movement displacement and velocity and reduced movement time with increases in rate. This does not, of course, rule out the possibility of a mechanism underlying stuttering which is based on aberrant sensorimotor interactions but does indicate that afference abnormality, if it does exist, is not in the terms Zimmermann proposed. The point to be made here is that on the basis of descriptive physiological data gathered during stutterers' fluent and stuttered speech, it may be possible to postulate neural mechanisms reponsible for stuttering and test hypotheses which are consistent or inconsistent with these postulations. The outcome of such hypothesis testing will then shape further model development.

Development of models which explain stuttering in terms of neuromuscular function, of course, requires a knowledge of the neurophysiological underpinnings of normal speech, for which it was stated earlier few concrete 'facts' are available. Even now, however, there are a multitude of findings and concepts regarding speech motor control which could be helpful in guiding thinking about abnormal speech motor function. Only one set of findings and the conceptual frame of reference they suggest will be discussed here. (For a more complete discussion of motor control and stuttering, see Armson, in preparation).

Earlier in this section, the adaptability of the speech system in dealing with external disturbance was described. Recall that one of the experimental tasks involved perturbation of the lower lip prior to or during movement onset for production of the phoneme /b/. In coping with a perturbation delivered before the onset of lower lip movement both upper and lower lips made movement adjustments to achieve bilabial closure; when perturbation was delivered after onset of lower lip movement it was the upper lip which provided the major compensation, by markedly increasing the extent of its movement downward. In behaving this way, the lips appear to be functioning as a unit coordinated to achieve a particular result, in this case closure for production of /b/. In another experiment Kelso *et al.*, (1982), showed that when the jaw was perturbed during the production of /b/, the lower lip compensated for the change, but when this same perturbation was applied during /z/, it was the tongue which compensated.

Clearly, during speech, articulatory reaction to perturbation is not stereotypic; instead muscles react so as to yield the appropriate or intended speech result. Thus, muscles appear to be recruited for the production of a speech goal as functional units, so that they are able to operate together with flexibility in meeting movement goals. The examples given so far have described interaction of articulators of the supraglottal system, but functional linkage of muscle groups also occurs across subsystems. For example, when oral closure for the production of a plosive is delayed because of unanticipated perturbation, compensatory adjustments are made in the larynx so that correct voicing is achieved. If the structures of the motor speech mechanism are marshalled as a unit for production of a particular speech goal, regardless of whether the outcome is fluent or stuttered production, it would not be surprising to find that during an instance of stuttering, movement abnormalities occur in each of the three speech subsystems. More importantly, given this sort of organization, stutterers would be expected to stutter with their whole systems even if the breakdown in speech flow were to originate as a problem in only one subsystem since the parts of the mechanism not originally affected would be expected to respond to the disrupted part. The response of the originally unaffected parts might take the form of the original disruption, e.g., tremor (an overflow effect) or alternatively could take the form of attempted compensatory adjustment. Such adjustments would be unlikely to be successful if the original disruption were sufficiently severe or maladaptive. This perspective presents an alternative to the discoordination hypothesis (Perkins, Bell, Johnson and Stocks, 1979) in which it is proposed that stuttering results from defective coordination among speech subsystems. No one would argue, of course, that the temporal relations among at least some of the events produced by the subsystems are disrupted during stuttering, since stuttering moments are manifest in this way. The issue, then, is not whether stuttering presents as discoordination among speech subsystem events but whether it is caused by this. The view of stuttering as inherently a disorder of subsystem coordination has been a popular one since it has been proposed, perhaps in part because it is consistent with the fact that movement abnormalities of some type during stuttering have been reported for every subsystem (See Van Riper, 1982, p. 402–3 for a review).

However as shown earlier such findings are not necessarily inconsistent with speech flow breakdown originating in a single system. To date there is insufficient empirical evidence to support either position since the study of the operation of the subsystems relative to one another has been undertaken only recently and work in this area is still quite scant. In addition, this study has been of the operation of two subsystems in concert rather than three. For example, Borden and Armson (1985) assessed supraglottal/laryngeal interaction of production of /f/ in the words 'four' and 'five' by measuring temporal intervals between functionally analogous articulatory events in the two systems (e.g., onset of lip raising and laryngeal abduction at initiation of consonant production; onset of lip lowering and laryngeal adduction for consonant release). Preliminary findings suggest that coordination of lip and laryngeal articulatory gestures, at least, is frequently normal at the onset of stuttered production. On the other hand, Watson and Alfonso (1986) in studying respiratory/laryngeal interactions have found that severe stutterers prepared for phonation in a reaction time paradigm in a maladaptive manner; specifically they began abdominal compression before vocal fold closure occurred. In comparison, normal speakers and mild stutterers generally attained vocal fold closure before the onset of respiratory compression. Clearly, cross-system coordination is an area ripe for study and will be necessary to settle the question of whether stuttering originates as an interaction problem between subsystems or alternatively originates in one subsystem with subsequent impact on the others.

Clinical Implications

It should be said first that the motor perspective on stuttering has not yet produced very many clear facts, and consequently it is really too soon to change clinical practices, either diagnostic or therapeutic. So, in that sense, there are no clinical implications. However, even if it is too soon to change clinical practices, it may not be too soon to begin looking at clients from a somewhat different perspective and to be thinking about how practices might change in the future, should the empirical data confirm the theoretical notions that are now being discussed.

Assessment

Starkweather (1981) has defined fluency as the capacity to move the speech mechanism rapidly and easily, and stuttering as a clinically recognizable disorder in which speech is produced with excessive effort. These are definitions which fit comfortably within the motoric perspective. The fit is evident when one considers that motoric discoordination may have both spatial and temporal aspects, that is, one can be discoordinated by failing to achieve spatial targets with sufficient precision, or one can be discoordinated by failing to achieve temporal targets with sufficient precision. But because of the imperative to communicate, the effect on speech output of either one of these types of discoordination would be a slowing of the rate at which speech is produced. This argument is advanced in more detail in Starkweather (1987). Consequently, the motoric perspective may imply that the assessment of fluency will include an assessment of the rate of speech, against which improvements in fluency during therapy can be objectively assessed. Many clinicians assess rate on intake anyway, but it is worth noting that this practice is consistent with the motoric perspective. It should be understood, however, that language formulation, and perhaps other nonmotoric factors also play a role in the determination of speech rate. Clinicians should not assume that a slow rate of speech production indicates a faulty motor system, although it might be assumed that a rapid rate of speech production does imply an intact motor system.

The rate of normal adult speech is typically 5 to 6 syllables per second in American English (Walker and Black, 1950; Miller, 1951), French (Malecot, Johnston, and Kizziar, 1972), and Japanese (Osser and Peng, 1964). A clinician interested in getting a baseline syllable per second rate can do so using simple equipment such as a digital stopwatch (Amster, 1984), although it is necessary to listen repeatedly to the recorded signal and anticipate the onset and offset of the utterance in order to minimize the effect of the clinician's reaction time. Unfortunately, reaction time is not entirely eliminated by repeated listening, and the reaction time to the onset of the utterance is somewhat less than reaction time to the offset of the utterance, which introduces an error factor that tends to lengthen the duration of the utterance and consequently reduce the rate measure. This systematic error is known, however, and can be compensated for mathematically (Amster and Starkweather, 1986).

The rate of speech will vary with the length of the utterance, longer utterances being spoken more quickly than shorter ones (Jones, 1944; Lindblom, 1968; Malecot *et al.*, 1972; Lehiste, 1972; Huggins, 1978). Amster (1984) found a similar rate-for-length adjustment in the speech rate or normal preschool children. For baseline measures of rate, it may be important to control for utterance length by sampling a variety of lengths and reporting the different rates for each.

In contrast to the rate-for-length adjustment in normal speakers, Meyers and Freeman (1985) found that in the fluent speech of the stuttering preschool children they studied, longer utterances were produced more slowly. This may be an indication that even the apparently fluent speech of stutterers is different from the speech of normal speakers. It may also be, however, that these samples of 'fluent' speech actually contain instances of what has been called 'subclinical stuttering' (Shapiro, 1980). The presence of abnormalities of muscle activity such as Shapiro described would be expected to slow the rate of the stutterers' speech, accounting perhaps for the many observations that stutterers' 'fluent' speech is slower than that of nonstutterers (Zimmermann, 1980b; Starkweather and Myers, 1979). If, indeed, it is subclinical stuttering that slows the speech of stuttering children, then we would expect to find longer sentences more influenced by this effect than shorter ones. Whichever interpretation is accepted of the reversal in stutterers of the rate-by-length interaction, it may be that children who are at risk for stuttering could be identified at earlier ages because they show this difference.

Much has been written about the importance of phonation, and the role that abnormalities of glottal movement may have in stuttering (Adams and Reis, 1971; 1974; Freeman and Ushijima, 1978; Starkweather, Hirshman, and Tannenbaum, 1976). Certainly, it is useful to assess glottal motor functioning in children who stutter or who appear to be at risk for stuttering. The presence of hard or abrupt glottal attacks or a voice quality that has deteriorated as a result of the habitual use of such attacks should be noted. Indeed, chronic tension in the vocal folds associated with frequent stuttering can produce a chronically deviant vocal quality as most clinicians who work with stutterers have seen. Similarly, it may be that chronic tension in the upper articulators also changes their physical properties in a way that diminishes their motor functioning. Adult stutterers have long been known to demonstrate slower and less regular diadochokinetic performance (Blackburn, 1931), slower reaction times (Starkweather, Hirschman and Tannenbaum, 1976), and slower speech (Zimmermann, 1980b). All of these findings may have resulted from the fact that components of coordinative structures may have been altered in their stiffness and/or mass by chronic muscle tension. It seems useful, at least when chronic tension seems present, to test for velocity and smoothness of movement through diadochokinesis or reaction time. Indeed, the latter test is one of the most reliably obtainable differences between stutterers and nonstutterers (Andrews, Craig, Feyer, Hoddinott, Howie, and Neilson, 1983). The possibility of its future use in the clinic, as a way of deriving information about the physical state of the client's speech motor system, should not be ignored. Of course, further data need to be gathered about the distribution of this variable and its predictive relationship with severity, prognosis, or other measure of clinical relevance. In fact, we do not even have a standard reference for it. Perhaps in the future, we will be able to use reaction time tests, diadochokinesis, or some other test of speech motor control as a way of determining to what extent the mass and stiffness of a child's speech mechanism has been affected by chronic tension due to stuttering.

Another important area which must be addressed during assessment is that of attitude. Negative thoughts and feelings interact with all motor functions, including speech, both stuttered and nonstuttered, in a complex and reciprocal manner. Stuttering, like other motor dysfunctions, will increase when a stutterer has negative attitudes about himself or when he is full of speech-related fear or anxiety. These attitudes need to be addressed in therapy, and are usually assessed before therapy begins. Typically these are attitudes assessed by client interviews, questionnaires, and sentence completion tests. With the help of the clinician, the client identifies attitudes which make him less able to cope with and work on his problems. Most clinicians are familiar with idiosyncratic situations or specific words that a client fears because of its frequency of occurrence or significance in his life. Many clients relate how difficult they feel their own names or addresses are to say. One former client, a meat cutter, had special fears about words dealing with his job such as 'gizzards', and 'giblets'. This kind of specific 'word fear' is interesting from a motor control perspective. An unusual focus of attention on a particular motor act may alter the mechanical properties of the system as it is used in performing that act. It may be that stutterers have word fears for good reason. Their focus on and dread of saying such important words may actually alter the stiffness of the muscles, or change the mechanism momentarily in some other way so that a particular word is more difficult to say. If this is the process by which word fears become a factor in a stutterers' speech, it simplifies our understanding of stuttering to the extent that we do not need to look for deeper psychological explanations of such phenomena. Consequently, obtaining a list of feared words from a client during an assessment procedure may be more revealing of the state of his motor system and its susceptibility to transient changes in muscle stiffness than it is of the state of his psyche.

Starkweather and Gottwald's 'demands and capacities' model of stuttering development (1986) works quite well with a motor dysfunction approach to stuttering. They believe that stuttering develops when a young child lacks the capacity to produce syllables as fluently as the environment demands. When assessing young children, it is important to assess the parents' rate of speech as well as the child's since the parents' speech rate can affect the child's fluency. 'Speakers tend to adopt the same rate when conversing, and children are inclined to model behaviour patterns after their parents, so there is a natural tendency for the child to speak more rapidly to an adult who speaks rapidly' (Starkweather and Gottwald, 1986). The parents' and child's rate should be assessed in fluent syllables per second. The difference in rate between parent and child rather than the absolute rate may be most demanding of fluency (Starkweather and Gottwald, 1986). Recently, Hutt (1986) has observed that the difference between parents' and nonstuttering children's speech rate is significantly larger for boys than for girls. In this pilot study, the girls tended to talk more rapidly, and although the parents adjusted the rate of their speech for age-related changes in the child's speech rate, they made no such adjustment for differences in rate attributable to gender. Interestingly also, Meyers and Freeman (1985) found that adults speak faster to children who stutter, and we have noted clinically that an increased rate of speech is one kind of reaction parents show to an instance of stuttering. These observations suggest that the child's dysfluency may actually precipitate the parents' faster rate.

In addition to rate, other demands on the child's fluency need to be addressed such as conversational interruptions, negative parental reactions to stuttering, the child's reaction to dysfluency, time pressure, rapid turn-taking style, not enough time set aside for conversation, parents asking many questions, and demand speech. The values obtained in each of these areas of assessment may reflect the motoric functioning of the child's speech mechanism. Some measures, such as time pressure or a rapid turn-taking style, have a direct influence on motor performance by increasing the child's rate; others, such as negative parental reactions or interruptions may alter the child's speech motor control by reducing his sense of confidence or increasing his apprehension about speech performance. Parental language level when speaking to the child should also be assessed, since it has been noted that children are more dysfluent when their syntax is more complex (Pearl and Bernthal, 1980; Haynes and Hood, 1978; Gordon, 1982). The effect of language on motor performance is complex, but it should at least be noted that sentences that are more complex syntactically are also longer and so tend to be produced more quickly. However, it may also be the case that the formulation of more complex language makes demands on the central nervous system that detract from or interfere with its control of motor performance.

Much of this information can be gathered during a family play session in which the family is instructed to play together for about 15 minutes. The play session is video-taped for later fluency and language analysis. Other information can be obtained from interviewing the parents.

Therapy

From the motoric perspective, stuttering is seen as a form of motor dysfunction, and the entire speech mechanism as a unit in which vocal, respiratory, and articulatory processes normally function together. Of course stuttering has been viewed as dis-coordination of phonation with respiration and articulation (Perkins, Bell, Johnson and Stocks, 1979). Whether this is true or not, there is enough reflexively based co-ordination among the three major systems of speech production that movements per-formed by one system are likely to influence the movements of the two others. For this reason, it is often sufficient to work on one system in order to produce effects in one of the others. Specifically, a concentration on vocal targets, which may be easier to teach, can influence the tension levels and velocity of movements in the respiratory or articu-latory system.

The goal of any therapy is normal sounding speech. Slowing articulatory rate and simplifying phonatory movements facilitate speech coordinations and contribute to fluency (Perkins, Bell, Johnson and Stocks 1979). Following this principle, a number of 'fluency-shaping' therapies have been described. In these programs, the client begins by producing speech at very slow rates and then through successive approximation is taught to produce fluent speech at a normal rate. An essential aspect of this, and other fluency shaping types of therapy, is training in the execution of specific speech motor targets to bring the flow of speech under the stutterer's control. One target is con-tinuous phonation, or blending, which is achieved by exaggerating the continuity of phonation within a breath group through emphasizing vowel production. When this is properly accomplished, several words produced on a single breath should sound like one long 'word'. Another target is easy onset in which voice is initiated in a gentle and gradual manner so that the voice begins at an almost inaudible level and gradually increases in volume to full voicing. Easy onset is used only at the beginning of a breath group. Easy onset and continuous phonation are practiced at slowed speech rates in various contexts. Throughout this practice, normal prosody should be maintained as much as possible. Once fluency is established the client is taught to evaluate and monitor his progress, then standard transfer strategies are instituted. Since some speaking situations are more difficult than others, it is not necessary to use the same rate for all situations. During the transfer period a client's speech fears as well as attitudes and fears related to social situations usually become apparent. These fears should be dealt with directly because they can interfere with the clients' ability to maintain speaking control and can affect his speech performance. For instance, he can be assisted in identifying and eliminating avoidance behaviour. Pseudostuttering in controlled situations may be helpful in confronting the desire to hide the disorder from others. Similarly it may be helpful to talk about the disorder with friends and family, so that time and energy are not spent trying to keep the disorder 'in the closet'. Word fears can be worked on through mass practice, until the fear around a specific word diminishes. Situation fears can be handled with role playing, relaxation techniques, or *in vivo* practice. Throughout therapy, transfer, and maintenance, the client should be encouraged about his ability to be in control of most speaking situations, so that he will be able to maintain fluency independent of his clinician.

In the case of young children, much of the therapy can be in the form of parent counseling, once the demands for fluency are identified in the child's environment. By reducing these demands, many children show increases in fluency, some of them dramatically in a few days; others may take a few weeks. In other children, usually those for whom the disorder is more advanced in its development, direct fluency-shaping techniques, such as slowed rate or easy onset, can be used to alter motor performance. If a child shows avoidance behaviours or negative reactions to stuttering, the clinician should try to reduce these reactions as much as possible. Pseudostuttering may be helpful, performed either by the parents or the child. A child who shows avoidance behaviours or negative reactions to stuttering can be counseled or directed not to perform these 'tricks', provided some other, more normal way of talking dysfluently is also demonstrated by the clinician as a substitute. This more normal nonfluency pattern, containing less tension, slower velocities of movement, and larger units of repetition (e.g., whole syllables in place of parts of syllables) takes up more time, and is typically accompanied by work on desensitization to time pressure.

In this discussion of assessment and therapy, we have not described a radically new approach. Instead, we have described a number of well-known approaches to stuttering that follow from principles derived from the motor perspective of the disorder.

II THE ASSESSMENT AND TREATMENT OF STUTTERING

The main focus of this book is upon the treatment of stuttering. Here, in the main body of the book, we have commissioned chapters from a variety of authorities on this central topic.

The first issue to be addressed here concerns the assessment of dysfluent speech. Progress in the treatment of any disorder requires the prior achievement of a fine grain of description of the problem. We have moved some way in the past decade from broad categorical classification systems of communication disorders to more precise multi-axial systems and this section opens with two papers which may well have far reaching implications for the multi-axial assessment of fluency disorders. William Hardcastle and Susan Edwards describe a new linguistic contribution to the assessment (and hence definition) of stuttering. Their analysis of the problem makes fascinating reading and could well become an indispensable tool in fundamental research and clinical practice. Ed Conture and Tony Caruso offer a series of proposals for the comprehensive assessment of childhood stuttering and in the process they discuss their own highly successful practice with this client group. Their paper sets new standards for the assessment of childhood dysfluency which, if universally adopted, would certainly lead to rapid progress in this area.

The remainder of this section is devoted to descriptions and discussions of the treatment enterprise. Hugo Gregory presents his own highly personal account of the development of treatments for stuttering. He offers an intriguing appraisal of where treatment is currently moving and how professional developments can speed up this process of change. Eugene Cooper, one of the most consistently innovative clinicians in the field, lucidly outlines his own *Personalised Fluency Control Therapy* programme and illustrates the treatment process with several practical case studies. Willie Botterill and Frances Cook discuss the value of *Personal Construct Theory* in the treatment of dysfluency and focus on their work with adolescent stutterers to highlight their practice. Lena Rustin describes the development of her intensive therapy courses for childhood stutterers where active family involvement in the treatment process is seen as the key to successful and durable treatment outcomes. Armin Kuhr discusses the relevance of *Paradoxical Therapy* to the problem of stuttering. This approach has received considerable attention in the behaviour therapy literature and may well have relevance to the clinical management of dysfluency. Bryan Hunt represents the consumers view here and discusses the ways in which stutterers can help themselves to cope with dysfluency through active support and self-help groups. Finally, this section closes with a unique document from St. Vincents Hospital in Sydney, Australia. Gavin Andrews and his colleagues introduce the treatment manual issued to patients on the intensive treatment courses for adult stutterers mounted at St. Vincents Hospital. We feel sure the manual will be of enormous help to clinicians who wish to move to an intensive model of treatment.

to syntactic information, each dysfluency is logged according to its position within the tone unit and the presence or absence of stress is marked. Thus in this profile both prosodic and syntactic information is available.

Other profiling schemes with which we are familiar do not attempt such a precise specification of the location of the dysfluency. For example, in the assessment protocol outlined in Wall and Myers (1984, p. 144) information on the loci and distribution of stuttering is confined to three rather broad categories: 'predominantly word bound, predominantly clause bound and both word and clause bound.' Van Riper's (1971) guidelines adapted by Peterson and Marquardt (1981) for differentiating stuttering from normal dysfluency include some measures relating to the location of gaps (silent pauses) such as 'within the word boundary and prior to speech attempt'. Here again no detailed syntactic analysis of the data is attempted. Among the measures proposed by Costello and Ingham (1984) in their assessment procedure there are none that relate to the actual location of the dysfluency. Their measures include global quantifiable categories such as percentage of syllables stuttered, duration of stuttering episodes, speed of speech, length of stutter-free utterances, and speech quality. One of the innovative features of our profiling scheme is that, by scoring each type of dysfluency in relation to its location at different levels we are able to assess whether a particular combination of phonetic, phonological, prosodic and syntactic features is more likely to predispose a stuttering behaviour than another. We may find for example for a particular stutterer that there is a very strong possibility of dysfluency occurring on a nuclear syllable involving a fricative and occurring on the head of a noun phrase functioning as the object element in the clause.

Profiling Procedure

The first stage of this profiling procedure is to obtain a sample of speech, which we do by video recording. Mindful that fluency is affected by subject matter, environment and audience (see, e.g., Costello and Ingham, 1985) but restricted by the recording process, we suggest that a minimum of three types of data should be collected: reading a set passage; a monologue, for example picture description and a sample of conversational speech. In order to standardise the data, it is obviously important to use the same eliciting material and to standardise the length of sample which is profiled.

An orthographic transcription is made of each recording, marking tone groups and each dysfluency (see Appendix). In each tone group we mark the nuclear syllable (the syllable containing the major pitch movement characterizing the tone group) and any rhythmical stresses in the head (that part of the tone group preceding the nucleus) and the tail (that part following the nucleus). Those tone groups which contain a dysfluency are then given a letter code and each dysfluency within that tone group is given a number code in the temporal order in which it occurs. Thus the number of dysfluencies within each tone group can easily be identified.

The present profile includes two primary features of stuttering, REPETITION and PROLONGATION, the elements involved, and the location of those elements (see sample profiles in Figs. 1–4). We define repetitions as multiple productions of phonemes, phoneme clusters, syllables, words, phrases or clauses. The segment that is reduplicated is of a similar length to the target segment. Prolongation is defined as an abnormal lengthening of a particular stage in the production of a phoneme. For stops and affricates, prolongation involves the closure phase and may or may not be accompanied by vocal fold vibration. For fricatives it involves the prolongation of the stricture phase. Prolongations may be accompanied by intermittent voicing or on occasions, oscillations of articulatory organs. Both these features are coded as ' + osc' in the profile. Although there is usually a clear distinction between the two main types of dysfluencies when this method of analysis is used, there are still some dysfluencies in which the distinction is less clear cut. Decisions in these instances are made on the length of the dysfluent unit and observed movements of the articulatory organs but a dysfluent incident in which, say, a prolonged initial bilabial nasal is reduplicated would count as both repetition and prolongation. Dysfluencies are logged under the target sound regardless of the phonetic realisation. For the majority of samples the repetition itself will be phonetically similar to the target phoneme although often with some minor distortion, but occasionally the distortion will be so great that another phoneme will be heard. In these cases the target phoneme is still the one logged. We appreciate that a precise specification of the phonetic characteristics of stuttering may be necessary for a deeper understanding of the nature of the disorder and we are currently carrying out research in this area using the instrumental techniques of electropalatography, laryngography and pneumotachography. In the light of results from this work it may eventually become necessary to refine our basic phonetic categories for the purposes of the profile.

'Location' in this profile includes the position of the dysfluency with reference to the structure of word, phrase or clause, and also the tone group. Thus linguistic and prosodic features of the location can be observed for any given type of dysfluency.

For each of the primary features we record the following:

1   the frequency per 100 words that each type of dysfluency occurs in each sample;
2   the type of target segment involved in the dysfluency;
3   the number of repetitions of each target sound and the duration of the prolongation;
4   the location of the dysfluency. Two levels are considered: the syntactic, and the prosodic. Within the level of phrasal description we note the word class.

We will start by describing how all these aspects apply to repetitions and then proceed to explain how the profile differs for prolongations.

Repetition features

1 The frequency refers to the total number of repetitions within the first 100 words for each of the three speech samples. It is also possible to obtain frequency scores of each of the types of repetition described below.

2 Type of repetition is sub-divided into: a elemental; b cluster; c syllable; d word; e phrase; f clause.

An elemental repetition is defined as a phoneme, a part of a phoneme, or a CV structure where V is a 'schwa' vowel. The elemental repetitions are further divided according to the phoneme target and grouped by manner of production; see Appendix: Text 2 and Fig. 3 where E1 on the profile logs the repetition of the initial consonant in the target word *to*. One justification for specifying the individual target phonemes is the suggestion in the literature that certain phonemes are associated with a higher incidence of stuttering than others (see, e.g., Johnson and Brown, 1935, for adults and Mann, 1955, for children). Also stutterers frequently report that they have more difficulty on a particular phoneme than others and our profile will reveal this. We have only one category for vowel targets but this will be enlarged if our research data suggests this might be a fruitful area for detailed investigation.

If more than one consonant phoneme is repeated for example: *br br broccoli* the repetition is logged under cluster. However, if a vocalic nucleus is involved, then the segment is logged under syllable. (There are no examples in the sample profiles: this example is taken from Sarah's picture description).

For the purposes of this profile a syllable is defined as a sequence of phonemes containing a vocalic nucleus and less than a word. For example: *lo... lodger* (E1 in Appendix: Text 1 and Fig. 1) is logged under syllable.

Whole words that are repeated are categorised according to their grammatical class and logged under the phrase level. We use categories based on Quirk's grammar (Quirk, Greenbaum, Leech, Svartvik, 1972) which are widely known and used in British speech therapy (e.g., in the linguistic profiling scheme LARSP, Crystal, Fletcher and Garman, 1976). Examples of word repetitions can be found in both sample profiles, e.g., in Appendix: Text 2 and Fig. 3, D1 logs >4 repetitions of *I*.

Phrases which are repeated are also described according to their constituent elements, as detailed above. This protocol permits some judgement of complexity, an important consideration which merits further investigation. It should be noted that at this stage we are omitting phrases which contain revision of content, although this may warrant further investigation at a later stage. Examples of phrase repetitions can be found in both sample profiles, for example see D4, (Appendix: Text 2 and Fig. 3) where *if you* is repeated twice.

Clauses that are repeated are logged under clause and all constituent elements in the clause which contain dysfluencies are underlined. There are examples in Andrew's sample (Appendix: Text 2 and Fig. 3) where F2: *find it* is repeated once.

3   Frequency or length of repetition.

The frequency or length of the repetition is logged according to whether the element, cluster, syllable, word, phrase or clause is repeated once, twice, thrice, four or more times. The rationale for including repetition frequency in our profile is the evidence from the literature that a pathological dysfluency as distinct from a normal non-fluency may be distinguished by the number of reduplications per stuttering instance (Adams, 1977, for example suggests three as the critical number). In addition the length of each repetition adds to the perception of severity. Thus we consider the number of repetitions per instance, and the duration of the repetition, i.e., whether the repetitions are slow or rapid. Assessments which only account for the numbers of incidences of repetitions cannot be used to distinguish between two stutterers both of whom have the same percentage of repetitions but differ in the severity of the repetitions. Repetitions which are considered to be unusually slow are distinguished by the entry being circled. Frequently the slow repetitions are accompanied by increased muscular tension, but we have not included tension in the present profile because of difficulties in quantifying it.

4   Location of repetition.

The location for each repetition is considered where appropriate at four levels of analysis: a prosodic; b lexical; c phrasal; d clausal.

a   Prosodic level.

Two aspects of prosodic information are considered: the position of the dysfluency in the tone unit, i.e., in the head, nucleus or tail, and the presence or absence of rhythmic stress ($\pm$ STRESS). If the dysfluency occurs in the head, the presence or absence of rhythmical stress is noted, while dysfluencies occurring in the nucleus will be assumed to be associated with stress. The tail of the tone group is normally very short in English and contains relatively few stressed syllables but until sufficient data is collected to justify omitting this section, it has a place in the profile with sections for stressed or unstressed elements.

b   Lexical.

The location of elemental and cluster dysfluencies in relation to the structure of the word is considered as occurring either word initially or within the word. WITHIN WORD is further subdivided into syllable initial or other. The grammatical word class (D, N, V, A, etc. see Appendix p. 75 [this text]) is specified under the phrase level.

c   Phrasal level.

The phrase in which the dysfluency occurs is logged under this section and the phrasal elements listed. If the dysfluency has occurred in a word, that element is under-lined. If the whole phrase has been repeated then the whole phrase is underlined.

d   Clausal level.

As in the phrasal section, the dysfluency is logged under the clause section and the element containing the repetition is underlined. We recognise five constituent elements of clauses. These are Subject (S), Verb (V), Object (O), Complement (C) and Adverbial (A). We have found examples where a single dysfluency affects more than one element of the clause. For example: the repetition *in a* which occurs in *to take in a lo ... in a a lodger* (E2, Appendix: Text 1 and Fig. 1) involves part of the verb element as well as part of the noun phrase object of the target clause. Thus these two clausal elements both of which contain the dysfluency are marked at the level of clause de-scription by a small curved line.

Examples of repetitions are given on the sample profiles in Figs. 1 and 3. It can be seen that totals can be gained of the types of elements which contain repetitions as well as the location of these dysfluencies. By inspecting the frequency column, it is also possible to gain an impression of the relative severity of the repetitions. If a weighting is assigned to each of these sub-totals we can gain an overall score of the severity of this type of dysfluency. For example, a repetition with a frequency of more than three will get a higher weighting than a single repetition. Thus the stutterer with many but slight repetitions will be distinguished from the stutterer who has the same or similar instances of repetitions but tends to exhibit multiple repetition of target sounds.

Prolongation features

Prolongations are the second primary characteristic of stuttering which we consider in the profile. Again four major aspects are recorded:

1   The total number of prolongations within the 100 word sample. As with repetitions, sub-totals can be scored for each of the types of prolongation.
2   The length of each prolongation is logged impressionistically, as either less or greater than one second. Instrumental analysis is essential for accurate measurement.
3   The type of each prolongation is recorded. A division is made between AUDIBLE and INAUDIBLE prolongations.
4   The location of the prolongation is recorded under the same format as that for the repetitions, noting position within the tone group, and within the word, phrase and clause as appropriate.

AUDIBLE PROLONGATIONS are grouped according to manner of production and individual target phonemes listed. Examples can be found on both sample profiles (Figs. 2 and 4). In Fig. 2, the reader will note that there are prolongations judged to be less then one second (E4 and F3) as well as some greater than one second (D1, C2, A1 and F1). Silent prolongations mainly involved the closure phase of stops and are further subdivided into place of articulation, labial, alveolar, velar and other. They may be accompanied by glottal closures. Again examples can be found on both sample profiles.

For both silent and audible prolongations we log the presence of audible oscillations of the vocal folds or supra glottal articulatory organs. The description of the location of prolongations is the same as for repetitions and totals for the type of element involved, the relative duration of the prolongation and the location can all easily be calculated.

Discussion of Sample Profile

Four sample profiles (Figs. 1–4) have been included in this chapter, two each from subjects we will call Sarah and Andrew. They are both normal healthy adults in their late twenties, work full-time and currently attend weekly group speech therapy. For the purpose of this chapter we include only the profiles of their spontaneous speech samples and discuss some of the information found on each of the profile sheets. Figs. 1 and 3 are the profiles for repetitions and Figs. 2 and 4 for prolongations.

The overall total number of dysfluencies for each subject (seen in the bottom right-hand corner of the page), gives one indication of the severity of dysfluency in the sample collected. The examples given show that Sarah, with an overall total of 14 (seven repetitions and seven prolongations) per 100 words, could be regarded as more fluent than Andrew with 41 dysfluencies (31 repetitions and ten prolongations). Furthermore, the total scores not only give information about severity, but we can also immediately see the type of dysfluency which is characteristic of the speaker. Whereas Sarah has an almost equal distribution of repetitions and prolongations, Andrew's dysfluencies are predominantly repetitions. The figures at the foot of the columns headed REPETITION FREQUENCY and DURATION on the prolongation sheets give further measures of severity. For example, scores in Fig. 4 indicate that although Andrew has 10 instances of prolongations compared with Sarah's seven (Fig. 2) all of Andrew's prolongations were judged to be less than one second whereas most of Sarah's were judged to be greater than one second. Thus in the overall totals it is possible to consider various dimensions, severity, number and type of dysfluencies, size of speech unit involved (i.e., element, syllable, words, etc.) and the intensity of each moment of dysfluency.

This basic information about the severity and type of dysfluency, which is potentially helpful in indicating suitable therapy, is not readily available from the traditional method of measuring the severity of stuttering. Also by collecting three types of speech samples, it is possible to investigate whether these measures hold in different speech conditions. Most clinicians would expect to find a difference on both measures and our data to date support this expectation. Some preliminary work suggests that not only does the number of dysfluencies vary depending on the type of data collected, but also on the type of dysfluency manifested.

The horizontal totals in Figs. 1 and 3 contain information about the type of element, syllable, word, phrase or clause that is repeated. For example, Andrew's profile shows that a high proportion of repetitions involve single words, (13 out of a total of 31). In addition we can see the types of phonemes that are repeated and how often each type is involved. In his data, the consonant phonemes involved in repetitions all belong to the obstruent class (/b/ /t/ and /θ/, occur twice, /d/ and /s/ once). The presence or absence of voice does not seem to be a very potent factor. No evidence of place, manner of articulation or voicing preference is apparent in Sarah's data although the number of dysfluencies is much smaller in this case.

At the prosodic level, we can observe that both subjects have repetitions involving both stressed and unstressed positions in the utterance. However, whereas Sarah's repetitions are predominantly involved with stress (five stressed; two unstressed), Andrew's distribution is the reverse, (11 stressed segments and words; 19 unstressed segments and words). Although our small sample cannot at this stage be used to support or refute theories concerned with the relationship between stress and dysfluency, it does demonstrate the diversity of such behaviour and hint at the complexity of the relationship. In contrast to the differences found at the prosodic level, we observe that both subjects are consistent in producing all repetitions at word initial position.

Inspection of the phrase level columns gives an indication of the types of phrases and word classes involved. For neither subject is it true that on the so-called 'information carrying', 'content' words are involved although there is a predominance of nouns in Sarah's data.

Although nouns are logged in Andrew's speech sample, other word classes are also repeated on several occasions: for example, C2 *the*, D3 *if*. In both subjects there were examples of phrase repetition. Sarah's phrase *in a* and one of Andrew's phrases involved more than one clausal element. Following Palmer (1974), we have described 'in' as a particle and therefore part of the verb phrase. Thus at clause level part of the verb phrase and the object element are involved. Similar features in Andrew's data occurs at D4 *if you* where both subordinator and subject are marked, F2 *find it* where both verb and object elements are indicated.

There are quite marked differences in the subjects' data at clause level. It can be seen that many of Andrew's responses were phrases and lacked the full clausal structure. This reflects the nature of the sample in that many of his utterances were responses rather than initiations. Thus he had a tendency to produce elliptical utterances which we do not credit with the full clause structure but log as phrases on the profile.

At clause level we can obtain information about the complexity of structure involved, in terms of clause length and expansion of the clausal elements. If we accept these two measures of complexity, then there is some evidence of a relationship between complexity and dysfluency in Sarah's data. Compare, for example, structures coded as E and F with those coded as B and C. There are four examples logged as E and F and only one in B and C. It can be seen that the E and F dysfluencies occur in much longer and more complex structures than those of B and C. It is also possible to observe the position of dysfluencies in relation to the verb phrase. For example, five out of the six repetitions on Sarah's profile occur post-verbally but the situation is less clear on Andrew's profile. On both profiles there are examples where the verb phrase is involved but there is yet no clear evidence that any one part of the clause is potentially more vulnerable than any other.

As observed above, the total columns in the prolongation section indicate the relative severity of this type of dysfluency. Whereas Sarah's dysfluencies are fairly equally divided between these two basic types, Andrew has considerably fewer prolongations (10) than repetitions (31). The duration of the prolongations gives another dimension of severity. Five out of Sarah's seven prolongations exceeded one second whereas Andrew's are all judged to be less than one second. Half of Andrew's prolongations are silent; only one of Sarah's is silent. The presence of oscillations also distinguishes these subjects, for all of Sarah's prolongations are accompanied by oscillations but only three of Andrew's.

At the prosodic level it can be seen that all Sarah's prolongations are situated in the nucleus but only one of Andrew's is similarly sited. The co-existence of stress and dysfluency varies quite considerably in these two profiles for it can be seen that Andrew has six instances in unstressed positions and two in the tail of the tone unit, positions not found in Sarah's data. It is evident that certain aspects of the profile are related. For example, we can predict that because all Sarah's prolongations are associated with the nucleus, the words are going to be 'information carrying' and indeed, the phrase level column indicates that six of the seven are nouns and the seventh, an adjective.

In the same way, in Andrew's data, the diversity of position in the tone unit is reflected by the variety of word class; as associated with prolongations (N twice, Neg twice, Pr, sub and A once each). At clause level there is, once again, a number of zero entries for Andrew, reflecting the type of utterance he favoured in this sample, as discussed above. It could be argued that this speaker is avoiding the verb form by the use of ellipsis. Indeed, as shown in Fig. 3, of the 16 clauses which contained repetitions, half involved the verb phrase. This is not seen in the prolongations but might be a useful area to investigate further in therapy. Most, but not all of Sarah's dysfluencies, both repetitions and prolongations, occur post-verbally. Again, this observation would warrant further investigation.

Concluding Remarks on the Sample Profiles

Inspection of the profiles permits an evaluation of not only the severity of the dysfluency but also the type of dysfluency, the elements of speech involved and the location of each dysfluency. We have discussed two subjects who vary not only in the amount of dysfluencies but also in the type of dysfluencies and the locations most often involved. Sarah's sample contains a small number of dysfluencies almost equally divided between repetitions and prolongations. Prolongations tend to be greater than one second; repetitions were equally divided between one and two repeats. Most of her dysfluencies tend to be associated with stress, the prolongations occurring on the nucleus, and there is some evidence of influence of both word class and position within the clause. Andrew produced a greater number of dysfluencies, 41 in a 100 word sample. In this sample there were three times more repetitions than prolongations and the prolongations tended to be less severe. No clear picture of stress preference emerged, neither was there any indication that word class or position within the clause was especially vulnerable. There was a suggestion, however, that the verb phrase might cause this speaker difficulties and there was evidence of a passive role in conversation.

A detailed profile such as this will give considerably more information than more traditional assessments. Clinically, the predominance of one type of dysfluency could have important implications, suggesting the type of therapy that might be most suitable. The types of location might also suggest to the therapist the most suitable type of material to be used at various stages of therapy. Finally, the detail of the profile provides a sensitive measurement of progress. This profile would indicate, for example, that a client had reduced the length of each repetition although overall, the number of instances of repetitions had remained the same. In the same way a shift of dysfluent behaviour, for example a tendency to repeat elements rather than single words would also be readily seen on this profile.

The profile is potentially a potent tool for both research and therapy for it permits a considerable amount of phonetic, prosodic and syntactic information to be portrayed. The profiles discussed above are given as samples and not to typify stuttering, for until a larger number of subjects have been studied it is not possible to judge whether this behaviour is characteristic or whether the differences shown here reflect different types of stutterers or perhaps different stages in recovery.

Future Directions

In this profile we have considered aspects of two of the so-called core types of dysfluency, repetitions and prolongations. We recognise, however, as mentioned above, that there are other speech characteristics of dysfluency which cannot be categorized under those two main types. Pausing phenomena, for example, may be a relevant feature to include in a more complete profile and in fact has been discussed elsewhere in the context of disorders of fluency (see, e.g., Dalton and Hardcastle 1977). The type of pause which would be relevant here is a perceived gap in the acoustic signal which cannot be easily accounted for in terms of articulatory activity. The prolonged closure phase of a stop, for example, would not score as a pause but would be regarded in terms of the present profile as a silent prolongation. 'Breath' pauses however, i.e., those gaps in the signal during which an inhalation occurs, would count as a pause and their location could be logged in the profile in the same way that the repetitions and prolongations are. Further research is needed to decide the most appropriate manner in which the type, duration and location of pauses can be scored in the profile.

In addition to pausing phenomena, there are a number of general quantitative measures which are potentially relevant for an assessment of the speech characteristics of stuttering and could be included as a supplement to the present profile. Temporal measures such as those relating to the overall rate of utterance and the duration of moments of stuttering could be included in a more comprehensive assessment as could those relating to respiratory activity such as Vital Capacity, use of lung volumes during speech etc. Research is continuing in these areas.

Acknowledgments

Thanks are due to Janet Pethyjohns, Ann Glavina, Sue Rant and Carolyn Letts for their assistance in this project.

APPENDIX

Sample texts

Transcription conventions:

Tone group boundary: / e.g. (from Text 1) /oh well it's in *Woodley*/

Nucleus of tone group: the stressed syllable carrying the nuclear tone is in italics e.g. *kit*chen

Syllable carrying rhythmical stress:' placed before syllable e.g. 'walk

Type and location of a particular dysfluency:

Each dysfluency is identified by the letter and number code described above (p. [page number on this text]). In the transcription, the location of elemental repetitions or prolongations are shown by an asterisk before the syllable on which the dysfluency occurs. Cluster, syllable, word, phrase and clause repetitions are shown by repeating the relevant part of the target item in the transcription.

The interviewer's utterances are written within brackets.

Text 1   Subject: Sarah (spontaneous speech)

(tell me about your new flat)

A1:P   B1:R

oh well it's in *Woodley/ um it's in um 'East 'East 'East

*Read*ing/ and I've been 'there 'now for 'two *months*/ and um it's

C1:R   C2:P

'quite 'near um * *South 'Lake/ um 'which is/ well I think 'that's

the *nic*est thing 'about it/ 'cause it's 'quite 'nice to go and

'walk 'round the *lake*/ um 'it's got um *kit*chen/ *sit*ting

D1:P

room/ and two *bed*rooms/ and um I 'hope e'ventually to take in a

E:1R E:2R E3:R E4:P   F1:P F2:R   F3:P F4:R

lo in a a a *lod*ger/ to 'help with the * to 'help with *mort*gage

'payments/ um um

(sorry)

G1:P

um the well/ the last *couple of 'weeks/ I've been um *cleaning*

the 'walls/ and now I'm 'trying to 'persuade myself to get 'round

to *painting* them/ be'fore they get *dirty* again/

Text 2   Subject: Andrew (spontaneous speech)

(how do you get on in Rickie's group)

A1:P

um *not so *bad*/ *yeah*/

(bit more point to the session?)

B1:R   B2:P   B3:R   B4:R

um *as a *'practice in in in in in in in in *speaking*/er not

C1:P   C2:R   C3:R   C4:R

par'ticularly *from the the 'point *of 'view of of er 'Speech

C5:R

Therapy/ um/ it was in*te*resting/ *yes*/

(in what way)

D1:R   D2:R   D3:R   D4:R   E1:R

in I I I I I *'think if if if if you if you if you *listen*/ *to

F1:R   F2:R   F3:R   F5:R

the *tape*/ um I I find it find it *difficult *to *concentrate* on

G1:R

on techniques/ and and *that* sort of thing/

(why)

H1:R   H2:P

er er *because the *subject* er *'matter 'takes 'over/

(we were using small talk)

                    I1:R   I2:P
em *yes*/ well 'almost a normal conversat *conversation*/

(do you see any use for that sort of talk)

        J1:P   K1:R   K2:R   K3:R
um er *not as *padding*/ but as as um as a way of learn of of of

K4:R   K5:R   K6:R   L1:P   M1:R
of of of learning *learning*/ about *the other *person*/ or or

explaining a 'point/

(how about the job? how's the work going at the moment?)

            N1:R   N2:R
oh er we're we're we're 'quite 'busy at at at the *moment*/ I've

                                    O1:P   O2:P
'done a few 'late 'night and early *mornings*/ 'which *which

            O3:P   P1:R
towards the *end* of the 'week/ er er *be'comes a bit *wearing*/

(and you've managed to sort all the problems with the tax?)

Q1:P   R1:R
*no/ *that's* 'that's still on the 'go/ *yes*/

Symbols used in profiles

A	adverbial	Neg	negation
Adj	adjectival	O	object
Aux	auxiliary	part	particle
c	coordinator	Pr	preposition
C	complement	Pron	pronoun
cop	copular	s	subordinator
D	determiner	S	subject
Int	intensifier	V	verb
N	noun	osc	oscillations

Figure 1.

PROFILE OF STUTTERING BEHAVIOUR
Section 1   Repetitions

TYPE	TARGET	REPETITION FREQUENCY (slow)					PROSODIC LEVEL						WORD LEVEL		
							HEAD		NUCLEUS	TAIL		WORD INITIAL	WITHIN WORD		
		1	2	3	4	>4	+ stress	– stress		+stress	–stress		syllable initial	other	
ELEMENTAL / STOP	/p/														
	/b/														
	/t/														
	/d/														
	/k/														
	/g/														
FRICATIVE	/f/														
	/v/														
	/θ/														
	/ð/														
	/s/		Cl						Cl			Cl			
	/z/														
	/ʃ/														
	/ʒ/														
	/h/														
AFF.	/tʃ/														
	/dʒ/														
APPROXIMATE	/w/														
	/r/														
	/l/														
	/j/														
NASAL	/m/	F2								F2			F2		
	/n/														
	/ŋ/														
	VOWEL														
CLUSTER															
SYLLABLE		E1								E1			E1		
WORD			B1 / E3					B1	E3						
PHRASE		E2 / F4						F4	E2						
CLAUSE															
TOTALS		4	3					2	2	3			3		

W. Hardcastle and S. Edwards, Department Linguistic Science, University of Reading

NAME: *Sarah*
AGE: *29*
DATE: *JAN 1986*
SAMPLE: *SPONTANEOUS*

LOCATION		TOTALS	
PHRASE LEVEL	CLAUSE LEVEL		
		/p/	
		/b/	
		/t/	
		/d/	
		/k/	
		/g/	
		/f/	
		/v/	
		/θ/	
		/ð/	
ⓒ₁ = /nt Pr N̲ N	ⓒ₁ = S V A̲	/s/	1
		/z/	
		/ʃ/	
		/ʒ/	
		/h/	
		/tʃ/	
		/dʒ/	
		/w/	
		/r/	
		/l/	
		/j/	
F2 = Pr O̲ N N	F2 = S V A O ((O: V O A (A: V A̲))	/m/	1
		/n/	
		/ŋ/	
		VOWEL	
		CLUSTER	
E1 = O N̲	E1 = S V A O ((O: V O̲ A (A: V A))	SYLLABLE	1
B1 = Pr N̲ N	B1 = S V A̲		
E3 = O̲ N	E3 = S V A O ((O: V O̲ A (A: V A))	WORD	2
E2 = part O̲ N	E2 = S V A O ((O: V O̲ A (A: V A))	PHRASE	2
F4 = V̲ part	F4 = S V A O ((O: V̄ O A (A: V̲ A)̲	CLAUSE	
		TOTALS	7

Figure 2.

PROFILE OF STUTTERING BEHAVIOUR
Section 2   Prolongations

TYPE	TARGET		DURATION		OSC.		PROSODIC LEVEL					WORD LEVEL		
							HEAD		NUCLEUS	TAIL		WORD INITIAL	WITHIN WORD	
			<1 sec.	>1 sec.			+stress	-stress		+stress	-stress		syllable initial	other
AUDIBLE	+VOICE STOP CLOSURE /b/													
	/d/													
	/g/													
	-VOICE FRICATIVE /f/													
	/θ/													
	/s/		C 2	C 2					C 2			C 2		
	/ʃ/													
	/h/													
	+VOICE FRICATIVE /v/													
	/ð/													
	/z/													
	/ʒ/													
	VOICE AFF /dʒ/													
	APPROXIMATE /w/		A 1	A 1					A 1			A 1		
	/ɹ/													
	/j/													
	/l/		E 4						E 4			E 4		
	NASAL /m/		F 3	F 1	F 1				F 3 / F 1			F 3 / F 1		
	/n/													
	/ŋ/													
	VOWEL													
SILENT	STOP CLOSURE LAB		D 1	D 1					D 1			D 1		
	ALV													
	VEL		G 1						G 1			G 1		
	OTHER													
	TOTALS		2	5	4				7			7		

W. Hardcastle and S. Edwards, Department Linguistic Science, University of Reading

NAME: *Sarah*
AGE: *29*
DATE: *JAN 1986*
SAMPLE: *SPONTANEOUS*

LOCATION			TOTALS	
PHRASE LEVEL	CLAUSE LEVEL			
		/b/		
		/d/		
		/g/		
		/f/		
		/θ/		
$C2 = Int\ Pr\ \underline{N}\ N$	$C2 = S\ V\ \underline{A}$	/s/	1	
		/ʃ/		
		/h/		
		/v/		
		/ð/		
		/z/		
		/ʒ/		
$AI = Pr.\ \underline{N}$	$AI = S\ V\ \underline{A}$	/w/	1	
		/r/		
		/j/		
$E4 = D\ \underline{N}$	$E4 = S\ V\ A\ O\ ((\ O:\ V\ \underline{O}\ A\ (A:V\ A\ ))$	/l/	1	
$FI = Pr\ O\ \underline{N}\ N$ $F3 = Pr\ N\ \underline{N}$	$FI = S\ V\ A\ O\ ((\ O:\ V\ \underline{O}\ A\ (A:V\ \underline{A}\ ))$ $F3 = S\ V\ A\ O\ ((\ O:\ V\ \underline{O}\ A\ (A:V\ \underline{A}\ ))$	/m/	2	
		/n/		
		/ŋ/		
		VOWEL		
$DI = N\ N\ Adj\ \underline{N}$	$DI = S\ V\ \underline{O}$	LAB	1	
		ALV		
$GI = D\ Adj\ \underline{Adj}\ Pr\ N$	$GI = \underline{A}\ S\ V\ O$	VEL	1	
		OTHER		
		TOTALS	7	

Figure 3.

PROFILE OF STUTTERING BEHAVIOUR
Section 1   Repetitions

TYPE		TARGET	1	2	3	4	>4	HEAD +stress	HEAD −stress	NUCLEUS	TAIL +stress	TAIL −stress	WORD INITIAL	WITHIN WORD syllable initial	WITHIN WORD other
ELEMENTAL	STOP	/p/													
		/b/	H1	P1						H1 P1			H1 P1		
		/t/	E1 F4							E1 F4			E1 F4		
		/d/		F3				F3					F3		
		/k/													
		/g/													
	FRICATIVE	/f/													
		/v/													
		/θ/	O2		C5			O2		C5			O2 C5		
		/ð/													
		/s/	B4							B4			B4		
		/z/													
		/ʃ/													
		/ʒ/													
		/h/													
	AFF	/tʃ/													
		/dʒ/													
	APPROXIMATE	/w/													
		/r/													
		/l/													
		/j/													
	NASAL	/m/													
		/n/													
		/ŋ/													
		VOWEL	B1C3							B1 C3			B1 C3		
CLUSTER															
SYLLABLE			I1 K3							I1 K3			I1 K3		
WORD			C2 C4 F1 F5 K6 M1 O2	K1 N2	O3		B3 D1 K4	O2		B3 C2 C4 D1 D3 F1 K1 K4 M1 N2	K6				F5
PHRASE			K2 K5	O4						O4 K2	K5				
CLAUSE			F2 R1	N1				N1		F2	R1				
TOTALS			20	6	1	1	3	4		19	7	1	12		

W. Hardcastle and S. Edwards, Department Linguistic Science, University of Reading

NAME: ANDREW
AGE: 28
DATE: JAN 1986
SAMPLE: SPONTANEOUS

LOCATION		TOTALS	
PHRASE LEVEL	CLAUSE LEVEL		
		/p/	
H1 = Sub P1 = V	H1 = Sub SV P1 = SubAVC	/b/	2
E1 = V Part F4 = Part V	E1 = Sub SVO F4 = SVOC(c:AVA)	/t/	2
F3 = A	F3 = SVOC (c :AVA)	/d/	1
		/k/	
		/g/	
		/f/	
		/v/	
D2 = V C5 = NegAPrDNPrNPrNN	D2 = SV Sub(Sub:c SVO)inc C5=∅	/θ/	2
		/ð/	
B4 = PrDNPrN	B4 = ∅	/s/	1
		/z/	
		/ʃ/	
		/ʒ/	
		/h/	
		/tʃ/	
		/dʒ/	
		/w/	
		/r/	
		/l/	
		/j/	
		/m/	
		/n/	
		/ŋ/	
B1 = PrDNPrN C3 = NegAPrDNPrNPrNN	B1 = ∅ C3 = ∅	VOWEL	2
		CLUSTER	
I1 = Int DAdjN K3 = cPrDNPrN PrDAdjN	I1 = ∅ K3 = ∅	SYLLABLE	2
B3 = DNPrN C2 = NegAPrDNPrNPrNN C4 = NegAPrDNPrNPrNN D1 = Pron D3=Sub F1 = Pron I=5=V Part K1=butasDNPrNPrDAdjN K4 = cPrDNPrNPrDAdjN M1 =or K6 = cPrDNPrN PrDAdjN N2 = PrDN O2 = Sub	B3 = ∅ C2 = ∅ C4 = ∅ O1 = SVSub(Sub:SubSVO)inc D3 = SubSVO F1 = SVOC(c:A) K1 = ∅ F5 = SVOC(c:A) K4 = ∅ K6 = ∅ N2 = SVCA O2 = SubAVC	WORD	13
O4 = Sub Pron K2 = cPrD K5 = cPrDN PrN PrDAdjN	O4 = SVb SVO K2 = ∅ K5 = ∅	PHRASE	3
	F2 = SVOC(c:AVA) N1 = SVCA A1 = SVC	CLAUSE	3
		TOTALS	31

Figure 4.

PROFILE OF STUTTERING BEHAVIOUR
Section 2   Prolongations

TYPE	TARGET		DURATION <1 sec	DURATION >1 sec	·OSC	PROSODIC: HEAD +stress	HEAD -stress	NUCLEUS	TAIL +stress	TAIL -stress	WORD INITIAL	WITHIN WORD syllable initial	WITHIN WORD other
AUDIBLE	+VOICE STOP CLOSURE	/b/											
		/d/											
		/g/											
	-VOICE FRICATIVE	/f/	C1		C1			C1			C1		
		/θ/											
		/s/											
		/ʃ/											
		/h/											
	+VOICE FRICATIVE	/v/											
		/ð/	L1					L1			L1		
		/z/											
		/ʒ/											
	VOICE AFF	/dʒ/											
	APPROXIMATE	/w/											
		/r/											
		/j/											
		/l/											
	NASAL	/m/	H2						H2	.	H2		
		/n/	J1 Φ1		J1	J1		Φ1			J1 Φ1		
		/ŋ/											
		VOWEL											
SILENT	STOP CLOSURE LAB		B2			B2					B2		
	ALV												
	VEL		I2					I2			I2		
	OTHER		A1 / O1 O3		A1			A1 / O1	O3		A1 / O1 O3		
	TOTALS		10		3	1		6	1	2	10		

W. Hardcastle and S. Edwards, Department Linguistic Science, University of Reading

NAME: *Andrew*
AGE: *28*
DATE: *JAN 1986*
SAMPLE: *SPONTANEOUS*

LOCATION		TOTALS	
PHRASE LEVEL	CLAUSE LEVEL		
		/b/	
		/d/	
		/g/	
$C1 = Neg A \underline{Pr} D N Pr N Pr N N$	$C1 = \emptyset$	/f/	1
		/θ/	
		/s/	
		/ʃ/	
		/h/	
		/v/	
$L1 = c A D N Pr N Pr \underline{D} Adj N$	$L1 = \emptyset$	/ð/	1
		/z/	
		/ʒ/	
		/w/	
		/ɾ/	
		/j/	
		/l/	
$H2 = D Adj \underline{N}$	$H2 = Sub \underline{S}VA$	/m/	1
$J1 = \underline{Neg} Pr N \qquad Q1 = no$	$J1 = \emptyset \qquad Q1 = \emptyset$	/n/	2
		/ŋ/	
		VOWEL	
$B2 = Pr D\underline{N} Pr N$	$B2 = \emptyset$	LAB	1
		ALV	
$I2 = \underline{Int} D Adj \underline{N}$	$I2 = \emptyset$	VEL	1
$A1 = Neg \underline{Int} Adj$	$A1 = \emptyset$	OTHER	3
$O1 = \underline{Sub} \qquad O3 = \underline{A}DN Pr DN$	$O1 = S\underline{A}VC \qquad O3 = S\underline{A}VC$	TOTALS	10

5 Assessment and Diagnosis of Childhood Dysfluency

Edward G. Conture and Anthony J. Caruso

Introduction

The purpose of this chapter is to present issues and procedures in the assessment and diagnosis of stuttering in children. Stuttering is viewed as a complex interaction between the child's environment and the skills and abilities the child brings to that environment. Within this interactionist framework past and present approaches to the diagnosis of stuttering are discussed. One diagnostic battery for assessing childhood stuttering and related concerns is presented with emphasis placed not only on deciding whether the child stutters, but whether the child is different from other youngsters who stutter. It is suggested that continued advances in the diagnosis of stuttering may indicate that childhood stuttering develops along different pathways and as a result, different groups of young stutterers may require different forms of speech therapy.

While clinicians all want to help their clients, there are some kinds of help they can do without. In too many situations therapy begins before the clinician has an adequate understanding of the breadth and depth of their client's speech and language difficulties. This is not to say that the clinician can and/or must know *all* there is to know about each and every client *before* therapy begins, but rather than assessment and evaluation is an integral, very necessary part of the therapeutic process. We argue that any meaningful therapeutic regimen for children who stutter should always be preceded by a thorough diagnostic evaluation. Fortunately, the general topic of the evaluation of stuttering has already been adequately covered elsewhere (Johnson *et al.* 1963; Williams, 1978; Hayhow, 1983; Pindzola, 1986) permitting the present writers to focus on the unique challenges presented in the diagnosis of stuttering in young children.

The following discussion begins with some general points about the diagnostic process followed by an outline of the authors' basic orientation to childhood stuttering. We will then present a brief review of the literature pertinent to the assessment and diagnosis of stuttering; a suggested battery of diagnostic tests will then be out-

lined. We conclude with a general description of three broad categories of stutterers
and   we believe are frequently encountered in the clinic.

! Stuttering

It   nicians have a great amount and variety of data available
to   evaluation. What is needed, of course, is the means to
w   mation and organize it so the clinician can arrive at three
b

it speech dysfluency of a frequency and type which
.e child a stutterer?

: above is yes, does the child appear to need therapy?

)th the above questions is yes, does the nature of this
roblem, suggest that therapy should be similar to, or
ffered to most other children who stutter?

It ..   ity to make these decisions should improve as our ability to
differenti.   gsters who stutter becomes more refined and precise. After
all, why shou.   add to their caseloads children who will, with time and some
simple changes in parental interaction, become better by themselves (Ainsworth, 1981;
Cooper, 1979b)? Likewise, why should we, as clinicians, allow some child to languish
without services for one to three years while we wait to see if 'he'll outgrow it'?
Further, why shouldn't clinicians try to identify, right from the beginning, those
children for whom concentrated, protracted therapy is going to be necessary, and make
this belief apparent to the child's parents as well as other interested parties (Conture,
1982a)?

Defining 'Who and What' is Stuttering

Bloodstein (1981) and Conture (1982a) have stated that it is very difficult, if not impossible, to develop *absolute* definitions of who and what is stuttering. However, it
does appear possible to develop *relative* definitions of stuttering based upon statements
of probability rather than certainly (Conture, 1982a). When attempting such definitions we need to bear in mind Wingate's (1964) suggestion: that definitions of stuttering need to capture the essentials of those speech units listeners are most apt to consider
stuttering.

A listener's ability to differentiate a stutterer from a nonstutterer appears to relate to a set of perceptual criteria that are used to make judgements about the speaker's type, number, and duration of speech dysfluencies (Bloodstein, 1981; Conture, 1982a; Van Riper, 1982). Research has consistently shown that part-word repetitions, sound prolongations and other within-word dysfluencies are most likely to be classified as 'stutterings' by listeners. On the other hand revisions, interjections and other between-word dysfluencies are more likely to be considered 'normal' dysfluencies (Boehmler, 1958; Williams and Kent, 1958; Johnson, 1961; Schiavetti, 1975).

The frequency of dysfluencies exhibited by young (non) stuttering children has also been studied (Davis, 1939, 1940; Branscom *et al.* 1955; Johnson *et al.* 1959; Winitz, 1961; Yairi, 1982; Yairi and Lewis, 1984). Johnson *et al.* (1959) have shown that almost 80% of children labeled as normally fluent produce 1.0 or less *within-word* speech dysfluencies, while only 20% of children labeled as stutterers produce so few within-word dysflencies. Conversely, these authors also reported that 50–60% of stuttering children produce 3.0 or more within-word dysfluencies, while less than 10% of normally fluent youngsters produce so many within-word speech dysfluencies. Thus, a grey area would appear to exist for these children who produce between one to three within-word dysfluencies per 100 words in terms of whether they are perceived to be stutterers or not. However, for clinical purposes a set of relative criteria for defining a 'stutterer' appears appropriate as well as adequate for many of these youngsters.

In essence, we begin to consider a child to be a stutterer (or 'at risk' of becoming one) if he or she meets *both* of the following criteria:

1   production of 3 or more within-word speech dysfluencies (e.g., sound/syllable repetitions and sound prolongations) per 100 words of conversational speech, and

2   people in the child's environment explicitly express concern regarding a. the child's speech (dys)fluency and/or b. the possibility that the child is a stutterer.

As we will discuss below, other variables and behavior clearly influence our judgements of whether or not the child is a stutterer; however, the above mentioned criteria are necessary, if not sufficient in some cases, for us to make such a judgement.

In our view there has been increased discussion in recent years about differential diagnosis (Gregory, 1973; Gregory and Hill, 1980; Williams, 1978). This discussion, we believe, is appropriate; however, even as we talk about 'individual differences' among stutterers we continue to make group judgements or generalizations about them. Although stutterers' frequency and type of speech dysfluencies may generally differ from normally fluent speakers, these *between*-group differences should not obscure the possibility that there may be significant *within*-group differences among stutterers in terms of the etiology of their stutterings. Moreover, stuttering may be manifest in significantly different ways for different clients (e.g., Van Riper, 1971; 1982; Conture, 1982a).

Simply put, there may be as-yet-undiscovered etiological, physiological and behavioral differences amongst youngsters who stutter which are as significant as the differences we observe between stutterers and normally fluent speakers (e.g., Caruso, Gracco and Abbs, in press; Daly 1981a; Schwartz and Conture, in press). Many different paths may be travelled by children on their way to developing a stuttering problem, and once the problem has developed they may continue along parallel, but separate routes (see: Daly, 1981; Preus, 1982; Schwartz and Conture, in press; St. Onge, 1963; Van Riper, 1971). Knowing something about the nature and number of these paths may assist us in different diagnosis and subsequently in remediation.

Basic Orientation to Stuttering: An Interaction Between the Child's Ability and the Child's Environment

The first author has stated elsewhere (Conture, 1982a) the belief that stuttering relates to a complex interaction between the child's environment and the skills and abilities the child brings to that environment. We will call this position, for lack of a better term, an 'interactionist' position. That is, we believe that stuttering can best be considered and treated in terms of how the client's skills and abilities *interact* with his or her environment. Thus, as we will try to show in this chapter, both the child *and* the child's environment should be assessed and considered during the diagnostic sessions.

The child's abilities

Somewhere between 3 and 5 years of age the typical youngster who is going to stutter begins to do so (Johnson *et al.* 1959). Our present assumption, based on clinical observation as well as empirical data (Conture, Rothenberg, and Molitor, 1986; Caruso, Conture and Colton, 1987), is that these children probably consist of three general groupings:

1   those who exhibit a subtle developmental delay and/or deviancy related to neuromotor maturation for speech production and related skills

2   those who are at the lower ends of normal, proficient oral communication

3   those who are within the 'mid-range' of normal, proficient oral communication.

While we have little idea how many young stutterers fall into each of the three groups above, it would seem that when young stutterers are considered together as a group, they 'spread out' along a continuum which starts from the upper end of developmentally delayed and/or deviant speech production and extends into the lower to middle ranges of normally fluent speech production. Whatever the reasons, we believe that many young stutterers are less than proficient oral communicators in the sense of being able to rapidly, correctly and smoothly initiate speech as well as move between sounds and/or syllables.

The environment's contributions

For some of these youngsters such difficulties would seem to be of little consequence as long as their environment is one where rapid, precise and overly mature oral communication is *not* required, emphasized or encouraged. However, we posit that when such oral communication is required, emphasized or encouraged by the adults in the child's environment, particularly for the child with a developmental delay or deviance, the child finds it difficult to control and/or stabilize fluent speech production.

In other situations the environment may appear appropriately facilitatory to fluent oral communication as we think it should be, but the child still stutters. We suspect that with this latter group of youngsters we would find children who exhibit speech production difficulties related to delays and/or deviances in neuromotor maturation for speech production. We further suspect that these children with slow and/or deviantly developing speech production systems would have the highest probability of continuing their stuttering into their latter childhood years and beyond (see Caruso, Gracco and Abbs [in press] for preliminary findings concerning adult stutterers' aberrant sensimotor processes associated with fluent speech).

The above discussion makes apparent that we believe both the child *and* his or her environment are germane to the problem of stuttering. It is logical, therefore, that we will suggest that clinicians try to assess, as thoroughly as possible, both the child *and* the child's environment. The means by which this is accomplished are numerous and provide the clinician with a variety of options. Indeed, the major difficulty lies not in developing a means to evaluate the young stutterer but in deciding which among the plethora of formal and informal tests best suit the child of interest. Before presenting our decisions about which of these tests might be most useful we will provide a brief review of the literature pertinent to the assessment and diagnosis of stuttering.

The Assessment and Diagnosis of Stuttering

As previously mentioned, there has been increasing discussion about the 'differential diagnosis' of stuttering. While such discussion is quite appropriate, there is a basic lack of objective diagnostic procedures whereby such 'differentiation' can be obtained, particularly with regard to young children. Johnson *et al.* (1963) provided some of our better criterion- as well as norm-referenced information regarding the assessment and evaluation of the speech dysfluencies and related behaviors of young children; information which Williams (1978) has since elaborated upon. With the apparent exception of the *Iowa Scale of Stuttering Severity* and *Stutterer's Self-Ratings of Reactions to Speech Situations* (Johnson *et al.* 1963), however, much of this objective information has not been further developed into formal standardized diagnostic tests. However, the *Iowa Severity Scale* appears more closely related to differentiating among levels of stuttering severity than different 'types' of stuttering and/or stutterers. Likewise, the *Self-ratings of Reactions to Speech Situations* test does not directly address the issue of differential diagnosis. Further it is unclear whether young children can provide the kind of meaningful 'self-reports' of situational concerns required by these instruments, and indeed whether such concerns are particularly germane to the problem of stuttering in the young child between 2 and 8 years of age.

Published guidelines

From these early beginnings clinicians have advanced various clinical suggestions regarding the diagnosis of stuttering, two of the more widely referenced articles on this topic being those of Adams (1980) and Gregory and Hill (1980). While both articles are based on the solid clinical experience of three noted speech–language pathologists, they provide rather informal, relatively subjective guidelines for evaluating youngsters who stutter. Further, the number and nature of the subjects, as well as the sampling procedures employed in these studies is unclear. In a similar vein, Cooper (1980) and Conture (1982b) reported to otolaryngologists and pediatricians further diagnostic guidelines and suggestions for the clinical management of stuttering. Once again, these guidelines represent rather informal and fairly subjective means of evaluating individuals who stutter. Such subjectivity is, of course, not an inherently serious problem, but warrants consideration while evaluating these guidelines. Similar types of informal diagnostic information have been made available to the parents of stutterers or suspected stutterers (Ainsworth, 1981; Cooper, 1979).

(In)Formal tests

Notable exceptions to the above concerns are two formal diagnostic procedures developed by Riley (1980, 1981). Riley 'standardized' his *Stuttering Severity Instrument* (SSI) on 109 children and 28 adults employing three major areas of information (frequency, duration and 'physical concomitants' of stuttering) to derive an overall severity score for children and adults. While the SSI's measurement of frequency of stuttering is reasonable and probably adequate in most cases, the test's means of measuring both stuttering duration and 'physical concomitants' is quite subjective and seemingly insensitive to some real differences among youngsters who stutter (Schwartz and Conture, in press). However, the SSI and its related test, the *Stuttering Prediction Instrument* (SPI), are important landmarks in the field of stuttering in young children and represent one of the better attempts to objectify criteria for the clinical assessment of stuttering in young children (see Riley and Riley, 1982).

A less formal diagnostic test for young stutterers is presented by the *Stocker Probe Technique* (Stocker, 1976; for a review of this test see Conture and Caruso, 1978). Stocker's test provides an intriguing approach to the assessment of stuttering frequency in association with different levels of communicative responsibility or demand. Although Stocker provides some criterion-referenced information that clinicians can use to compare their young clients, it is not clear how this information relates to the child's typical speaking behavior. Further, it is doubtful whether some of its administrative procedures are appropriate for obtaining the best insights into the nature and degree of dysfluency in young stutterers. For example, if a child answers a test question with 'I don't know', the test scores this response as an instance of stuttering.

More recently Thompson (1983) has developed the *Assessment of Fluency in School-Age Children* (AFSC) test which attempts to assess child, parental and teacher reactions. While the current authors have not had as much clinical experience with the AFSC test as with the SSI, SPI or Stocker Probe, the basic rationale and approach of the AFSC test appears sound. Furthermore, the AFSC directly attempts to assess classroom teacher reactions to the child, making it unique among tests of childhood stuttering and apparently giving this test a degree of face validity for use by school-based speech and language pathologists.

Parent interview questions

In terms of interviewing the parents or caregivers of young stutterers, Tanner and Cannon (1978) have developed a commercially available series of diagnostic questions that may be asked of the mother and father of a youngster who is (or who is suspected of being) a stutterer. Conture (1982a) and Zwitman (1978) have also presented similar questions; however, the usefulness of all three sets of questions rests with the practising clinician since none of these authors provide norms or criteria to help the clinician assess the significance of the parents' responses. The present writers wish to emphasize that what is perhaps more important than the use of these 'pre-packaged' questions is the clinicians' flexibility and creativity during the interview process to generate 'follow-up' questions to probe for further areas of particular concern for a certain family, for example, a child's *strong and chronic* fears of loud noises, fire and the dark; a family that *frequently* encourages and requests their child to give speeches, verbal performances, 'dramatic' readings and the like to visiting friends and relatives; or a family where the father and/or mother *routinely* watch television while eating dinner rather than verbally interact with the child.

Assessment of stutterers' attitudes

Erickson (1969) provided a scale for measuring the communication attitudes that distinguish stutterers from nonstutterers and a revised version of this scale was successfully employed by Andrews and Cutler (1974) to measure attitude change during the course of therapy. While the relationship between stutterers' attitudes and changes in their speech behavior as a result of therapy are less than clear (see Guitar and Bass, 1978; Gregory, 1979; Ingham, 1984b), Erickson's scale provides a solid beginning for a diagnostic instrument capable of assessing the attitudes of stutterers. Unfortunately, the salience of such attitudes to youngsters who stutter (and whether these questions could even be asked of them) makes the application of this test to children quite problematic. Along these lines, Guitar and Peters (1980) discuss a modified experimental version of the Erickson scale the *Nineteen item A-scale* which they have successfully used with children. It is unclear whether such a test would be practical to administer to preschool and early elementary school youngsters, and whether the findings of such a test will ultimately prove valid and reliable for this population.

Recently, Brutten (1982), expanding upon and refining a clinical procedure originally developed by Shumak (1955), reported on a children's form of the *Speech Situations Checklist* (SSC). The SSC is a self-report questionnaire procedure which has been shown capable of differentiating the self-reports of adult stutterers from those of their normally fluent peers in terms of negative emotion and speech behavior (Hanson *et al.* 1981). Brutten reported that the children's form of the SSC appears to have promise for delineating between the self-reports of young stutterers and those of their normally fluent peers in terms of negative emotion and speech disorganization. However, it is again by no means certain whether such a self-report questionnaire procedure could be readily and reliably administered to pre-school and early elementary school-age children (between 2 and 7), the ages when most children actually begin to stutter.

Summary

The above literature review highlights three important issues:

1   There is both clinical and theoretical interest in the need for formal, objective diagnostic tests pertinent to youngsters who stutter.

2   Most presently available tests are either:
   a   informal without criteria or norms, or
   b   formal but containing aspects not sufficiently sensitive, objective nor quantitative to be useful in some clinical situations, or
   c   simply nor relevant nor feasible to administer to young stutterers.

3   Therapeutic regimens for children who stutter more than likely suffer from a lack of clarity about who is and who is not a stutterer; and whether or not there are significant differences observable among those youngsters diagnosed as having the problem, or being highly at risk for developing it.

While the 'ideal' test(s) for assessing and diagnosing stuttering in children are still not available, those that have been developed clearly provide a great deal of useful information. Nothing, of course, can take the place of a clinician's experience in the use and interpretation of tests. However, the longest journey starts with a single step and clinicians must begin somewhere if they are ever to arrive at a group of tests that fit their particular diagnostic needs. Below we outline a number of tests and procedures that we have found useful in assessing childhood stuttering together with comments on their interpretation and limitations. For additional insights into diagnostic testing procedures for young stutterers see Riley and Riley (1982) and Wall and Myers (1984).

Diagnosing Stuttering in Children — Practice

The following will reflect our basic philosophy towards the assessment and diagnosis of stuttering: evaluate the clients' fluency in as much detail as time and circumstances permit but also assess, as best as possible, all other variables which may contribute and/or relate to the speech fluency problem. Therefore, after we discuss below the assessment of fluency, we will also describe some of the assessment procedures we use to evaluate the client's expressive and receptive language abilities, their articulation/phonological processes, word-finding skills, neuromotor (non)speech behavior, voice, reading, and, with children, parental attitudes. Although not every client will need to have all these variables evaluated, many will. It is now clear, for example, that more than a few stutterers have concomitant speech articulation concerns (Thompson, 1983) and that for some clients these concomitant difficulties may have significance for the nature, duration and success of therapy. In fact, for some clients, their stutterings are of secondary or tertiary importance relative to their other problems and it behooves the clinician to examine, as best he/she can, the entirety of the client's abilities and not simply focus on their fluency difficulties.

Frequency of stuttering

One of the first things the clinician will try to define about dysfluency is the average number of stutterings per 100 words (or syllables) as well as the range observed. Assessing stuttering frequency raises the questions of the size of the speech sample required and whether stuttering frequency should be measured in percentage of *words* versus *syllables* spoken.

There is no easy, straightforward way to make either decision. With regard to sample size, our experience suggests that a corpus of 300 words spoken by the child in conversation with the parents or primary caregiver is quite sufficient for most clinical purposes (although some might feel more comfortable with collecting up to 500 spoken words of conversation). Certainly, one sample of 100 words or syllables is barely, if at all, adequate to assess the average number and variability of a child's frequency of stuttering. If the judgement of who is and who is not a stutterer is based *solely* on assessment of conversational speech, then the larger the size of the sample the greater the confidence one would have in the judgment.

Regarding the measurement of stuttering frequency in terms of percentage of stuttered *words* versus percentage of stuttered *syllables*, there is no conclusive published evidence that we are aware of that indicates that one procedure surpasses the other in terms of precision in estimating stuttering frequency. Another way to view this issue is to ask whether one would come up with *significant* differences in percentages of stuttering, across most stutterers, using one method versus another. One can, for most stutterers, convert percent stuttered words to percent stuttered syllables by multiplying the former by 1.5 (Andrews and Ingham, 1971). While this means of conversion only provides a rough approximation of percentage of stuttered syllables, it is probably close enough for diagnostic assessment purposes. For further discussion of this issue see Ham (1985).

Besides overall stuttering frequency, we've found it *very* helpful to list, from most to least frequently occurring (i.e., the rank order), the dysfluency types expressed as a percentage of the total number of speech dysfluencies produced in a sample of 100 words spoken. In this way, the clinician can assess the child's most frequently occurring dysfluency types as well as their relative contributions to the total number of dysfluencies. Detailed descriptions and examples of various dysfluency types can be found in Johnson *et al.* (1963) and Conture (1982b). It is not usual to find a young stutterer producing sound/syllable repetitions, audible and inaudible sound prolongations, whole-word repetitions, revisions, phrase repetitions, interjections, etc., all within the same conversation of 100 to 300 words in length. What does differ amongst these young stutterers, however, is the percentage or proportion of their total dysfluencies represented by each of these different dysfluency types. Since Schwartz and Conture (in press) reported that the percentage of sound prolongations in a sample of stutterings is one important feature in distinguishing among youngsters who stutter, we believe reporting the rank order of *each dysfluency type*, as well as their proportion of the total dysfluencies, is an important clinical observation.

Duration of stuttering

We routinely measure the average (and range) of the child's stuttering duration across a sample of 10 randomly selected stutterings. Doing this should help the clinician realize that many youngsters' apparent stutterings are *shorter* than 1000 msec (1 sec) in duration. For example, it is not at all unusual to have a young stutterer with a mean stuttering duration of 600 msec and a range of 230 to 1025 msec. Clinicians should try to learn how to measure and be sensitive to stuttering duration because it is often the first thing to change in therapy, even before frequency of stuttering and like behavior. It should be noted that we produce, and are thus used to hearing, an average of 10 or more sounds per second (Darley *et al.* 1975); therefore, we are used to hearing at least one sound every 1/10th of a second (or every 100 msec). Any sound segment which extends appreciably beyond this 100 msec 'time window' will probably be 'noticed' by most listeners (Lingwall and Bergstrand, 1979).

For the young stutterer, these 'extensions' (prolongations) or 'reiterations' (repetitions) of sound segments (stutterings) will often be well below 1000 msec (1 second) in duration. The clinician can only become sensitive to hearing, measuring and recording these rather brief dysfluencies if she/he uses a stopwatch to time the duration of the child's stutterings. As the clinician gains experience timing the duration of the child's stutterings during the diagnostic, he/she should become better at 'tuning-into' the child's behavior quickly and precisely, and consequently becoming better able to identify behaviors that need change during actual therapy.

Consistency of stuttering

Although we recommend trying to assess 'consistency' we often find it problematic. To adequately assess consistency the child has to say the identical thing at least three times in a row — no small task for a pre-reading 5-year-old! We've used sentence repetition procedures (Neely and Timmons, 1967; Williams *et al.* 1969) for eliciting consistency samples in children and have found some success; but there are a number of children who become extremely fluent when repeating back to us age-appropriate sentences or find this task apparently boring, silly or difficult to the point where their cooperation, attention and performance all but nullify the diagnostic usefulness of such procedures.

(In)Formal tests of stuttering

In the previous literature we already mentioned the *Iowa Scale for Rating the Severity of Stuttering* (Johnson *et al.*, 1963), the *Stuttering Severity Instrument* (Riley, 1980), the *Stuttering Prediction Instrument* (Riley, 1981) and the *Stocker Probe Instrument* (Stocker, 1976). We routinely use all four of these 'tests' in our fluency diagnostic, but for quite different purposes. For example, on the first page of our diagnostic report which describes the 'Summary Statement' (see Figure 1), where we mention the 'Tentative Diagnosis' or 'Diagnosis' or 'Diagnostic Category', we might mention that the child is a 'moderate stutterer' with an asterisk (*) after the word stutterer.

Then, as is illustrated in Figure 1, on the bottom of this first page of the diagnostic report, which lists both the identifying information as well as summary statement, we insert a footnote stating: *Rating = 4 on the (no stuttering) to 7 (very severe stuttering) *Iowa Scale for Rating the Severity of Stuttering* (Johnson *et al.*, 1963). In this way the child's parents, teachers, physicians and so forth, who may *only* read these first one or two pages of the diagnostic report, get some sense of what we mean by 'moderate' in a loosely objective way.

For the practicing speech and language pathologist, and others who ever read further, we report in some detail the results of the *Stocker Probe Technique*, the *Stuttering Severity Instrument* and the *Stuttering Prediction Instruments*. The clinician should be forewarned that it is not unusual for the child to rate 'moderate' on the Iowa Scale but 'mild' on the SSI and vice versa. These discrepancies, we now believe, do not reflect so much on the relative validity of the various tests as they do on the fact that the child's behavior is variable, and will be evaluated differently depending on the speech task and measures employed. Using the *Stocker Probe Technique*, as we've pointed out elsewhere (Conture and Caruso, 1978), results in an estimate of 'stuttering frequency' which is typically about twice that observed during conversation; however, this difference is instructive, we believe, because it suggests to the clinician how 'severe' the child's stutterings might become given certain circumstances, for example, when the child tries to answer a complex question or describe a previously occurring event to an impatient or inattentive listener.

Expressive/Receptive language

Given the fact that our main responsibility in a fluency evaluation is evaluating fluency we must expend most of our energies in that direction. However, some of these children *do* have other concerns and these need to be considered wherever possible. While language, particularly the expressive component, would appear salient, we tend to be more impressed with articulation/phonological problems (more on this below). Regardless, we routinely assess the child's mean length of utterance (MLU) in morphemes and delineate the presence/absence of various grammatical morphemes. If these rather molar judgements of expressed language suggest problems, then more formalized tests may be used (for example, the *Preschool Language Scale* (Zimmerman *et al.*, 1979), the *Test of Early Language Development* (Hresko *et al.*, 1982). The clinician should try, if at all possible, to sort out language concerns which are: a. relatively independent of the fluency concerns versus those which are b. secondary to the fluency problem, for example, the child who is habitually avoiding and substituting words and/or phrases in attempts to avoid stuttering. As an aside, sometimes when a highly dysfluent child becomes more fluent an expressive language difficulty will emerge. It is as if the child's formerly severe stuttering 'masked' or made relatively insignificant his language concerns. Although the relation between this child's dysfluencies and language concerns is not particularly clear, it is probably safe to say that therapy will initially have to focus on the stuttering and then as that improves, shift primary attention to language difficulties.

There are two tests of receptive vocabulary which are easy to administer and provide norm-referenced measures: the *Peabody Picture Vocabulary Test* (PPVT) (Dunn and Dunn, 1981) and the *Quick Test* (QT), Ammons and Ammons, (1962). We typically use the PPVT with pre-school and early elementary school children, reserving the QT for older children, teenagers and adults. One of our uses of the QT with older children is, perhaps, a bit unorthodox since we use it to provide us with some rough index of a child's general intelligence. Obviously, (in)formal testing of intelligence is the province of the clinical psychologist. However, because of our practical need to know at the time of the diagnostic whether the child's IQ is roughly within normal limits, we use the QT as a crude approximation. It should be noted that the QT as well as WISC vocabulary sub-test are both highly correlated with the full scale WISC IQ. Further, while some young stutterers may score very well on the PPVT, a number of them will score six months and more below the age norms. Children with low PPVT scores may also exhibit language and/or articulation difficulties in addition to frequent within-word speech dysfluencies.

Articulation

We have observed varying degrees of speech sound misarticulations in young stutterers. In one recent sample of 30 youngsters nearly 50% of them had some degree of misarticulations/phonological difficulties. This figure is not that dissimilar to the 35 to 45% incidence of 'suspected (articulation) deficits' Thompson (1983) observed in two samples (N = 31 and N = 17) of young stutterers. Clearly the correlation between within-word dysfluency (stuttering) and phonological difficulties needs careful, objective scrutiny. At the very least, we recommend that the clinician informally but carefully observes the child's sound system and then administers the 'Sounds in

REPORT OF SPEECH AND LANGUAGE EVALUATION

I. IDENTIFICATION

Name:	Rob Bunker	Date of Current Evaluation:	March 30, 1987
Address:	2.5 Main Street	Date of Initial Evaluation:	June 2, 1986
	Syracuse, NY	Date of Birth:	April 29, 1978
Phone:	(315) 999–9999	Age at Current Exam:	8 yrs., 11 months
Parents:	Archie and Edith	Referral:	John Clinician
Siblings:	Second born age 4		Speech/Language Pathologist
	Third born age 1 yr.		Any elementary school
	6 months		Syracuse, New York
Faculty Supervisor:	Edward Conture, Ph.D.	Tentative Diagnosis:	Moderate stutterer*

II. SUMMARY STATEMENT

On March 30, 1987, Rob Bunker, accompanied by his parents, was seen at the Syracuse University Gebbie Speech and Hearing Clinics for a speech and language reevaluation. During the reevaluation, Rob produced an average of 15 speech disfluencies per 100 words of conversational speech (range: 7 to 25 speech disfluencies per 100 words) which included the following disfluency types (listed in order from *most* to *least* frequently occurring): audible sound prolong-ation, whole-word repetitions, phrase repetitions, sound/syllable repetitions and revisions. Mean duration of Robert's speech disfluencies was 0.48 seconds (range: from examiner's reaction time to 0.78 seconds).

Examination of Rob's oral peripheral speech mechanism revealed no gross structural or functional abnormalities. Rob's vocal pitch variability was judged to be somewhat limited and monotonous during isolated as well as connected speech tasks. His speech articulation was characterised by interdental productions of /s/ and /z/. The client's receptive/expressive language and reading abilities were judged to be within normal limits for his present chronological age (eight years, eleven months). Bob exhibited marginal abilities during informal tests of fine and gross motor movement and balance.

During a forty minute interview, Mr. and Mrs. Bunker provided information regarding Rob's speech and language development, and his medical, social and familial history since his last evaluation (6/2/84). Mr. and Mrs. Bunker reported that 'Rob's stuttering has gotten worse (more frequent and of greater duration) since the previous evaluation'. Further, Mr. and Mrs. Bunker stated that 'Rob is becoming frustrated with his speech' and says, 'I wish I could talk right'.

Based on the results of the present evaluation (3/30/87), it was recommended to Mr. and Mrs. Bunker that speech therapy for Rob's fluency problem is presently (3/30/87) *indicated*. It was also recommended to Mr. and Mrs. Bunker that Rob receive an evaluation to assess his current level of psycho–social adjustment. Detailed suggestions (see Recommendations) were provided to Mr. and Mrs. Bunker for facilitating Rob's speech fluency at home.

*Rating a 4 on the 0 (no stuttering) to 7 (very severe stuttering) Iowa Scale for Rating the Severity of Stuttering (Johnson, Darley, and Spriesterbach, 1964).

Figure 1 Report of Speech and Language Evaluation

Words' subtest of the *Goldman–Fristoe Test of Articulation* (Goldman and Fristoe, 1969) for any and all sounds suspected as problematic. The clinician should not only note the number and type of sounds in error, but also indicate the presence of any 'unusual' phonological processes: for example, glottal replacement (e.g., /be?/ for 'bed'). For detailed discussion of such processes see Edwards and Shriberg (1983). While this type of informal testing can become rather extensive and complex, it is best considered as only the beginnings of documentation of the child's possible phonology/fluency difficulties.

Word finding

The relation of word-finding to language abilities has been adequately explored elsewhere (Kail and Leonard, 1986). Relative to fluency, word finding difficulties would appear to be a contributing factor. However, with stutterers it is extremely difficult to separate out 'latencies' due to 'word finding' difficulties and those related to stuttering. Recently, German (1986) introduced the *Test of Word Finding* as an objective means of assessing word finding and related abilities. To date this test appears to be one of the best indices of word-finding abilities in children that we have used in clinic. However, we still believe that in common with other tests, it cannot readily distinguish response latencies due to difficulties with word finding from those due to stutterers' hesitating/pausing because of a reluctance to say a particular sound, syllable or word.

Neuromotor (non)speech behavior

Until recently the ability to assess and evaluate rate, range and force of motion during speech and nonspeech tasks was largely dependent on clinician experience. Rates of alternating oral motor movements (diadochokinesis) could be assessed for uni-, bi-, and tri-syllabic productions and then compared to published norms (Fletcher, 1972). Recently, Riley and Riley (1985) introduced the *Oral Motor Assessment Scale* (OMAS) which not only provides some norms against which to evaluate the child, but also attempts to assess the 'quality' of various oral motor productions. It is unclear whether empirical research will ultimately determine which aspects of the OMAS are most salient to our understanding and remediation of youngsters' oral motor (dis)abilities. However, it does seem that the OMAS, and the others like it that will surely follow, point in the direction of more sophisticated, thorough assessment of youngsters' speech motor proficiency.

Another more comprehensive test of neurological integrity, the *Quick Neurological Screening Test* (QNST) (Mutti *et al.* 1978), explores gross and fine body movement, balance, coordination and related abilities. It scores individuals as 'normal' (0–24), 'suspicious' (26–35) and 'impaired' (35 and above). It is our experience that the QNST should not replace, but rather supplement and elaborate oral motor testing. While its assessment of oral/speech motor movement is limited, its assessment of basic hand co-ordination and movement, as well as the client's ability to 'translate' visual and auditory instructions into hand movements, is quite informative.

Voice

Most youngsters who stutter, in our experience, exhibit voice usage roughly or grossly within normal limits. Youngsters' voice 'problems' whether or not they stutter, usually present either in the form of low-pitched, monotonous voice and/or hoarseness related to hyperfunctional voice use (for example, excessive yelling inside and outside of home, frequent use of 'monster' or animal noises, frequent singing in accompaniment to loud music or noise, habitual loud talking, and so forth). Typically by listening to the child's conversational voice both the above voice problems become apparent, with the latter usually justifying a referral to an ENT specialist, particularly if it is a persistent problem.

Informal tests we've found helpful in this area include having the child copy the examiner's model for changing pitch from low to high (and vice versa) in both discrete and continuous steps. Sometimes these youngsters will respond better to (that is, imitate) models like 'a baby kitty', 'the daddy kitty', 'a wolf howl', 'a siren', and the like. We've also employed the s/z ratio (Eckel and Boone, 1981) with these youngsters but found that many of them (under 7–8 years of age) have difficulty understanding and/or cooperating with the task in terms of prolonging the /s/ and /z/ for sufficient durations. However, most of them, even when they shorten the duration of these fric-atives (typically preschoolers and early elementary children produce /s/ and /z/ between 3 and 7 seconds) sustain these sounds for approximately equal lengths, which results in a s/z ratio of approximately 1.00 (roughly $+/-1$ SD $= 0.37$), which is well within normal limits. In essence, the clinician computes the s/z ratio by timing the duration (in seconds) that the client can sustain the /s/ on one exhalation and then dividing this temporal measure by the length of time the client sustained the /z/ on one exhalation. Generally, the client is given several chances to sustain each of the two sounds with the longest duration of each used to compute the ratio. The s/z ratio re-presents an indirect, rather 'rough' means of assessing the client's efficiency of vocal fold approximation or functioning during phonation.

Reading

It is generally not necessary nor possible to assess the reading abilities of pre-schoolers; however, assessment of reading obviously becomes more relevant for the beginning reader in early elementary school, particularly for the clinician who wishes to use reading material with the child during speech therapy. We have had extensive experience administering the *Woodcock Reading Mastery Test* (Woodcock, 1973) to children and have found that most stutterers are well within normal limits (Conture and van Naerssen, 1977). Of the five subtests of this test, the 'Passage Comprehension' component gives the examiner the best overall view of reading skills. If concerns are apparent here, referral to a reading specialist may be in order. If a specialized reading program is recommended, the speech and language pathologist should work closely with the reading teacher to develop procedures that are sensitive to the child's speech and will not unduly influence the child's fluency *or* detract from his or her interest in oral reading.

The parents

We and others have discussed elsewhere the role of parents in the problem of stuttering (Bailey and Bailey, 1982; Conture, 1982a, 1982b; Conture and Schwartz, 1984). Indeed, one of the reasons we take an interactionist position relative to the problem of stuttering, particularly in the young child, is that we have found that parents can make subtle changes in their own speech that will benefit their child's fluency. We closely study the parents' interactions with their child during a 10–15 minute parent/child conversation and with us during our interview of the parents (Conture, 1982a, Appendix A). While the information they provide and the content of their questions is definitely of interest, we pay particular attention to three things:

1   The parents own rate of utterance

2   The length of time parents pause between the end of the speaker's statement and the beginning of their own (turn-taking pause)

3   The parents' relative tendency to interrupt or talk while the speaker is talking (simultalking).

It is not at all unusual to find the parents of young stutterers talking well in excess of 190–200 words per minute (median 'normal' adult rate of utterance = 170 words per minute, Fairbanks, 1960). It is also not uncommon to observe these parents interrupting the speaker, beginning their own utterance before the conclusion of the speaker's utterance, or using turn-taking pauses of 500, 250 msec or less. We hasten to add that we are not trying to increase the parents' guilt about 'causing' the child's stuttering, but we are interested in understanding those behaviors the parents may exhibit which provide less than a fluency–facilitating environment.

Depending on the results of our observations during this assessment of parental speaking behavior we may proceed by having the child's parents or primary caregivers examine, for a one-to-three week period of time, the following points:

1   Their own rate of utterance

2   The pause time between the end of their child's utterance and the beginning of their own (turn-taking pause) and

3   Their tendency to interrupt or talk simultaneously with the speaker ('simultalk') or the tendency of the adult to interrupt the child or spouse until they 'relinquish the floor'.

We employ, as one 'ideal' model, Fred Rogers (of 'Mr. Roger's Neighborhood') to show the parents or caregivers one example of an adult who speaks with children by using a 'slower paced' manner of speech containing more appropriate lengths of turn-taking pauses and less 'simultalk', but who maintains a linguistic/intellectual content which is still stimulating and holds the attention of young children.

The child's parents will almost without exception remark that these changes in speech/language behavior are difficult to make. However, we have found that with patience, guidance and *modeling* on the clinician's part, many of these parents can and will make the necessary changes; subsequent improvements in their child's fluency are usually noted. We stress to the parents that making these changes 5 minutes a day, every day, is far better than 35 minutes on one day in the week.

Once again the clinician must exhibit patience for the rather slow nature of human growth, but with encouragement and guidance many parents can learn, in the course of conversations with their children, to change those aspects of their own speech production which provide a less than optimum environment for their child's developing oral speech.

After the Diagnostic is Over

Parents of young stutterers typically want to know several things: Is my child OK?; If he/she is not OK, will he/she 'outgrow' the problem?; If he/she won't 'outgrow' the problem, does he/she need therapy? If therapy is needed what kind and how am I to be involved? These questions relate, to some degree, to the three broad categories of young stutterers the clinician usually encounters. What follows is a brief description of these three categories as they may present themselves after a thorough diagnostic evaluation.

Category One: Children with frequent within-word dysfluency (stuttering) having few other problems and whose parents may (or may not) be concerned.

These children frequently exhibit within-word dysfluency (i.e., 3 or more within-word dysfluencies per 100 spoken words), with sound/syllable repetitions being the predominant dysfluency type. However, rarely do these youngsters exhibit other speech, language or related concerns and it is our speculation that they represent the low- to mid-range of 'normal', proficient oral communicators regarding their ability to rapidly, correctly and smoothly initiate speech as well as move between sounds and/or syllables.

Some of these youngsters' parents may talk too fast (190–200 words per minute or faster), may use complex vocabulary/linguistic structures that are too sophisticated for the child's level of development, and usually exhibit brief (below 500 msec) turn-taking pauses. Many such children will probably be 'OK' with time and 'best practices' on the part of the parents (i.e., a supportive, facilitatory environment where patience and tolerance is exhibited for the child's unique rate of development).

Formal tests like the SSI and Stocker Probe may identify these children, but some of them will probably score as 'sub-clinical' on the SPI (a test of stuttering chronicity). We believe that children in this grouping probably have the highest chance of spontaneous recovery, (that is, 'outgrowing' their stuttering problem), particularly if the parents modify their speech/language behaviors to facilitate their child's fluency as previously discussed. It is not unusual for these youngsters' problems to improve significantly during the course of 2 to 4 successive evaluations (each evaluation separated by 3 to 6 months) *without* any direct therapeutic intervention.

Category Two: Children who stutter with(out) other problems and whose parents clearly are concerned.

These children may be frequently producing sound/syllable repetitions or even beginning to produce sound prolongations. Fixed articulatory postures along with associated nonspeech behavior (e.g., frequent closing of eyelids, breaks in eye contact with the listener, movements of the head to the side, and so forth) may also be present. They may also have one or two other difficulties, for example, sound misarticulations, expressive language problems, etc. (Blood and Seider, 1981).

We speculate that this group of children have oral communication skills which range from the upper ends of developmentally delayed/deviant to the lower ends of normal limits for oral communication. One of the main clinical concerns here is modification of the parental speaking model if it consists of rapid, complex utterances where the child is frequently interrupted and turn-taking pauses are quite brief (500, 250 msec or less). These parents may also give the child the impression, in one way or another, that rapid, precise and mature speech and language is desired and expected. These children may (in)formally test like the previous group, but many of their parents will clearly indicate in word and deed that they have a role in the problem. These parents, with patient assistance by the clinician, can and do make significant progress and often do well in a parent/child fluency group. Many of these children positively benefit from therapy and generally no harm is done by evaluating them twice (3 to 6 months between evaluations) *prior to* initiating therapy.

Category Three: Children who frequently stutter, have other problems and whose parents may (or may not) be concerned.

These children clearly stutter. Sound prolongations predominate or are one of the child's chief dysfluency types. Further, associated nonspeech behaviors are noticed. They typically have other speech and language problems such as subtle difficulties in (non)speech sensorimotor coordinations, phonological difficulties, word finding difficulties, and so forth. We suspect that these children represent the upper end of the range of those who exhibit developmentally delayed and/or deviant speech production in terms of being able to rapidly, correctly and smoothly initiate speech, as well as move between sounds and/or syllables.

Some parents may present speech and language models that are quite facilitatory, while others exhibit the opposite. Formal tests like the SSI and SPI would clearly identify these children as stutterers. It is our guess that those whose concurrent difficulties (e.g., language, articulation, etc.) seem primarily related to slow development would have the best prognosis for positive change. Conversely those whose problems appear more deviant (i.e., irregular phonological processes) will probably require longer, rather protracted therapy. If the clinician's therapy caseload is full then this type of child should be referred to another clinician experienced in remediating childhood stuttering, or at least scheduled for re-evaluation in 3 to 6 months, with therapy being indicated if there is no improvement, or indeed if the problem seems to have deteriorated.

A Few Last Words

As we mentioned at the beginning of this chapter, we take an interactionist position on childhood stuttering. This can be seen in our diagnostic approach to the problem as well as in the three broad categories of young stutterers and their parents outlined above. Further, our therapy for these children (Conture, 1982a; Conture and Schwartz, 1984) typically involves the parent and the child to the point where we believe the parent has either become appropriately facilitatory to the child's fluency, or at least is no longer inhibitory to the child's fluency development.

We believe, in many of these cases, that the child clearly has a role (after all, the child is the one that stutters) but so too do some parents. It is a truism that if you 'look, ye shall find' and one cannot discover parent/child interactions if one never tries to observe them. We hope the above discussion helps those interested in furthering their understanding of these interactions and encourages others to give these variables greater consideration in their assessment and diagnosis of childhood stuttering.

gory

ıngster with a developing problem of stuttering, then at
was a client in therapy, and after that a student in
pathology, followed by my professional career. The
ration of the recent history of stuttering therapy, leading to
ontemporary issues, will be approached using my own ex-
these periods as a frame of reference.

Experiences as a Stutterer

Many adult stutterers have said to me that even though they have been told that they
stuttered during preschool years, their first memories of stuttering were at 8 or 9 years
of age, often in a classroom reading situation. This was true for me. An accompanying
memory is that of laughter by some young friends, confirming a childhood attitude
that stuttering is strange and amusing, and therefore to be inhibited or avoided.
During elementary school, it seems that I always enjoyed talking, telling stories before
my class and acting in plays. As junior high school (ages 12–14) came along, I became
more sensitive about stuttering and began to withdraw from classroom discussion.
When a new girl came to my school in the ninth grade, I was determined to conceal
my stuttering, feeling that this was necessary if I was to have a chance of friendship
with her. I have a vivid memory of the day in class when I stuttered and realized that
Mary Alice was looking at me. My attitude was that all was lost, that she would not
want to be seen around with me and risk relating to some of the teasing I received.

I had never heard of speech therapy. There was none available in 1944 in my home
state of Arkansas in the USA. Fortunately, I did read about an institution 1500 miles
away in the State of Rhode Island. With the support of my family, I went there for
therapy in the summer of the year I turned 15 years of age.

At Martin Hall, I learned that stuttering was due to a faulty reaudiorization and revisualization of words (Martin, 1926), a theory I was later to associate also with Bluemel (1930) and Swift (1915). Faulty imagery was the basic problem, but we were also told that with time a fear-motivated conditioned inhibition of speech developed. The vicious cycle: stuttering, increased fear, increased tension, increased stuttering, was described.

Therapy at Martin Hall consisted of being on silence (no conversation) for periods of time in which we practised syllables, words and sentences from a drill manual. We learned a rule for the production of each consonant, then as we said a word we thought of the rule for each other consonant and called up strong auditory and visual images. This first step was known as word analysis. I practised analysing words all over that beautiful landscape on Mount Hope Bay in Rhode Island. In word analysis, transitions between sounds were very smooth, but words were spoken one at a time. At the end of two weeks, we suspended our period of silence for the weekend and were allowed to speak, using careful word analysis. To a girl, with whom I had been writing notes while on silence, I was now able to say, 'P-A-T, W-O-U-L-D Y-O-U L-I-K-E T-O G-O T-O T-H-E M-O-V-I-E S-A-T-U-R-D-A-Y N-I-G-H-T?' After that weekend we went back on silence to practise phrasing in which we analysed only the first word of a phrase and then blended the remaining words smoothly without analysis. However, we could revert to word analysis when difficulty was expected. At the end of two more weeks, I was able to say, 'Pat / would you like to go / to the Biltmore Hotel / in Providence / for dinner / Saturday night?' In addition to the improvement in speech, the jump up from a movie in Bristol to dinner at the Biltmore in Providence in two weeks was pretty exciting. Not bad for a 14 year old.

This was my introduction to what we now designate as the speak-more-fluently approach to therapy. I viewed word analysis and phrasing as the way to break the habit of stuttering and to learn to speak fluently. I hoped to substitute word analysis and phrasing for stuttering.

Although I was conscientious in practising words and sentences every day, utilizing my rules, a few months after returning home I began to slip, to have increasingly more trouble. However, I never had as much difficulty again as before that first summer of therapy. Today, we would say that I did not have an adequate transfer and maintenance experience. I often think of this when I see stutterers who have gone away from home for concentrated one to six week therapy programs and who then return to the stimulus conditions of home without systematic help in transfer and without adequate follow-up assistance.

Without realizing it at the time, I was beginning to understand Wendell Johnson's (1948) idea that individuals should not evaluate themselves as 'either or', either they are stutterers or not stutterers. I began to view myself more and more as a person who stuttered sometimes as he talked, and who was going through a process of change. I began to see that I needed to change from an attitude of 'beating stuttering' to one of 'working with it'. As I felt more hopeful about speaking, I learned that others did not think of my stuttering nearly as much as I thought that they did. Later, after studying psychology, I could label this as projecting my attitude toward myself onto others.

My own experience as a stutterer, as a person in therapy, and finally as my own therapist, impressed upon me the beliefs that a stutterer's speech habits have to be modified and that attitude exploration and change is a reciprocally interacting aspect of therapy. I saw that just as stuttering had developed over a period of years, successful therapy was a process involving changing, evaluating, changing again, etc.

Experience as a Student: Learning about Theories and Therapies

In 1949, I went to Northwestern University to study 'speech correction'. As we all did then, I learned the principle theories of stuttering, an approach that until recent years was almost always used in teaching courses on stuttering. I began my long association with the sequential editions of Van Riper's *Speech Correction: Principles and Methods* (Van Riper, 1947, 1954, 1963, 1971) by reading in the 1947 edition about six principle theories of stuttering: developmental, psychoanalytical, neurological, neurotic, imagery, and inhibitory. Recall that I had become acquainted with the last two at Martin Hall, five years earlier (see p. 106).

The *developmental theory* held that stuttering had its origin in the natural hesitations of childhood and was learned behaviour that resulted when penalty and fear were associated with dysfluency (Johnson 1934, Heltman 1938, Johnson 1944). Treatment of children focused on helping parents to understand speech development and to have realistic expectations about their children's speech–language development.

Coriat (1943), who adhered to a *psychoanalytic-theory* believed that stuttering was a pyschoneurosis 'caused by the persistence into later life of early pregenital oral nursing, oral sadistic and anal sadistic components' (p. 27). Coriat (1943) and Glauber (1958) wrote many articles on stuttering between 1928 and 1958, recommending psychoanalysis as the treatment for stuttering and inferring that a healthy psychosexual development for a child was the way to prevent stuttering.

The *neurological theory* grew out of Orton's speculations about cerebral dominance for language (Orton, 1927, 1937). Travis (1931) in his classic research based book, *Speech Pathology*, hypothesized that the paired speech musculatures of stutterers receive poorly timed neural impulses due to a weak motor lead control in one cerebral hemisphere that was related to handedness. Change in handedness was associated with stuttering because the change disrupts natural dominance. The lack of dominance could also be inherited or be associated with minimal brain damage. Psychological factors in stuttering occurred as the problem developed. Therapy consisted of training proper handedness, as determined by extensive testing, analysis of the stuttering pattern and speech modification, and mental hygiene techniques emphasizing an objective attitude about the problem. One of my instructors recalled seeing stutterers at the University of Iowa Speech Clinic with one arm bound in a sling, a procedure for enforcing the use of the hand that it had been determined should be dominant.

Fletcher (1928) and Gifford (1943) viewed stuttering as a *neurotic difficulty* rooted in the way in which the child related to environmental figures during childhood social development. This neurotic theory in which stuttering was seen to be a symptom of an emotional problem was vague and difficult to define. The treatment involved speech modification, but it also had to include social readjustment, the latter being the key objective.[1]

Van Riper (1947) spoke of predisposing factors that could be physiological, precipitating factors mainly related to the environment, and maintaining factors related to a learned fear of stuttering and the vicious spiral effect, 'The more he stutters, the more he fears stuttering, and then the more he avoids speaking' (Van Riper, 1947, p. 277). We students appreciated, as have students and clinicians around the world throughout the years, Van Riper's concrete descriptions of therapy for children and adults including lists of suggested steps. For example, a few years later (Van Riper, 1954) he provided a detailed description of the sequence-cancellation, pull-out, and preparatory set for preventing symptom reinforcement and for modifying stuttering. Cancellation consists of learning to stop after a stuttered word and then to say it again with less struggle or using some type of voluntary stuttering. The cancellation is not successful until the word is produced under voluntary control. After a satisfactory degree of success with cancellation, the stutterer learns to 'pull out' by modifying the stuttering behavior as the word is spoken. The last step in the sequence is the preparatory set in which the adaptive, altered behavior moves forward in time, and the person is able to approach the word more appropriately in terms of a normal speech response.

Just as my therapy at Martin Hall, emphasizing word analysis and phrasing, had introduced me to speak-more-fluently procedures, becoming acquainted with Van Riper's thinking introduced me to anxiety reduction, avoidance reduction, stutter-more-fluently concepts. In my own speech I began to experiment with voluntary stuttering. I became fascinated with the idea of 'playing with my speech pattern', 'do-doing thi-thi-this or thaaaat'. My subjective evaluation was that voluntary stuttering, what I now more properly designate as voluntary dysfluency, helped to reduce my fear of speaking and my sensitivity about dysfluency. I began to perceive a conflict between techniques based on avoidance reduction as the way to improve fluency and the use of direct fluency-enhancing procedures.

Johnson (1946) emphasized that the misevaluation of children's dysfluency by parents and others led to an apprehensive, anticipatory, hypertonic, avoidance reaction, resulting in the learning of stuttering. He could not see how organic conditions, about which there was speculation, could account for the development of stuttering and the variability of the behavior (Johnson, 1948, 1956). In preventing stuttering, Johnson informed parents about normal dysfluencies in children's speech, helped them to modify their evaluation of their child's speech appropriately, and counseled them about activities that were conducive to building fluency, or stated as Johnson may have preferred, keeping fluency within normal limits.

At the 1950 convention of the American Speech and Hearing Association (ASHA), John Black from Ohio State University and Grant Fairbanks of the University of Illinois, demonstrated delayed auditory feedback (DAF) equipment and the effect of DAF on speech. When one of my professors introduced me to them, I spoke under DAF for the first time. Apparently I did better than most people, i.e., DAF did not disturb my speech flow as much as Black and Fairbanks expected. They concluded that this was due to my concentrating on tactile–kinaesthetic monitoring as I spoke, one thing I had learned to do in therapy. Lee (1951) wrote an article, 'Artificial Stutter', which along with reports by Black (1951) and Fairbanks (1954) on how DAF disturbed speech flow, led to much research focusing on the functional integrity of peripheral and central auditory processes in stutterers (Gregory and Mangan, 1982) of which my doctoral dissertation (Gregory, 1959) was one of the first.

During this period, it was also found that the speech of moderately severe to severe stutterers improved when speaking under DAF (Nessel, 1958) and that masking noise had an ameliorative effect on stuttering (Cherry and Sayers, 1956). We will see later how continued work in this area has affected present clinical procedures.

In the early 1950s we began to apply learning theory to the understanding of the nature of stuttering and to the formulation of treatment (Wischner, 1950; Sheehan, 1953). Wischner related learning theory to Johnson's diagnosogenic explanation of the development of stuttering, and Sheehan applied approach–avoidance conflict theory (Miller, 1944) to understanding the development and maintenance of stuttering. From Sheehan and Wischner, I learned that the momentary reduction of tension and anxiety that follows the occurrence of stuttering probably reinforces unadaptive stuttering behavior. Since we were so focused upon the punishing nature of stuttering (Van Riper, 1937; Frick, 1952), it was difficult to comprehend how the occurrence of stuttering could be rewarding or reinforcing in this way. Van Riper's cancellation procedure, mentioned earlier, was viewed as a way of diminishing this reinforcement, since stutterers stopped and cancelled their blocks before proceeding. In cancelling, the stutterer repeats the word modifying the tension in a controlled manner. A modified response is reinforced. This is in harmony with the stutter-more-fluently avoidance reduction model of therapy.

Professional Career: Dealing with Controversial Issues

In the late 1950s and early 1960s, as I began my career as a clinician, researcher, and teacher, I had two main goals related to stuttering therapy. First, I wanted to generate procedures for the evaluation and treatment of stutterers. Secondly, I wanted what I did to be based on research about the nature of stuttering and its treatment. In connection with the second goal and my role as a university teacher, I focused upon defining and clarifying issues about stuttering therapy, attempting to understand, evaluate, and integrate established as well as new ideas. In the remainder of this chapter, I will draw upon this experience in describing the present status of controversial issues about stuttering therapy. I will relate current developments to the historical theories and therapies described previously in this chapter.

Intervention with Children

Contemporary issues pertaining to the prevention and/or treatment of stuttering in children include:

1   When should we be concerned about the fluency of a child's speech?

2   What factors are considered in the evaluation of children aimed toward the prevention of stuttering, the management of early developmental stages, or the treatment of a more advanced or confined stuttering problem?

3   What are appropriate intervention strategies?

When to be concerned about a child's fluency

We have made considerable progress in understanding children's dysfluencies and thus we can make much better judgments about when to be concerned than we could ten years ago. Research has shown that there is a great intersubject and intrasubject variability in the occurrences of dysfluency (DeJoy, 1975; Haynes and Hood, 1977; Yairi, 1981; Wexler and Mysak, 1982; Yairi, 1982; DeJoy and Gregory, 1985). Dysfluency in children's speech, as well as stuttering, is cyclic. Thus, we are cautious about judgments made during only one evaluation. Breaks in fluency at the word level (sound and syllable repetitions and prolongation of sounds) occur less frequently than non-repetitious dysfluencies and one syllable word dysfluencies in the speech of most children (Brownell, 1973; Haynes and Hood, 1977; Bjerkan, 1980; Wexler and Mysak, 1982). Therefore, in general, we are more concerned about increases in these breaks at the word level in a child's speech. In addition, we are more concerned about one syllable word repetition or part-word syllable repetition if there is a high frequency of repetition per instance (two or more) and more so if the tempo among repetitions is irregular (Gregory and Hill, 1980; Gregory and Hill, 1984; Yairi and Lewis, 1984).

There is even more concern if there is a disruption of air flow or phonation between repetitions or if a schwa-sounding vowel is substituted for the correct one in the repetition of a syllable (Cooper, 1973b; Adams, 1977; Curlee, 1980; Gregory and Hill, 1980; Van Riper, 1982; Gregory and Hill, 1984). Some children's speech is characterized by signs of increased tension in the lips, jaw, larynx, or chest, and of course, these signs create more concern and point more definitely to a problem. A few children (nonstutterers, beginning stutterers, and confirmed stutterers) manifest rapid, slurred, and jerky patterns, typified by the running together of words, known as cluttering. Cluttering has been discussed more in Europe (Freund, 1952; Weis, 1964) than in the United States, but most clinicians who see stutterers report seeing children with 'cluttering components'.

These observations about the quality of dysfluency, along with available quantitative guidelines (Adams, 1977; Gregory and Hill, 1980; Van Riper, 1982; Gregory and Hill, 1984; Yairi and Lewis, 1984), have increased the clinician's ability to make decisions about the types of dysfluency that signal more unusual fragmentation and disruption of vocal tract dynamics during speech production. Notice that I did not say, ability to define stuttering.

As Perkins (1983) has reminded us, defining stuttering can still produce considerable debate. Stuttering takes its place along with other behavioral problems that involve overt and covert features and that are dimensional disorders, not an 'either or' matter. Thus, we have moved away from attempting to determine whether a child is, categorically, normally dysfluent or a primary stutterer. Most often, the clinician describes the child's speech precisely and then, based on the quality and quantity of dysfluency and other manifestations of tension present, state a degree of concern or lack of concern about the child's speech. Since there are situational differences in the occurrence of dysfluency and stuttering, evaluations are based on recordings made in different circumstances such as monologue, dialogue, play, and play with pressure. A sample made in the natural home environment is obviously valuable.

Differential evaluation

Sometime in the future we may be precise in stating the cause or causes of stuttering. Presently, the best we can do is to describe as definitively as possible the characteristics of the person's speech and the subject and environmental variables that research has shown may be related to increased dysfluency and stuttering. Then, based on these observations, we formulate a treatment program in which these variables are manipulated where possible. Our rationale for this strategy is strengthened by our clinical experience showing that there is improvement when we deal with these contributing factors.

The following series of statements pertains to the variables, which, based on clinical experience and research, are considered in the evaluation of a child:

1 *Family history of stuttering*

The development of more precise genetic models has led Kidd (1980, 1983) and Andrews, Craig, Feyer, Hoddinott, Howie, and Neilson (1983) to conclude that a genetic factor functions to predispose some children to stuttering. Kidd (1983) states that for some individuals a primary problem of unknown etiology may exist and that stuttering, late talking and articulation difficulties are different manifestations of what is in all probability an inherited condition. Thus, a family history may alert us to the possible existence of this syndrome. The clinician also considers the possibility that family history has influenced the parent's evaluation of the child's speech.

2 *Auditory processes in stutterers*

Studies of middle ear muscle activity and the functioning of the central neural auditory system in stutterers have been inconclusive (Gregory and Mangan, 1982; Rosenfield and Jerger, 1984; Gregory, 1986a, b). The most positive findings have been the results of dichotic listening procedures, using meaningful words, in which stutterers show more reversals and smaller between-ear-differences scores. Whereas Travis (1931) was interested in cerebral dominance and speech production, those findings are interpreted as being related to cerebral dominance and speech perception.[2] Very few centers utilize such auditory tests routinely, since individual test results are not sufficiently reliable.

3 *Speech motor processes in stutterers*

In describing earlier theories, we saw that speech motor control factors were related to cerebral dominance and handedness (Travis, 1931). After about 1950, as our society became more tolerant of handedness differences and as new research contradicted previous findings, there was less interest in speech motor factors in stutterers. However, since about 1970, there has been a renewed research interest in motor factors and stuttering. Although findings are somewhat mixed, the motor speech reaction time differences in which stutterers show slower voice initiation times implies the possibility of a slower reacting speech motor system in stutterers (Adams and Hayden, 1976; Cullinan and Springer, 1976; Starkweather, Hirschman and Tannenbaum, 1976; Luper and Cross, 1978; McFarlane and Prins, 1978; Cullinan and Springer, 1980; MacFarlane and Shipley, 1981; Reich, Till and Goldsmith, 1981; Till, Reich, Dickey, and Seiber, 1983). Positive evidence of a difference is stronger in adults than in children (Cullinan and Springer, 1980). Common sense implies that differences, if existent, are very small, and there is still debate about the influence of emotional conditioning in the small differences found. However, since we have a long history in speech and language pathology of experience with speech motor testing, those procedures are often routine in the evaluation of stutterers (Gregory and Hill, 1980; Riley and Riley, 1980; Riley and Riley, 1983; Gregory and Hill, 1984). In addition to evaluating diadokokinetic rates and the sequential chaining of syllables, we should study the clinical use of reaction time procedures, voice onset time measures, and electroglottographic procedures (Adams, 1984a, Conture, 1984).

4 *Language factors in stutterers*

The information we have about language and dysfluency (Muma, 1971; DeJoy, 1975; Haynes and Hood, 1978; Colburn and Mysak, 1982a; Colburn and Mysak, 1982b) and the higher incidence of articulation and language disorders in stuttering children (Berry, 1938; Bloodstein, 1958; Andrews and Harris, 1964; Pratt, 1972; Wall, 1980; Blood and Seider, 1981) provide some general direction to us in understanding the nature of stuttering, and the latter findings may point to an underlying disorder of language, articulation, and fluency that is genetic (Kidd, 1983). Although much research will be done in future years looking at dysfluency and stuttering as related to semantic, syntactic and pragmatic aspects of language, even now we appear to be in a relatively strong position to look at these factors clinically (Gregory and Hill, 1980; Riley and Riley, 1980; Riley and Riley, 1983; Gregory and Hill, 1984; Wall and Myers, 1984)

5 *Environmental factors*

All contributors to our understanding of the nature of stuttering have acknowledged the influence of environmental factors. We have mentioned the long history of this interest dating back to the theories of stuttering as a neurotic difficulty or a problem of psychosexual development. In more recent years, clinicians and researchers such as Glasner (1970) and Sheehan (1975) have emphasized the child's interpersonal relationships in the family as primary in the development of the problem. Others believe that environmental factors interact with physiological predispositions in some cases (Van Riper, 1973; Van Riper, 1982; Riley and Riley, 1983; Gregory, 1985a). Even those who have investigated the genetics of stuttering (Kidd, 1983), assume that environmental factors interact with physiological predispositions. Johnson (1959) hypothesized in one of his last contributions that stuttering resulted from an interaction between three major variables: 1 the child's degree of dysfluency, 2 the listener's sensitivity to the child's dysfluency, 3 the child's sensitivity to his own dysfluency and his sensitivity to his listener's evaluation. Shames and Sherrick (1963), utilizing Skinner's (1953) behavioral principles, have postulated the way in which normal dysfluency can degenerate into stuttering in certain environmental circumstances.

A careful case history is a source of information about the environment that is used by most speech clinicians. This is often supplemented by information from questionnaires such as those developed by Cooper and Cooper (1985b). Parent-child interaction evaluation procedures (Kasprisin-Burrelli, Egolf and Shames, 1972; Mordecai, 1979; Gregory and Hill, 1980; Gregory and Hill, 1984), enabling us to make more objective observations, appear to be a promising way to add to or to confirm case history reports. Rustin and Cook (1983) describe the way in which a child's speech environment is subjected to a careful functional analysis to ferret out characteristics of the child and the environment that may be related to increased dysfluency or stuttering.

These brief statements cover a great deal of territory in providing an overview of subject and environmental variables that are assumed to interact with each other to bring about the development of stuttering.[3] The most basic subject variable is the genetic predisposition that may exist. Others may include auditory, motoric, and linguistic factors that could be a reflection of genetic variables. Environmental influences are the many communicative and interpersonal stimuli that children experience. Clinicians should consider the possibility that new research, such as that by Conture (1984) on the use of electroglottography to study laryngeal functioning or Moore's electroencephalographic findings (Moore, 1984c) related to cortical hemispheric functioning of stutterers, may suggest additional assessments that should be added to the differential evaluation. We must constantly question whether we are applying the knowledge we have as effectively as possible.

Differential therapy

Differential evaluation focusing upon the above factors results in decisions about therapy that differ somewhat for each individual. This approach reflects a general agreement among clinicians and researchers that, in terms of what we are able to observe and measure at the present time, stutterers are a heterogeneous group (Andrews and Harris, 1964; Gregory, 1973; Riley and Riley, 1979; Preus, 1981; Van Riper, 1982).

This present point of view has had an impact on the way in which degree courses about stuttering are taught. As mentioned in the previous section about my student experience, courses during the 1940s and the 1950s covered the major theories about stuttering and then considered therapy. Often, the relationship between theory and therapy involved reasoning that was difficult to follow. Today, professors tend to de-emphasize complex theories, and instead, stress the relationship between information we have about stuttering and stutterers from research and clinical studies and what we do in evaluation and subsequent treatment. In 1957, Ainsworth wrote about integrating theories of stuttering. Today, we attempt to synthesize information we have about factors involved in stuttering (Gregory, 1979a, 1979b; Van Riper, 1982; Wall and Myers, 1984; Gregory, 1986a, 1986b).

In intervention with children, clinicians are focusing upon the following four areas of activity (Gregory, 1984a, 1984b, 1986a):

1 Communicative stress in the environment, e.g., the way in which parents and others talk to the child including the rates of the parents' speech;

2 Interpersonal stress, e.g., the general interaction between family members;

3   Linguistic (including articulatory) and motor developmental differences;

4   Speech fluency.

It is assumed that the first three of these influence the fourth, but consideration is also given to using procedures that help young pre-school children, as well as older elementary school-age children, modify speech flow.

Almost all authors writing about stuttering therapy recommend counseling of the parents aimed toward reducing communicative and interpersonal stress (e.g., Van Riper, 1973; Cooper, 1979a; Williams, 1979; Rustin and Cook, 1983; Gregory, 1984b; Gregory, 1985a). In addition to establishing a comfortable relationship and offering verbal descriptions of needed behavioral changes, clinicians have begun to model specific changes for parents and then reinforce them for appropriate responding (Gregory, 1973; Shames and Egolf, 1976; Stes, 1979; Gregory and Hill, 1980; Gregory and Hill, 1984). Parents have responded positively to this modelling, stating that they profited from the observation of clinicians and from receiving feedback about their attempts to change. Gregory (1985b, 1986a) believes that clinicians should think of themselves as models in every therapeutic interaction, from drills using a word list to the conveying of an attitude.

There seems to be general agreement that the effectiveness of environmental modification should be evaluated before it is decided to use more direct speech modification procedures, even the modelling of 'easy relaxed speech' or 'easy speech' by the clinician (Gregory, 1979b), to improve a child's fluency. However, there has been an obvious trend during the last fifteen years toward the use of more specific fluency enhancing procedures with pre-school children. These procedures range in directness from Ryan's gradual increase in length and complexity of normally fluent utterances (Ryan, 1974), to the modelling of a slightly slower, more easy relaxed speech pattern by Gregory and Hill (1980, 1984), a soft vocal production by Shine (1980a, 1980b) or Nelson (1984), to what appears to be the most direct procedure, Cooper's use (Cooper, 1979a) of fluency initiating gestures (slow speech, easy speech, deep breath, loudness variation, smooth speech, and stress variations). My experience indicates that it is wise to obtain normal fluency by focusing on the minimal number of parameters necessary. The clinician can always decide to increase the number of parameters of speech attended to depending on the vocal tract dynamics of the child's stuttering and what is effective (Adams, 1984b). Desensitization, as first described by Van Riper and England over twenty years ago (Van Riper, 1973) can be used as the child's fluency becomes more stable. Fluency disruptions, such as rushing the child, interrupting, or not paying attention are introduced and withdrawn as the child's fluency is observed carefully. This procedure increases the child's tolerance of factors that once disrupted fluency.

With reference to research findings that there may be minimal motoric differences of the speech mechanism (slowness of vocal reaction time and voice onset) or measurably longer glottal adduction per glottal cycle in some children who stutter (Adams, 1984a; Conture, 1984), these procedures that provide a vivid model for the child and that usually involve the slowing of speech production and an increasing of the length of speech segments with smoother blending would seem to be appropriate. Since motor responses do improve with practice, this may be involved in these fluency enhancing procedures. Also, in terms of findings that speech reaction times are slower in stutterers, Gregory (1986a, 1986b) has suggested giving stutterers, both children and adults, practice in the rapid initiation and termination of speech segments, vowels and consonant vowel combinations. I have seen improvement in children's ability to sequence sounds more rapidly as a result of practice. Assuming that fluency of speech, particularly when under linguistic or environmental stress, is related to some of these basic skills, it could be important to improve these skills. On the other hand, if we are only dealing with maladaptive learning, these exercises and the previously mentioned speech production procedures aimed toward increased fluency are still appropriate.

An issue usually considered when discussing fluency problems in children, is the way in which we should work with the child who also manifests a language, articulation, or cluttering problem. During recent years, clinicians appear to have resolved this issue by recognizing that therapy to facilitate fluency is best carried out in the context of a language activity program proceeding from shorter to longer utterances and from less meaningful to more meaningful content. Specific semantic and syntactic aspects of language can be improved as indicated. As a child is responding positively and fluency is improving, articulation can be focused upon using a relaxed developmental approach. A cluttering element can be treated by slowing the rate, correcting articulation and attending to phrasing and blending when needed.

Gregory (1979b) concluded that there is essential agreement among clinicians such as Bloodstein, Cooper, Gregory, Perkins, Ryan, Van Riper, Webster, and Williams that procedures should be used with confirmed school-age stutterers (ages 6 or 7 to around 14) that enhance fluency and the child's confidence to speak easily and enjoy talking. Analysis of stuttering behavior is, in general, viewed as counterproductive, although it might be used to the extent that the child does not respond to fluency-changing approaches. In recent years, Rustin and Cook (1983), Adams (1984a), Costello (1984b), Gregory and Hill (1984), and Shine (1984a, 1984b) have described sequences of procedures for improving the school-age child's fluency. All of these methods, in one way or another, focus on the proper initiation of voice and articulation and breath stream management for the blending of speech. Gregory (1986a) describes his method, easy relaxed approach, smooth movement (ERA–SM), as involving a somewhat slower phonetic rate and transition between sounds at the beginning of a word or a phrase. A smooth transition from sound to sound and word to word is practised. It may be necessary to use a somewhat slower general speech rate at first, but Gregory stresses keeping changes in rate and prosody to a minimum. Just as with pre-school children, this age group may be found to have concomitant language problems, articulation problems, below average motor control of the speech mechanism, and communicative or interpersonal stress factors needing attention. Parent counseling is important, and modelling as well as verbal interaction procedures may be employed. Parents and teachers learn when to reinforce the child's modified speech.

Attitudes of elementary school-age children are dealt with by being concrete about their feelings and by talking about speech change and other behavior change in behavioral terminology (Williams, 1971; Gregory, 1973; Williams, 1979; Gregory, 1980; Williams, 1980; Rustin and Cook, 1983; Gregory, 1985a). Almost all contributors (Gregory, 1979a; Gregory, 1979b) emphasize that a positive rapport between a child and the clinician is crucial to successful therapy. On occasion, this relationship will help the clinician to understand a child's need for a related service such as psychotherapy.

In stuttering therapy for younger and for older children and adults, we have increased the effectiveness of therapy by employing behavioral principles more systematically (Gregory, 1968; Ryan, 1974; Shames and Egolf, 1976; Ryan, 1979). The most systematic therapies involve the use of programmed learning formats in which stimulus, response, reinforcement, and criterion variables are carefully planned, allowing for branches in the progam as progress is assessed (Ryan, 1974). I have found this beneficial in the initial training of clinicians, but I have observed that most practising clinicians follow these principles in a less formal, albeit effective way.

Several commercially produced programs for the evaluation and treatment of stutterers are also available (e.g., Stocker, 1976; Shames and Florance, 1980; Shine, 1980a; Cooper and Cooper, 1985b). Wall and Meyers (1985) advise clinicians to realize what various programs cover or do not cover. In other words, the clinicians still must meet children's unique needs in a way in which particular programs may not do.

Therapy for Upper School Age and Adult Confirmed Secondary Stutterers

In contrast to stuttering in the early stages of development, factors that contributed to the onset and development of stuttering are not as apparent at this stage as are learned secondary speech behaviors, acquired attitudes, and learned ways of behaving that reflect the person's past life, including experiences with stuttering. There does not appear to have been as much specific attention to differential evaluation at this older age level, and this is viewed as a critical area for clinical research. Many clinicians, especially some of those who offer short term fluency shaping programs, seem to follow essentially the same steps with all clients, and quite often those therapies give little direct attention to the attitude component of therapy (e.g., Webster, 1979).

One of the best ways of discussing therapy for confirmed secondary stutterers is in terms of the controversy, described by Gregory (1979a), between those who adhere to a stutter-more-fluently or a speak-more-fluently model. Briefly, clinicians such as Bloodstein (1958), Johnson (1967), Sheehan (1970b), and Van Riper (1973), who based their work on a stutter-more-fluently frame of reference, stressed that the stutterer should not be given some method to stop stuttering and readily produce fluency, but that stutterers should attend to their stuttering, learn to monitor it, and then gradually learn to modify their speech by thinking of and seeing how they can stutter more easily. In this way, stutterers do not avoid stuttering as much because they are studying and modifying it. Sheehan (1970b, 1979) emphasized that stutterers need to perceive more realistically their dual roles as people who stutter sometimes but who also speak normally.

Replacing stuttering with various forms of fluent speech has been taught by several contributors during the last twenty years (Goldiamond, 1965; Brady, 1969; Ryan, 1974; Adamczyk, Sadowska and Kuniszyk-Jozkowiak, 1975; Wingate, 1976; Perkins, 1979; Ryan, 1979; Webster, 1979). Fluency initially obtained by using such procedures as delayed auditory feedback or instruction in the modification and practice of various parameters of speech (such as slower rate, easier and more relaxed onset, more continuous air flow, and smoother blending), is usually shaped to accomplish speech that is considered normally fluent. Gregory (1979a) classified the works of such contributors as Brutten and Shoemaker (1967), Cooper (1968), Gregory (1968), Williams (1971), and Shames and Egolf (1976), as not being closely associated with either model and as combining, in various ways, ideas from the two schools of thought.

When *Controversies About Stuttering Therapy* (Gregory, 1979a, 1979b) was published, this was perhaps the most controversial issue examined. In my most recent analysis of contemporary issues for a main report at the XX Congress of the International Association of Logopedics and Phoniatrics in Tokyo (Gregory, 1986b, 1986c), I observe that this issue has been clarified and the intensity of the controversy diminished. While there are clinicians who follow one or the other models rather closely, many now combine procedures based on the stutter-more-fluently and the speak-more-fluently models. Gregory and Gregory (1984) have shown how the identification, monitoring, and gradual modification of stuttering and associated unadaptive speaking behaviors (rapid rate, erratic prosody, etc.) can be combined with fluency building skills such as easier initiation of the words and phrases, blending, and variations in rate, loudness, and inflection. Practising delayed reponse is used to reduce time pressure. Voluntary dysfluency, like that emitted by most normal speakers, is used to continue the process of desensitization begun in the earlier stages of identification and monitoring. There is a paradox here that stutterers should recognize. 'Acceptance of stuttering' as a part of therapy contradicts 'building fluency' and vice-versa. Insight into this paradox is a part of the attitudinal aspect of therapy.

Guitar and Peters (1980) and Cheasman (1983) have also described methods for combining stutter-more-fluently and speak-more-fluently techniques, or for using procedures based on one model or the other depending on the assessed nature of a stutterer's problem.

In describing adjuncts to speech therapy, Lees (1983) refers to the use of the Edinburgh Masker, the use of biofeedback, hypnosis and drug therapy. She could also have included delayed auditory feedback (DAF). In my experience, the masker has been especially beneficial to those who have attempted behavior modification procedures with minimal success. The use of EMG biofeedback (Guitar, 1975; Lanyon, 1977) is a reasonable procedure to use in conjunction with speech modification work, since one of the obvious characteristics of stuttering is increased tension. Lees (1983) concludes that hypnosis may provide the stutterer a feeling of deep relaxation and thus result in enhanced fluency just as does relaxation therapy (Jacobson, 1983). Drugs have been found to reduce the severity of stuttering, probably because the ones used have a calming, relaxing effect (Aron, 1965). Finally, DAF is useful to some stutterers as they strive to modify their speech because DAF forces the person to use a pattern characterized by units of longer duration and slower transitions. Present information indicates that these adjuncts have different effects on individual stutterers, but that masking and DAF are the most useful. In general, today's clinician believes it is important to be informed about various methods and techniques, and while most follow a developed frame of reference, certain adjuncts are found useful with certain clients.

Attitude change

Briefly, attitudes may be defined as dispositions to respond to stimuli in certain ways on emotional conditioning and experience. Dealing with attitudes remains a controversial area. In general, clinicians accept the concept that attitudinal responses are involved in a stuttering problem, that attitudes influence a stutterer's response to therapy, and that therapy brings about attitudinal changes (Gregory, 1979a, 1979b; Dalton, 1983b). The controversy about attitudes is related to the extensiveness of procedures used *directly* to change affective responses and beliefs and how we assess attitudes.

Those who adhere to a speak-more-fluently model are likely to emphasize that improving speech is one of the most effective ways to alter feelings and thoughts (Ryan, 1979; Webster, 1979). Certainly, they say, we should observe the client's response to an effective speech modification program before spending valuable time on these more difficult to define entities. Advocates of stutter-more-fluently approaches and those who combine these basic models in one way or another, often integrate speech modification activity with verbal interaction procedures aimed at expanding the clients' understanding of the nature of stuttering and gaining added insight into their problem. However, practically speaking, all clinicians, by information and instructions given, influence clients' beliefs about the problem, about themselves as stutterers, and about therapy. In a subsequent chapter, Kuhr describes paradoxical treatment procedures that are related in conceptualization to stutter-more-fluently techniques and that should be explored with reference to the bringing about of desired attitudinal changes.

It has been my experience that the clinician who focuses on attitudes as a planned activity in therapy is more likely to recognize stutterers, or parents of children who stutter who have more pervasive needs or specialized concerns indicating a referral for psychotherapy. In some clinics, this possibility is recognized at the beginning of therapy by including a psychological consultation in the evaluation (Gregory, 1973, 1968a).

Attitudes cannot be measured as objectively as overt stuttering behavior, although there are problems with the definition and measurement of both (Gregory, 1979a, 1979b; Curlee, 1984; Ingham, 1984b; Young, 1984). Recently, Ulliana and Ingham (1984) have questioned the independence of responses representative of attitudes and response describing speech behavior in a situation. Using an instrument such as the widely known S–24 version of the Erickson Communication Attitude Scale (Erickson, 1969; Andrews and Cutler, 1974; Guitar, 1976; Guitar and Bass, 1978), Ulliana and Ingham concluded that responses to S–24 items are so positively related to stuttering behavior that the S–24 does not add information.

The Repertory Grid Technique (Fransella and Bannister, 1977), a procedure based on Kelly's psychology of personal constructs, is rather widely used in England to assess attitudes. Dalton (1983b) and Hayhow (1983) have described the uses of this assessment procedure with stutterers and Dalton provides a concise description of Kelly's theory. This is a very individualized approach to attitude assessment that is readily useful in the attitude change aspect of therapy. Cook and Botterill discuss this method in another chapter.

Barber (1981) has designed the Inventory of Communication Attitudes which reflects the multidimensionality of interpersonal attitudes by differentiating reports of behavior, cognition, and affect. Scale 1, 'Affective', obtains ratings of the subject's enjoyment of speaking in various situations. Scale 2, 'Behavioral', involves rating one's speech skills in the various contexts. Scale 3, 'Cognitive A', and Scale 4, 'Cognitive B', reflect the respondent's perceptions of most people's enjoyment of speech and most people's speech skills in speaking situations. The comparison of these scales is a key assessment idea in Barber's procedure. This tool has promise for providing more valid and clinically useful information about communication attitudes.

Transfer and maintenance

Increased planning for the effective transfer of change and the clinician's reponsibility for providing a maintenance program has been a major development in stuttering therapy during the last decade (Gregory, 1979b; Shames and Florance, 1980; Boberg,

1981; Dalton, 1983a; Gruss, 1983). Stimulus generalization enhances transfer, but clinicians and clients plan together activities in which responses made successfully in one situation are practised in progressively more difficult situations. With children, transfer can be accomplished as the parents join in the therapy process, changing their way of interacting with the child towards the model provided by the clinician. With school age children, parents and teachers can learn how to reinforce the child for speech change. Transfer activities in the classroom can be planned.

Therapy should progress from being fairly intensive during the beginning stages and gradually taper off to less intensive and finally infrequent, depending on the requirements of each individual. Based on my own experience, I want to place strong emphasis on how essential it is for the clinician to stay involved during what I prefer to call a follow-up period in which progress is not only maintained, but in which there are new positive developments based on the client's experience. As therapy gets under-way, I tell parents of the children who stutter and school-age or adult stutters that this continuation for 12–18 months following the core period of therapy is essential to success. About eighty per cent of the adults we see are willing to follow through in this way.

Measurement of change

We all agree on the advantages of having objective data regarding speech and other behavioral or attitudinal changes in assessing the success of therapy. Some contri-butors, such as Sheehan (1980, 1984), have expressed concern that clinicians may over-emphasize the importance of measures that are easier to make e.g., speech measures versus attitudinal measures. Speech and attitudinal measures should both be inter-preted with reference to known limitations (Gregory, 1979a, 1979b; Shames and Florance, 1980; Bloodstein, 1981; Ingham, 1984b, 1984c; Sheehan, 1984).

Ingham (1984b, 1984c) provides a rationale for making a time series of speech assessments outside the clinic twice weekly for at least four weeks before therapy, at the same frequency during therapy including the transfer phase, and finally, at the same frequency during maintenance. Observations and reports indicate that most clinics now make speech measures at the time of initial evaluation, at the beginning of therapy, at varying times during therapy and at the end of therapy. There is still a need for more attention to follow-up measures.

Clinicians recognize that there are differences between overt measures (the subject knowing a recording is being made) and covert measures (the subject not knowing that a recording is being made). However, the difference is probably minimal for pre-school children. According to a study by Howie, Woods, and Andrews (1982), overt and covert measures appear to differ the most immediately following treatment when the presence of a tape recorder is most strongly associated with therapy.

Finally, Williams (1979) cautions that even though speech change is obviously the goal of treatment, we must remember that criteria of 'success' and 'failure' are evaluative statements. He emphasizes that we should give 'due thought, respect, and understanding to the goals of the client' (p. 268). In other words, the clinician's desire to be objective about success has to be tempered by consideration of the way in which the client's goals evolve.

Specialist in Stuttering

In this chapter, I have described the way in which the evaluation and treatment of stuttering has evolved during the last fifty years, and have indicated the way which developments in therapy have been related to research pertaining to the nature of stuttering.

Clinicians offering service to stutterers must have an understanding of the complex nature of the problem and of the various therapeutic strategies. During formal training, students who identify stuttering as an area of particular interest should take advantage of as much course work and practicum experience in stuttering as possible. It is my opinion, our field being so broad, that clinicians in practice should identify several disorder areas for concentration, e.g., stuttering and voice disorders, or childrens' language and fluency. They should seek as much opportunity to work in these areas as possible, realizing that we all develop increased expertise as we have added experience. They should take advantage of as many continuing education opportunities as they can. What I am describing and advocating is a clinician who wishes to be identified as a 'specialist in stuttering' and who accepts referrals as such. Although we all often cringe a little when some of our former clients describe what they did in therapy, it is sometimes apparent when talking with a stutterer that stuttering therapy has been attempted by an inadequately prepared clinician. I believe that the designation of 'specialists in stuttering' is one of the best ways to improve service. I would like to see specialist certification programs approved by professional organisations or government agencies.

Notes

[1] For additional information about theories of stuttering during this period, see Hahn, E., Stuttering: *Significant theories and therapies*. Stanford University, CA: Stanford University Press (1943; Revised 1954).

[2] Travis (1957) moved to a more psychodynamic conception of stuttering, but he was always very interested in these dichotic listening differences in stutterers as these results may reflect less lateral brain dominance in stutterers.

[3] For additional discussion of these variables, see Bloodstein (1981), Van Riper (1982), Fiedler and Standop (1983), Curlee and Perkins (1984), Wall and Myers (1984), Shames and Rubin (1986).

7 The Cooper Personalized Fluency Control Therapy

Eugene B. Cooper

Introduction

Personalized Fluency Control Therapy (PFCT) was first described in the literature in Barbara's (1965) *New Directions in Stuttering*. At that time the process was entitled 'Inter-personal Communications Therapy for Stutterers' (Cooper, 1965). Subsequently the development of the therapy process was chronicled in a series of articles (Cooper, 1968, 1969, 1971, 1973a) that led to the publication of the PFCT program in 1976 in the form of a kit containing a manual, assessment instruments, and reproducible therapy materials (Cooper and Cooper, 1976). Four years later, (Cooper and Cooper, 1980), the kit was expanded to include Individual Education Program forms for clinicians working with dysfluent children in public school environments. The *Personalized Fluency Control Therapy — Revised* (PFCT-R) kit, published in 1985, includes assessment instruments, a clinician's handbook, reproducible therapy materials and therapeutically-oriented games for pre-school and school aged children.

Throughout more than a twenty-five year period, and continuing to this day, the authors have focused on developing principles, procedures and materials to assist clinicians in conducting comprehensive behavioral and cognitively-oriented and integrated fluency enhancement programs for children and adults.

This chapter begins with a statement of the author's current assumptions regarding the nature of stuttering and its treatment. Following a definition of stuttering, the chronic stuttering syndrome and dysfluency, issues with respect to the assessment of stuttering, early intervention programs, the significance of metalinguistic skills to early intervention, and the incurable stutterer are discussed. The chapter concludes, following an overview of the PFCT-R program, with five brief illustrative case histories of individuals having been treated with the PFCT-R program.

124

Assumptions

PFCT-R is based on the following assumptions about the nature of stuttering and its treatment:

1   Most chronic stuttering behavior is the result of multiple-coexisting physiological and psychological factors.

2   Central neurological deficits are among the major physiological factors involved.

3   Learning and anxiety are among the major psychological factors involved.

4   Stuttering may be viewed, for intervention purposes, as being the discoordination of the processes of phonation, articulation, and respiration.

5   Most forms of stuttering observed in early childhood are amenable to early intervention.

6   Certain forms of chronic stuttering are resistant to voluntary control and while alterable, are essentially incurable.

7   Comprehensive stuttering therapy programs include activities for the modification of fluency as well as fluency facilitating and impeding feelings and attitudes.

Stuttering, the Chronic Stuttering Syndrome, and Dysfluency

Stuttering refers to an abnormal lack of fluency of speech typically characterized by sound, syllable, or word repetitions and prolongations, or an inability to initiate or terminate phonation within a normal time frame. In its chronic form, stuttering is also characterized by the individual's reactive cognitive, affective, and behavioral responses all of which become significant aspects of the chronic stuttering syndrome. The term dysfluency refers to any disruption in the normal fluency of speech and may or may not be normal. The determination of whether any single dysfluency is an indication of stuttering (an abnormal lack of fluency of speech) may be difficult. However, by determining the types of dysfluencies, their frequency, and the individual's cognitive, affective, and behavioral reactions to the dysfluencies, clinicians are able to discriminate between normal dysfluencies and stuttering (for a discussion of this process, see 'Differentiating between the Developmentally Disfluent and the Chronic Stutterer', Chapter 4 in the Cooper PFCT-R Handbook, 1985b)

Assessing Stuttering

A comprehensive assessment of stuttering includes both the behavioral components of the dysfluencies observed and the individual's cognitive, affective, and behavioral reactions to the dysfluencies. For too long, too many clinicians have judged client progress in therapy on the basis of what may best be termed the 'frequency fallacy' (Cooper and Cooper, 1985c). The frequency fallacy is that the single most reliable and valid measure of stuttering severity is dysfluency frequency counts. During the last decade, in the rush to identify things to count, behaviorally oriented clinicians fixated on the frequency of stuttering. Despite the unreliability of such measures and their obvious lack of validity in indicating the significance of the problem to the individual involved, professionals continue to perpetuate the obsession.

Stuttering assessment instruments developed for use in conjunction with the PFCT-R program were constructed with an awareness of the frequency fallacy and of stuttering's multiplicity. The instruments were designed to assess the more critical elements of the stuttering syndrome: the types of dysfluencies, the physiological correlates of dysfluencies, the consistency of the dysfluencies, the variability of dysfluency types, the semantic, syntactic, and pragmatic features of the fluency failures, and finally, and perhaps most importantly, the individual's dysfluency-related affective and cognitive responses.

Without wishing to belabor the issue, a restatement of our position with respect to the assessment of stuttering severity appears warranted: the measurement of stuttering severity must include not only its behavioral components in all their complexity, but the client's cognitive and affective responses as well. Until the profession's technologies develop far beyond the present state we must rely on the very ancient, but time-honored tradition of making professional judgments. Such judgments must be based on our own cerebral analysis of data which are often nominal at best. Thus at the end of PFCT-R stuttering assessment instruments, clinicians are asked to make an overall judgment of stuttering severity. Such informed judgments are more reliable and reflective of reality than stuttering frequency counts. Unfortunately, some behaviorally-oriented purists persist in focusing on stuttering frequency counts noting that 'overall judgments' defy precise measurement while the number of dysfluencies can be counted with precision. They are like the man searching beneath a street-lamp for a coin he had dropped half-a-block away. When asked why he was searching there for a coin he had dropped down the street, he replied: 'The light is better here'.

Children's Assessment Digest

The PFCT-R program contains a children's and adolescent and an adult assessment instrument. The children's version of the PFCT-R Assessment Digest is a 12 page booklet containing the following assessment instruments:

Chronicity Prediction Checklist
Parent Assessment Inventory
Teacher Assessment Inventory
Frequency Assessment
Duration Assessment
Concomitant Behaviors Checklist
Attitudinal Indicators of Significance of Stuttering Checklist
Situation Avoidance Reactions Checklist
Child's Perceptions of Severity Rating Scale
Clinician's Perceptions of Severity Rating Scale

The first page of the assessment booklet, in addition to providing client identification data, is for summarizing the data obtained in each assessment activity. At the bottom of the first page, the clinician, after completing the assessment activities, judges the extent to which the child's fluency problem is socially and *educationally* handicapping.

Chronicity Prediction Checklist. This checklist consists of 27 questions which the clinician answers with 'yes' or 'no' responses after consultation with the child's parents and after observations of and interaction with the dysfluent child. Responses to the questions provide historical data (such as onset, family history of stuttering) and information concerning the parents' and child's attitudes toward the stuttering (for example, 'Do prolongations last longer than one second?'). 'Yes' responses are interpreted as predictors of stuttering chronicity, but no individual question weighting for predictive value is attempted. Information is obtained about variables which either have been found to relate to chronicity (for example, severity) or have been suggested as being related (for example, self-concept as a stutterer). The checklist is scored on the basis of the number of 'yes' responses obtained. Two to six 'yes' responses are termed as being predictive of recovery, seven to 15 'yes' responses as requiring vigilance, and 16 to 17 'yes' responses as being predictive of stuttering chronicity. The reader is referred to the following articles describing the development of this checklist: Cooper, 1972, 1973b; Lankford and Cooper, 1974; and McLelland and Cooper, 1978.

Parent Assessment Inventory. This inventory, used either in conjunction with the Chronicity Prediction Checklist or alone, assists the clinician in determining the parents' perceptions of the problem and their attitudes and feelings about it. The single page 16-question inventory determines if parents observe dysfluencies, and if they do, what kind of dysfluencies are observed, in what conditions, and with what consistency. In addition, the inventory includes items to assist the clinician in determining how the parents respond to the dysfluencies and what parental suggestions have proven helpful.

At the end of the inventory, parents are asked to make a stuttering severity judgment ranging from mild to severe.

Teacher Assessment Inventory. This single page 13-question inventory, similar to the Parent Assessment Inventory, determines if teachers observe dysfluencies, and if they do, what kinds are observed, in what conditions, and with what consistency. Teachers are asked if they discuss the dysfluencies with the child, and if the child has difficulties in other areas such as reading, spelling, and language. Finally, teachers are asked to make a severity judgment ranging from mild to severe.

Frequency Assessment. The PFCT-R Children's Fluency Assessment Digest includes the determination of stuttering frequency counts while the child is reciting, responding to questions, repeating phrases, reading aloud (if able), identifying pictures, and spontaneous speech.

Duration Assessment. Clinicians, using a stopwatch, are asked to estimate the typical duration of a moment of stuttering during the recorded two to three minute segment of the child's spontaneous speech elicited by having the child respond to the picture stories included in the Children's Fluency Assessment Digest.

Concomitant Behaviors. In this single page checklist, clinicians are asked to check which of the listed 32 behaviors frequently accompanying the act of stuttering are observed in the child being evaluated. These behaviors are listed under five categories: Posturing, Respiratory, Facial, Syntactic and Semantic (judged to be stuttering avoidance behaviors) and Vocal. To be checked by the clinician, these behaviors need not occur during every moment of stuttering, but should be in the child's current repertoire of concomitant behaviors.

Attitudinal Indicators of Significance of Stuttering Checklist. This single page form to assess the child's attitudes toward fluency is omitted with pre-school children for whom clinicians judge it to be inappropriate. The form consists of 20 attitudinal statements which are read aloud to the child. Children are asked if they agree or disagree with the statements. Clinicians modify or omit statements they feel are not appropriate for the children with whom they are working. Agreement with a statement suggests the child holds an attitude suggestive of a problem needing attention.

Situation Avoidance Reactions Checklist. Ten speech situations common to school-age children are listed in this brief section of the assessment digest. Additional spaces are provided for other speaking situations which might be identified by the child or the clinician. Children indicate which of these situations they avoid or would prefer to avoid because of their fluency. This section is omitted for pre-school children for whom the clinician thinks it would be inappropriate.

Child's Perceptions of Stuttering Severity Rating Scale. Children are asked in three ways to indicate how much of a problem they believe their fluency to be. Their responses are placed on a three-point severity scale.

Clinician Perceptions of Stuttering Severity Rating Scale. Upon completion of the assessment instruments, clinicians are requested to make five-point scale severity judgments on five aspects of the child's fluency: frequency, duration, consistency across speech situations, concomitant behaviors, and handicapping reactive attitudes and feelings.

Adolescent and Adult Assessment Digest

The first page of the adolescent and adult version of the PFCT-R Fluency Assessment Digest contains client identification information and a form for summarizing the assessment data obtained on the following six pages. At the bottom of the first page, the clinician, after completing all assessment activities, judges the extent to which the client's fluency problem is socially and *vocationally* handicapping. On the succeeding six pages of the form, the following dimensions of the client's fluency are assessed:

Frequency of Stuttering. Stuttering frequency counts are made while the client is reciting, repeating, reading, responding to questions, and speaking spontaneously for two to three minutes.

Duration of Stuttering Moments. The clinician, using a stopwatch, estimates the average duration of the client's moments of stuttering during the recorded two to three minutes of spontaneous speech. The spontaneous speech is elicited through topics of conversation suggested to the clinician in the Digest.

Situation Avoidance Reactions. On a single page form, 50 common speech situations are listed. Clients indicate which of the situations they avoid or would prefer to avoid because of their fluency.

Concomitant Behaviors. Similar to the children's version, clinicians check which of the listed 32 behaviors frequently accompanying the act of stuttering are observed in the client.

Attitudes Toward Stuttering. Clients indicate whether they agree or disagree to 25 statements concerning stuttering. The inventory is scored by adding the number of statements to which the client agrees. Agreement with the statements (for example, 'I think if I could stop worrying about my stuttering it would go away') is interpreted as indicating the client's attitude is undesirable with respect to that issue. A significant number of 'agree' responses is interpreted as indicating the client possesses fluency impeding attitudes.

Client Perceptions of Severity. Similar to the children's version except that it employs a five-point rather than a three-point rating scale, this form requires the client to judge the severity of the fluency problem by completing three sentences concerning the significance of the fluency problem.

Clinician Perceptions of Severity. Identical to the children's version, clinicians, using a five-point severity rating scale, make judgments with respect to the client's stuttering frequency, duration, consistency, concomitant behaviors, and handicapping reactive attitudes and feelings.

The Efficacy of Early Intervention

Early intervention with the very young dysfluent child became a controversial issue in the United States following the popularization of Johnson's (1955) theory that stuttering was caused by normal dysfluencies being labeled stuttering. Johnson's hypothesis came to be referred to as the 'diagnosogenic', 'semantogenic', or 'evaluative' theory. Although waning in popularity among professionals, its influence continues to be felt in America. Cooper and Cooper (1985a) studied the attitudes of 674 American speech-language pathologists toward stuttering, stutterers, stuttering therapy, parents of stutterers, and related issues during the years 1973 to 1983. Clinician attitudes were found to shift away from support of the Johnsonian concepts which suggest that parents cause stuttering and that early intervention is potentially detrimental. Despite this shift, Johnson's hypotheses still appear to have an inordinate influence on clinician attitudes toward stutterers, parents of stutterers, and early intervention procedures with young stutterers. Wingate (1976), noting the lack of data in support of the theory, suggests that its popularity continues to exist primarily because of its simplicity and because it has generated a considerable amount of research effort.

Cooper and Cooper's (1985a) finding that fewer clinicians in 1983 than in 1973 held parents responsible for their child's stuttering, were fearful of words like stuttering and were opposed to the early intervention procedures is perceived as a positive development. Unfortunately, as a review of the findings of the 1985 study reveals, clinicians continue to hold parents responsible for stuttering and continue to be hesitant in initiating intervention procedures with the very young stutterer. As Prins and Ingham (1983, p. 145) note:

> No issue concerning the treatment of stuttering is as tied to the disorder's folklore as the case for, or against early intervention. The impact of Wendall Johnson's theory, as interpreted by the profession and laity, has had an immobilizing effect. In spite of no clear cause-effect evidence to support it (and considerable evidence to negate it), the belief remains intransigent that calling

attention to dysfluency in a young child may 'cause' a problem of stuttering to emerge ... when a young child shows persistent and unusual signs of dysfluent speech ... intervene ... We believe the profession should embrace this information and thereby transmit it to the public and other professions that provide services to young children.

For the past decade we have recommended an aggressive intervention approach with the very young dysfluent child (Cooper, 1979b), based on the following assumptions:

1 Typical parental reactions generally facilitate the development of fluent speech in very young children.

2 Parents are the primary factor in the significant number of spontaneous recoveries from stuttering observed in young children.

3 Very young dysfluent children can be taught to use fluency initiating gestures efficiently and effectively.

4 Clinicians are responsible for assisting the very young dysfluent child in identifying and developing fluency-enhancing attitudes and feelings.

The Significance of Metalinguistics to Early Intervention

In our development of strategies to facilitate early intervention, we became aware of the significance of metalinguistics. Metalinguistics refers to an individual's ability to talk about language. According to Blodgett (1985), the term *metalinguistic* serves to distinguish between two essentially different types of linguistic abilities: primary or automatic language abilities and metalinguistic or self-conscious language abilities. Primary language abilities are used in comprehension and production of language for communication. Metalinguistic abilities are used when language itself becomes the subject of communication or thought.

Speakers exhibit metalinguistic awareness when they attend to some part of what they know about the language, and also are consciously aware that they possess that knowledge. Once children become aware of language and can manipulate it as an object of thought, they can use their metalinguistic skills for different purposes. For example, they can laugh at puns which play with the sounds or meanings of words, they can participate in reading, writing, and spelling activities, all of which require metalinguistic understanding of the sound system of language. At the highest levels, metalinguistic abilities are necessary for aesthetic appreciation of prose and poetry (Van Kleek, 1981).

Gleitman, Gleitman and Shipley (1972), deVilliers and deVilliers (1972), and Clark (1978) note the growth of metalinguistic ability as a process. Children begin to reflect on certain properties of language at an early age. They comment on their own growing linguistic abilities. For example Clark (1978) reports a child of 2 years 10 months said, 'When I was a little girl I could go "geek-geek", like that. But now I can go "this is a chair" ' (p. 17). It appears difficult for adults to conceptualize being able to use an aspect of language without being able to talk about that use. We assume a 2-year-old who can apply the past tense ending must be aware of it at some level in order to be able to identify and select it rather than other possible verb endings to denote completed actions. However, Clark's (1978) research indicates it is not until after 5 years of age that children identify the -ed ending explicitly as being the linguistic unit adding a past time meaning, or make judgments about the appropriate past forms of irregular verbs. In language development, there is often a lag between the possession of a particular skill in the context of natural speech and the self conscious, or meta-linguistic use of that skill (Fox and Routh, 1975). Implicit knowledge of language is virtually automatic and unconscious. This must be contrasted with the later gradual increase in active, conscious control over knowledge already acquired.

Blodgett (1985) reports that recently attention is being directed to questions about when and how metalinguistic abilities arise in children during the course of language acquisition. Van Kleek (1981) notes that for most aspects of language there appears to be a developmental sequence beginning with comprehension, proceeding to pro-duction, and then to metalinguistic ability. Blodgett (1985), in her study of the development of metalinguistic skills in children, found, as others have, a significant increase in metalinguistic skills after the age of 6 or 7. Authors such as Van Kleek (1981), Hakes (1980), Smith (1976) and Nippold and Fey (1983) suggest that the reason for the age factor may be related to the development of cognitive skills. Others, including Liberman, Shankweiler, Fischer and Carter (1974) and Read (1978) suggest that metalinguistic skills require instruction.

Whichever is the case, as Blodgett (1985) observes, there is a need for teachers and clinicians working with young children whose language development is deviant to be aware of the distinction between primary linguistic ability and metalinguistic ability and to be able to evaluate that metalinguistic ability. Too frequently, in therapy with communicatively disordered children, terms such as 'word', 'sound', and 'slow speech' are used with children with insufficient metalinguistic skills to understand what is being discussed.

As we focused on the very young dysfluent child and as we attempted to instruct them in altering various aspects of their speech, we found ourselves becoming language instructors. As we did so, we began to appreciate the relevance of the children's metalinguistic abilities to our intervention activities. Before we ask children to use slow speech, or easy speech, or deep breath, or easy onset, we need to ascertain if the child has sufficient metalinguistic skills to process such a request. The procedures and materials for very young dysfluent children included in the PFCT-R program were developed with an awareness of the significance of the child's metalinguistic skills. We describe our metalinguistic activities with young children as 'teaching the language of fluency'.

Incurable Stuttering

During the past ten years I came to accept something I resisted for the first twenty years of my professional life. Not all stutterers can become fluent speakers. Certainly we all hope that the day will arrive when we are able to cure stuttering in everyone. Realistically, however, we know that such a time is not within the foreseeable future. Until we can cure all stutterers, our goal is to communicate to those stutterers, for whom normal fluency is an unrealistic goal, the real sense of success that comes from being able to modify fluency. I have never known individuals for whom stuttering was the major disability who were unable to alter their fluency pattern. While many experienced clinicians report they can predict those stutterers for whom the control of stuttering will require a lifetime of vigilance, we have little research to assist us in identifying the predictor variables. Hopefully, such a body of knowledge will be developed in the decade ahead.

We are aware of the significance of accepting the fact that we cannot realistically assume that all stutterers can be fluent. Daly (1985) speaks compellingly and movingly of the danger of destroying stutterer's dreams of being fluent and of many stutterers' life-fulfilling quests for fluency. We need to be sensitive when that dream or that quest is present in the clients we serve. Our clinical skills will be challenged as we make difficult decisions as to how to respond to such clients. Nevertheless, we must not reinforce clients making unrealistic demands of themselves when our judgment is that normal fluency, for whatever reason, is beyond their grasp.

As we grappled with the realization that all stutterers cannot be fluent, we grasped the significance of support groups for chronic stutterers. We are referring to something more than a self-help group. We are hopeful that in the next decade we will see the development of support groups assisting not only those seeking to improve their fluency but also those lifelong chronic stutterers who, having accepted the level of fluency they have attained, are seeking nurturance from understanding others. The professional community's involvement in the development of support groups should be encouraged. Establishing support groups can be an effective and economically efficient method in bringing support services to the largely neglected population of lifelong chronic stutterers.

The STAR Therapy Process

The Cooper PFCT-R program features a four-stage intervention process labelled as

Structuring, Targeting, Adjusting, and Regulating. In the first stage the clinician structures the therapy process. In the second stage, the client's attitudes, feelings, and behaviors which impede or facilitate therapy are targeted. In the third stage, the client adjusts feelings, attitudes, and behaviors to maximize the enhancement of fluency. In the fourth and final stage of therapy, clients regulate attitudinal and behavioral patterns for the long-term maintenance of fluency.

Structuring Stage

The long term goals and short term objectives for the Structuring Stage are as follows:

1 To help the client identify the feelings, attitudes, and behaviors that constitute the stuttering problem:

   a To enable the client to identify and describe the concomitant stuttering behaviors: posturing, respiratory, facial, syntactic and semantic, and vocal,
   b To enable the client to identify and describe situation-avoidance behaviors,
   c To enable the client to identify and describe attitudes toward the stuttering,

2 To help the client understand the goals and the process of therapy:

   a To enable the client to describe the final long-term goals of therapy,
   b To enable the client to describe the therapy process.

In the Structuring Stage the clinician assists the client in identifying behaviors occurring during moments of dysfluency and behaviors adopted as a result of the dysfluencies. The clinician informs the client of the procedures to be followed in the therapeutic process. With older clients, the clinician discusses the rationale for focusing on the client–clinician relationship to assist the client in modifying fluency-facilitating attitudes and behaviors. In addition to the Children's and the Adolescent and Adult Fluency Assessment Digests, the PFCT-R kit includes therapy materials to assist the clinician in meeting the goals and objectives of therapy. The PFCT-R *Blackline Master Booklet* (102 pages of therapy forms, activities, and lessons for copying), provide materials the clinician can use with both children and adults. The kit also includes board games for helping young children learn the language of fluency and to understand the therapy process and its goals.

Targeting Stage

The long term goals and short term objectives of the Targeting Stage of therapy are as follows:

1 To eliminate distracting body and facial movements occurring during stuttering moments:

    a To reduce and/or eliminate distracting and extraneous facial behaviors such as loss of eye contact, flaring nostrils, and excessive eyelid movements occurring during the moments of stuttering,

    b To reduce and/or eliminate distracting and extraneous posturing behaviors such as hand, finger, trunk, or leg movements occurring during the moments of stuttering,

    c To reduce and/or eliminate distracting and extraneous respiratory, syntactic, semantic, and vocal behavior occurring during the moments of stuttering.

2 To establish a client–clinician relationship that will help the client explore feelings and attitudes and make changes in speech behaviors:

    a To create a client–clinician relationship in which the client feels free to express positive and negative feelings about the stuttering, the therapy, and the clinician.

3 To assist the client in targeting attitudes, feelings, and behavior patterns that impede or facilitate fluency changes:

    a To identify and label the client's attitudes and feelings that facilitate or impede changes such as, 'I don't think I have a speech problem', 'I like therapy', and 'I am dumb because I stutter',

    b To identify and label the client's behaviors that facilitate or impede fluency changes, such as appearing late for therapy, completing all the speech assignments, and forgetting a speech assignment notebook.

The Targeting Stage begins when the clinician asks the client to modify behaviors identified in the first stage of therapy. The clinician observes client behavioral patterns. Having targeted the client's behavioral and attitudinal patterns which impede and facilitate therapy, the clinician makes the client aware of these patterns. The goal of the clinician's confrontive behavior is to lead the client into an effectively dynamic helping relationship. The client reinforces expressions of feelings in response to the clinician's confrontations. Even the client's expressions of negative feelings (verbal or nonverbal) are accepted and rewarded to reinforce the client's honesty in the relationship. Through shaping client affective responses to the verbal mode, the clinician creates a therapeutic milieu conducive to client identification and evaluation of feelings and attitudes pertaining to the modification of the client's fluency problem.

The PFCT-R kit contains materials to assist the clinician in achieving the goals of the Targeting Stage of therapy including a daily 'Assignment and Evaluation Worksheet', a series of 'Stuttering Attitude Stimulus' and 'Speech Situation Discussion' pictures, and a 'Client Readiness for Fluency Control Inventory'. In addition, gameboards and activity sheets are included for assisting clinicians in working with the young stutterer who lacks the language skills to identify or discuss feelings and attitudes. Again these materials are presented to assist the clinician in teaching the child the language of fluency.

Adjusting Stage

The long term goals and short term objectives of the Adjusting Stage of therapy are as follows:

1   To help the client in adopting fluency-enhancing feelings, attitudes, and behaviors:

    a   To shape and reinforce the client's accurate and fluency-enhancing perceptions,

    b   To shape and reinforce fluency-enhancing behaviors.

2   To help the client in becoming an effective self-reinforcer:

    a   To identify and develop the client's self-reinforcing activities such as expressions of positive feelings toward self.

3   To help the client in identification, development and use of fluency initiating gestures:

    a   To identify the client's self-developed fluency-initiating gestures, such as 'slowing down', 'changing words', and using 'starter words',

    b   To identify fluency-related speech changes under various speech conditions, such as delayed auditory feedback,

    c   To develop the use of the Universal FIGs (Slow Speech, Easy Onset, Deep Breath, Loudness Control, Smooth Speech, Syllable Stress) in clinical situations.

In the Adjusting Stage of therapy the clinician reinforces client expressions of affect to facilitate client self-evaluation and to maintain client commitment to change. The clinician reinforces accurate, self-appreciative, and productive verbalized client cognitions and also reinforces behavioral expressions of adequacy. The clinician instructs the client in self-reinforcement procedures for the maintenance and continued enhancement of the individual. Concomitantly, the clinician instructs the client in manipulating speech behaviors in the therapy environment to determine which fluency initiating gestures (for example, speech rate change, the easy onset of phonation, or breathing pattern changes) appear most appropriate for the client. The Universal FIGs are defined as follows:

Slow Speech: a reduction in the rate of speech (typically involving the equalized prolongation of syllables),

Easy Onset: a gentle superimposition of phonation on a gentle exhalation,

Loudness Control: a conscious and sustained effort in varying vocal intensity,

Smooth Speech: a reduction in the frequency of phonatory adjustments in conjunction with the use of light articulatory contacts (plosive and affricate sounds being modified to resemble fricative sounds),

Deep Breath: a consciously controlled inhalation prior to the initiation of phonation (typically used in conjunction with Easy Onset),

Syllable Stress: a conscious variation of loudness, pitch, and rate to alter the prosody of speech. Initially taught with the use of a metronome resulting in a repetitive syllable stress pattern, the client subsequently learns to vary the stress of syllables and the rate of syllable production in a random manner in connected discourse. Clients learn to 'play' with their speech.

The Adjusting Stage is brought to a close when both the clinician and the client mutually agree that the client has made sufficient adjustments with respect to fluency-related attitudes, feelings, and behavior to enable the client to begin to strive for the feeling of fluency control in situations outside of the clinic or the home environment. The PFCT-R kit includes over 60 FIG practice sheets to assist the clinician. In addition activity sheets and gameboards for each of the Universal FIGs are included for work with the very young client.

Regulating Stage

The long term goals and short term objectives of the Regulating Stage are as follows:

1   To assist the client in developing the feeling of fluency control,

    a   To enhance and regulate client attitudes and behaviors that indicate the client possesses:

        i   an accurate perception (as judged by the clinician) of the stuttering behavior and the interpersonal ramifications of that behavior,

ii   a realistic emotional and intellectual appreciation of self,

iii   a capacity of self-reinforcement, and

iv   a knowledge, feeling, and belief in the capability to gain the feeling of fluency control.

b   To regulate the client's use of fluency initiating gestures in speech situations outside of the therapy situation varying from the least difficult (in terms of maintaining the feeling of control) to the most difficult.

In the Regulating Stage, the clinician assists the stutterer in planning and using FIGs in the kinds of speech situations that had previously resulted in fluency problems and a loss of the feeling of control. The primary goal in this stage of therapy is the development of a *feeling* of fluency control. Regularly scheduled therapy may be terminated when stutterers feel that no matter how difficult the speaking situation may be, they are capable of employing FIGs to obtain a level of fluency acceptable to themselves for the particular speech situation involved.

Perhaps the only truly unique feature of the PFCT-R progam's STAR therapy process is that of its ultimate goal; the feeling of fluency control. Others have developed programs in which arbitrarily established stuttering frequency rates during pre-determined speech activities in prescribed situations are set as the goals of therapy. Taking frequency counts of dysfluencies in controlled situations may be less difficult and demonstrably more precise than assessing a hypothetical construct such as 'the feeling of fluency control'. However, the latter is perhaps the key variable in determining if a stutterer will maintain an acceptable fluency level upon termination of therapy. Our clients are not asked to evaluate their progress in terms of how fluent they are in various situations. Rather, they are asked to evaluate their speech attempts in terms of whether they did or did not experience a feeling of fluency control. If stutterers report they felt able to modify their speech during the situation, the speaking experience is judged as being successful even if they were dysfluent. The focus remains on the feeling of control and not on fluency itself.

Illustrative Case Histories

Following are five brief case histories of individuals having received therapy based on the STAR Therapy Process in which materials included in the PFCT-R kit were utilized to assess as well as to instruct.

Clark

Clark's parents first called the Center expressing concern over his dysfluent speech behavior when Clark was 2 years and 9 months of age. During the initial speech–language evaluation, it became apparent that although Clark's speech was characterized by frequent sound, word, and phrase repetitions, his language skills were advanced for his age. The length and complexity of his utterances were indicative of a child of 4 years rather than a child of 3. Clark was a spontaneously verbal child and although appearing annoyed at his 'getting stuck' on words, enthusiastically continued his vocalizations. His father, an electrical engineer, and his mother, an elementary school teacher, are both articulate and verbal individuals with rapid speech rates. Upon administration of the Chronicity Prediction Checklist (now a portion of the PFCT-R Children's Assessment Digest), it was found that Clark's father perceives himself as having been a stutterer at a very young age but as having 'grown out of it' by the time he reached first grade at about the age of 6. The results of the Chronicity Prediction Checklist were predictive of recovery rather than of chronicity. In addition, responses to the Parent Assessment Inventory, now a portion of the PFCT-R Assessment Digest, indicated Clark was able to modify his rapid rate of speech upon parental correction and that the type of dysfluencies was limited to repetitions rather than to prolongations or involuntary vocal tract closures.

The parents were provided a copy of the pamphlet *Understanding Stuttering: Information for Patients* (Cooper, 1979b) and a family counseling session was scheduled. Approximately one week later, the clinician met with the family to review the findings, to model fluency enhancing responses for the parents, and to discuss material covered in the pamphlet. At the conclusion of this session, an appointment was made for a three-month re-evaluation. Just prior to that scheduled appointment, Clark's mother called to report that they did not feel the need to come to the Center because Clark's dysfluencies appeared to be 'less disruptive', and that they were 'not panicked' about the problem anymore. Three years later, Clark was seen by the clinician during a routine speech and hearing screening program in the public schools. Clark's speech was judged to be normal and subsequent discussions with the mother revealed that Clark's fluency improved gradually between the ages of 3 and 6, and that he experienced no problems with his speech by the time he entered first grade in school after having attended a nursery school and kindergarten.

Chris

Chris was referred to the speech–language pathologist by his first grade teacher when he was 7. She expressed concern about his stuttering, indicating that 'he can hardly get a word out'. She indicated his stuttering interfered with his classroom performance. A fluency assessment using what is now the PFCT-R Children's Assessment Digest which includes both parent and teacher assessment inventories was supplemented by observing Chris in the classroom situation. Christopher's fluency disorder was rated as being moderately severe on both the social and the educational summary severity rating scales. The PFCT-R Dysfluency Descriptor Digest indicated his speech pattern to be characterized by repetitions of initial sounds, a rapid articulatory rate, the use of superfluous sounds such as 'uh, uh, uh,' and shallow breathing. In addition, there was a distracting loss of eye contact during moments of stuttering.

At the initial parent conference, a Parent Attitudes Toward Stuttering Checklist as well as the Parent Assessment and the Chronicity Prediction Checklist (instruments now included in the PFCT-R) were administered. Initially both parents indicated they did not want Chris to be enrolled in therapy. They stated their son was 'not retarded' and his speech did not warrant therapy. Later in the conference, Chris' mother recalled that when she was in school, children in therapy were considered to be retarded and others made fun of them. By the end of the conference, after the clinician's treatment plans were reviewed with the aid of the PFCT-R Parent Guide, the parents agreed, reluctantly, to Chris' enrollment in therapy. They did acknowledge concern about their son's stuttering and, reassured enrollment in therapy did not signal retardation, they were willing to enroll their son in therapy.

When Chris began therapy, he told the clinician he 'stuttered'. He said he knew he stuttered because his parents and others told him so. He was not able to describe his stuttering nor to imitate it. He said, when questioned about his 'stuttering' that 'I just don't talk good'. He stated he did not care about his speech although he frequently talked about other children making fun of his speech. At one point, he commented, 'I just beat them up when they make fun of me'.

Therapy initially focused on increasing Chris' metalinguistic skills to provide him with the language of fluency. The Stuttering Apple (a PFCT-R therapy guide) was used to assist Chris in conceptualizing the stuttering problem. Using the Stuttering Apple to initially structure therapy, Chris was taught to maintain eye contact during moments of stuttering. When he was able to describe his stuttering with some accuracy and to use such terms as 'stuttering', 'slow speech', 'fast speech', and 'deep breath', Chris was taught the FIGs (Fluency Initiating Gestures) using FIG Sheets (over one hundred of these single page practice sheets are provided in the PFCT-R). Gameboards included in the PFCT-R kit and therapy activity sheets from the *Blackline Master Booklet* assisted the clinician in maintaining Chris' motivation to alter his speech behavior. The results of the Dysfluency Descriptor Digest indicated Deep Breath and Slow Speech were the most appropriate FIGs for Chris.

At the same time, Chris was instructed in self-reinforcement and in the development of fluency-enhancing attitudes and feelings. His teachers were provided the PFCT-R Teacher Guides and their assistance was sought in helping Chris attain therapy goals. Chris remained in therapy over a four year period. During the first two years, for each of the nine months of school, Chris was seen individually for thirty minutes twice weekly. During the next year, he was seen once weekly for thirty minutes for nine months. During the fourth year he was placed on a maintenance/monitoring program, being seen once a month during the school year. Three years later, at the age of 15 Chris perceives himself as being essentially a normal speaker with 'a little help from my friends, the FIGs'. The end goal of therapy, that of achieving the feeling of control of fluency, appears to have been reached and maintained.

Nathan

Nathan, at the age of 15, asked his father to get him help with his stuttering. The family was completing plans to move and Nathan, faced with having to enter a new high school, was anxious about his speech. He had been seen by a speech–language pathologist in school when he was 11 and in the fifth grade. Nathan is unable to recall anything about that experience other than that he saw the clinician only a few times. Nathan has one brother five years younger. His father is an industrial designer for an architectural firm and his mother is employed in a secretarial/administrative assistant capacity. There is a history of chronic stuttering in the mother's immediate family. Nathan has experienced excellent health except for a number of allergies. Nathan describes himself as being an average student. He played on the high school junior varsity football team and had been lifting weights for body building on a regular schedule for almost two years.

At the initial interview, Nathan's speech was characterized by sound, word, and phrase repetitions and hesitations in the flow of speech. These dysfluencies occurred as frequently as on 20 per cent of the words spoken. During these moments of stuttering, Nathan would blink his eyes, look away from the listener, flare his nostrils occasionally, and move his arms and legs randomly. Frequently, it appeared the moments of dysfluency were occurring near the end of his exhalation of air for speech. His stuttering pattern included both hard articulatory contacts and what appeared to be laryngeal spasms. Perhaps the most attention-getting aspect of his stuttering pattern (other than the repetitions and prolongations) was the frequent and consistent use of 'um, um, um', or 'well ah, well ah, ah'. Nathan noted his speech during the interview was typical of his speech with his parents, teachers, and strangers, but that he is generally fluent with his friends in informal situations. On the PFCT-R Adolescent and Adult Assessment Digest, Nathan rated himself a severe stutterer while the clinician judged his stuttering to be moderately severe.

Nathan and his parents were advised that the end goal of therapy would be the development of Nathan's feeling of fluency control and not fluency. With this understanding, therapy was initiated on a once-a-week basis for an hour and continued so for 10 weeks. Following that period, Nathan was seen every other week for 6 weeks and then once a month for 3 months for a total of 16 sessions. The clinician spoke with either Nathan's mother or father at every session and met with the entire family as a unit on three occasions. The parents' responses to the PFCT-R Parent Attitudes Toward Stuttering Checklist were discussed with the clinician. In addition, the parents received a copy of the PFCT-R Parent Guide. The clinician telephoned Nathan once during each of the weeks he was not seen for therapy. Nathan's assignments were discussed and, as he was working on one or more the FIGs at the time, he was asked to use them during the conversation. The clinician evaluated Nathan's use of the FIGs during the telephone conversation. Therapy was structured in keeping with the goals and objectives in the PFCT-R Treatment Plan and by using materials such as the Stuttering Apple, the Dysfluency Descriptor Digest, the Fluency Analysis Checklist, Stuttering Attitude Stimulus Sheets, and Speech Situation Discussion Sheets (all included in the PFCT-R Blackline Master Booklet).

Perhaps as a result of his desire to have his speech under control when he arrived at his new high school, within the first 2 weeks following the initiation of therapy, Nathan had learned to establish and maintain good eye contact and to control extraneous facial and body movements during moments of dysfluency. Nathan was able to express his feelings openly and a significant portion of each therapy session was spent in identifying Nathan's therapy-impeding as well as facilitating behaviors, attitudes, and feelings. The importance of an open and honest relationship between Nathan and the clinician was a significant topic of discussion. Because of Nathan's willingness and ability to explore and express his feelings and attitudes openly, it quickly became evident that Nathan perceived his stuttering and the interpersonal ramifications of his stuttering accurately. It also became evident that Nathan possessed the capability of being an excellent self-reinforcer.

FIGs had been mentioned in the initial interview and described for Nathan and his parents in the first therapy session. In view of the rapid progress Nathan made in controlling the stuttering-related behaviors and in view of his therapy facilitating feelings and attitudes, the clinician moved quickly (during the fourth session) to have Nathan begin practising FIGs. Based on the results of the Dysfluency Descriptor Digest, Nathan was instructed to begin with the Slow Speech and the Deep Breath FIGs using the Fig Practice Sheets provided in the PFCT-R Blackline Master Booklet. For the next 6 sessions over a 2 month period Nathan used the practice sheets to develop skill in using the six FIGs. Each day he would use his cassette tape recorder to record samples of his practicing, give a report of his day using the FIG or FIGs on which he was concentrating at that moment, and rate himself (on a one to ten scale) as to the extent of the overall feeling of fluency control he experienced that day. He brought the tape to the next therapy session. The clinician listened to samples of Nathan's using the FIG practice sheets and to the daily reports and discussed with Nathan his reactions concerning what he heard.

By the tenth session Nathan had control of his eye contact and other distracting hand, arm, and facial movements. He continued to practice being a good self-reinforcer. Nathan had begun to experiment (as clients typically do) with his FIGs in several speech situations outside of the home. He was now ready to 'go for the feeling of fluency control'. Beginning with the eleventh session, Nathan was given a 'contract' covering the period until his next scheduled visit. The contract specified on a day-by-day basis what FIG he was to use, in what situations he was to use it (for example, calling a movie theatre and asking for the time of the feature film). In addition, the contract required him to describe 'Today's best situation', and to judge (on a one to ten scale) 'Today's Overall Feeling of Control Rating'.

Nathan's 16 therapy sessions were conducted during a 6 month period. During the third month of therapy, after 9 therapy sessions, Nathan began to express feelings of having achieved the 'feeling of control' in various speaking situations. When he worked on the Syllable Stress FIG, Nathan expressed pleasure that he could now go into speaking situations and 'play' with his speech by varying the stress patterns. He found that listeners were unaware that he was consciously altering his speech pattern (the rate was not abnormally slow or the articulation slurred), yet he felt he could manipulate his speech freely. Nathan experimented with using the various accents typical of southern speakers and even began to imitate the stress patterns of well known television evangelists. Nathan thrives on his ability to manipulate his speech through altering the stress and rate patterns.

Just prior to entering his third year in high school, it was agreed that regularly scheduled therapy sessions no longer appeared necessary. By that time Nathan no longer considered his fluency disorder to be his 'number one problem'. He now (one year following termination of therapy) terms the severity of his problem as being mild. Although he continues to experience dysfluencies in many situations, the dysfluencies are without tension, are not accompanied by loss of eye contact or other distracting movements, and Nathan no longer experiences the feelings of a complete loss of control even in his most dysfluent situations. Whereas he avoided the telephone altogether prior to therapy, he uses it with ease and with pleasure. His mother noted she never thought she would be grateful that her friends could not reach her by telephone. Now, however, with Nathan calling and being called all the time, she reports she feels good every time a friend complains that her line is always busy.

Larry

Larry, a 26-year-old husband and father of two, has been employed by a large heat and air conditioning contractor since his high school days. There he met his wife who serves as a secretary and radio dispatcher for the company's many service trucks. Larry has become one of three foremen for the company and his expertise in diagnosing problems and in designing alternative repair procedures is highly valued by his employers and respected by those under his supervision. His wife called the clinician to make the initial appointment for a speech evaluation.

During the initial evaluation, Larry stuttered on 75 per cent of the words spoken on each of the five frequency-of-stuttering sections of the PFCT-R Assessment Digest. The dysfluencies consisted primarily of sound repetitions spoken with an abnormally rapid rate of articulation and frequent but brief pauses indicating struggle to initiate phonation. Eye contact with the listener was practically nonexistent and during moments of stuttering, unusual eye movements and facial movements were observable and distracting to the listener. Larry's responses to the Situation Avoidance Reaction and the Attitudinal Indicators of Significance of Stuttering Inventories included in the PFCT-R Assessment Digest indicated that Larry preferred to, or did, avoid most common speaking situations such as using the telephone, ordering in a restaurant, and initiating conversations. His responses to attitudinal statements indicated his stuttering was his 'biggest problem' and that it 'is my own fault'. His stuttering was judged to be severely handicapping on both the social and the vocational PFCT-R stuttering severity rating scales.

Larry reported he had asked his wife to call for the speech evaluation because he was aware that his continued success at work was becoming increasingly dependent on his ability to communicate effectively. He had never received therapy for his stuttering. He described himself as being 'a quiet person' because of his stuttering. At the conclusion of the initial evaluation the clinician described the PFCT-R STAR therapy process to Larry and recommended that he be seen for therapy one hour weekly. It was explained that the duration of therapy would be determined subsequently when both the clinician and Larry would be able to talk more knowledgeably about the matter.

At the beginning of the second session, the clinician used the PFCT-R Stuttering Apple therapy guide to help Larry conceptualize the things he did when he stuttered (for example, looking away from the speaker, wrinkling his brow) and the things he did because he stuttered (for example, avoiding answering the phone, asking his wife to make calls for him). The PFCT-R Readiness for Controls Inventory was completed to assist the clinician and Larry to identify therapy-impeding and facilitating behaviors and attitudes. In addition, the Dysfluency Descriptor Digest was used to assist in determining which of the FIGs might be most helpful for Larry. In keeping with the PFCT-R Treatment Plan, Larry was instructed to reduce or eliminate the distracting and extraneous facial and body movements occurring during stuttering. In addition, over the next two therapy sessions, Larry's fluency-impeding feelings and attitudes were identified and discussed. It quickly became evident that Larry focused on his stuttering to such an extent that he had little appreciation for what he was (a husband, father, valued employee). Before the end of the second session, Larry agreed that he needed to initiate a program of self-reinforcement. One of his assignments after the second session was to set aside five minutes each day for 'self-appreciation'.

FIGs were described and discussed with Larry during the initial therapy session. However, it was not until the fifth session that the clinician and Larry agreed he had made sufficient progress in controlling extraneous behavioral components of his stuttering and in altering his attitudes about himself and his stuttering to begin using the FIGs outside of the therapy situation. As was predicted by the Dysfluency Descriptor Digest, Larry found the Slow Speech, Deep Breath, and Smooth Speech FIGs to be most helpful in gaining the feeling of fluency control. During the tenth session (three months following his initial contact with the clinician), while expressing his delight with how much better he felt about himself and his speech, Larry noted: 'Before I came here and learned FIGs, every time I was in a speech situation, I felt like I was in the middle of a four lane highway going the wrong way dodging cars'.

Larry continued seeing the clinician on a once a week basis for four more sessions. Following that, he was seen once a month for three months. Larry terminated therapy feeling he had gained the feeling of fluency control. Although still experiencing dysfluencies in a number of speech situations, Larry reported that he was no longer 'obsessed' about his speech problem and that although he assumed he would have 'to attend to it' for most of the rest of his life, he said 'I'm in control now and that means everything'.

Richard

Richard, a 34-year-old foundry worker, married and the father of two children ages 11 and 8, made an appointment to discuss his stuttering problem. During the initial interview, Richard reported he could remember stuttering since he entered school at the age of 6. He noted his stuttering varied in severity over the years and was particularly severe during his high school years. He described himself as an outgoing individual who does not allow his stuttering to keep him from entering speech situations even though he continues to be conscious of the problem. Richard described himself as 'always having lived' with the problem. He was seeking help now only because he had been made a foreman at the foundry and was concerned that his speech would begin to interfere with his work. When asked if he had any indications from those with whom he worked that his speech was causing trouble, Richard noted that he could not recall any instances in which his stuttering had been a factor. He noted he was generally able 'to do things to be fluent when it is important'. He had never received therapy. Upon administration of the PFCT-R Adolescent and Adult Assessment Digest, Richard's stuttering was judged as being not at all socially handicapping and mildly vocationally handicapping.

In discussing how he had learned to cope with his problem throughout his life, Richard described how he had slowed the rate of his speech, substituted words in his speech to avoid words on which he anticipated stuttering, altered his breathing pattern, and forced himself to enter situations he would have preferred to avoid because of his stuttering. He noted he found all of these techniques to be useful but was uncertain as to whether he was doing the right things. At this point in the interview, the clinician told Richard how impressed he was with Richard for having so successfully developed, on his own, procedures for controlling his fluency. The clinician emphasized the need for Richard to be appreciative of his accomplishments and a second session was scheduled.

During the second session, the clinician described the clinical process for achieving the feeling of fluency control, emphasized the importance of self-reinforcement, and introduced each of the fluency initiating gestures (FIGs). Richard noted he had used each of the FIGs at one time or another and that he found the Slow Speech and the Deep Breath FIGs to be most helpful to him in maintaining fluency. He also noted that, since the first session, he had 'done a lot of thinking' and had concluded that he *should* feel 'damn good' about himself and how he had overcome his own problem. Richard expressed appreciation for being made aware of just what he had accomplished and for having the goal of 'the feeling of fluency control' defined for him. He concluded that knowing he was doing a good job in handling his stuttering and that he was able to self-reinforce his use of controls made him feel he was already doing what needed to be done with his speech. He was dismissed from therapy.

It was agreed that Richard would call the clinician if he once more became concerned with his stuttering. Richard has never called. On the two occasions the clinician has met Richard accidentally in the community, Richard has expressed appreciation for the clinician's guidance. In the experience of this clinician, Richard's story is not uncommon. It is for this reason his story is reported here.

8 Personal Construct Theory and the Treatment of Adolescent Dysfluency

Willie Botterill and Frances Cook

Introduction

The treatment of fluency disorders in adolescence is a continuing concern for speech clinicians. Virtually all adolescent stutterers have a relatively long history of dysfluency and as they approach the final years of their schooling it is vitally important that renewed efforts are made to help them bring their speech under control. We know that a high proportion of untreated clients go on to develop the chronic adult syndrome of stuttering. Further, although many adolescents have received treatment in childhood their dysfluency persists. We feel that a different approach to the problem of adolescent dysfluency based on Kelly's (1955) personal construct theory (PCT) and further developments by Bannister and Fransella (1986) and Evesham and Fransella (1985) could hold the key to further progress for many stutterers.

Fransella (1972) described a series of experiments in the treatment of adult dysfluency where the principles of personal construct theory were brought into play. This work continues to generate a great deal of interest amongst UK clinicians and the training of PCT therapists has grown dramatically in the last ten years. The popularity of the approach lies in a growing awareness that the solution to stuttering is not simply a matter of establishing fluency in the clinical setting. Rather, the challenge lies in helping the individual achieve fluency in their own social world. This is a much less predictable and controllable environment than the confines of the treatment room. Perhaps the only way to ensure that fluency gains won in treatment transfer adequately to the real world is by addressing the personal issues that concern the dysfluent individual. In our experience many stutterers develop psychological as well as physical coping devices as a direct consequence of their speech problem. By including a phenomenological psychological appraisal as a fundamental component of the treatment process the therapist acknowledges the *personal* dimension of speech dysfluency.

It seems to us that PCT offers a framework within which the therapist can help the client to understand him/herself and the personal issues that might be impeding

147

further progress towards the goal of fluency. Our work in this area began several years ago when we were treating adult patients on an individual basis. We have gone on to apply the same principles to the treatment of adolescents within the *Hampstead, Bloomsbury and Islington* dysfluency treatment projects, and in this chapter we will try to give the reader some idea of the philosophy and treatment techniques that are typical of Personal Construct Therapy.

We believe that people with speech dysfluency (or indeed any other handicapping condition) inevitably develop a very extensive personal construct system built around their problem. For example, predictions about the likelihood of stuttering in particular social encounters are usually based on a past history of communication failure. Past experience may far outweigh the rapid, almost magical fluency gains that are possible with modern motor speech therapy techniques. The failure to maintain new found fluency may have its roots in the *psychological* status of the individual rather than any 'deterioration' of the treatment effects. In what follows we try to outline the essence of PCT in order to stimulate others to explore personal construct theory and therapy principles further.

Personal Construct Theory – PCT

Kelly's (1955a,b) seminal work *The psychology of personal constructs* had at its core the philosophical assumption of *constructive alternativism*. This fundamental of PCT suggests that:

> All of our present interpretations of the universe are subject to revision and replacement . . . we take the stand that there are always alternative constructions available to choose among in dealing with the world. No one needs to paint himself into a corner; no one needs to be completely hemmed in by circumstances; no one needs to be the victim of his biography (Kelly, 1955a, p. 15).

There can be no question that this is a highly optimistic view of man. Kelly's psychology is based on the assumption that man has the ability to change every aspect of his thought, emotion and behaviour. Man is able to achieve this level of adaptation because he creates, for his convenience, an interlinked network of *personal constructs* which are based on past experience of life situations. Constructs are bi-polar; for example, *good–bad* is a personal construct. It is like a rating scale along which people, institutions, societies, problems and even therapists may be judged by the construing client. Typically an individual brings many personal constructs to bear on the interpretation of his social world. Constructs tend to cluster around particular aspects of living. Therefore we can conceive of individuals as having many elaborate *construct subsystems* which have a primary role in the development of attitudes and values, hopes and fears, thoughts and behaviour.

Construct systems are developed primarily from past experience (both direct and vicarious) but their prime aim is the prediction of the future. Man actively tries to anticipate what may happen in the future and formulates plans to help him cope effectively in a variety of alternative scenarios. He is not the passive recipient of the unfolding future. He plans long term goals and makes preparations in advance for the inevitable pitfalls that will arise in the course of pursuing his goals. Our personal construct systems form the basis for planning and anticipation and they are never (or at least *should never* be) static. As new experiences and events confront a person his or her construct system should be evolving. By having an 'up to date' construct system we can predict future events and experiences far more accurately. We go further by actively trying to *elaborate* our construct systems concerning particular aspects of our interpersonal world. We behave in ways aimed at gathering further information about particular situations. We seek out information that will enhance our construct systems knowing that this is our best chance of predicting and controlling future events.

The phenomenological emphasis in construct psychology highlights the importance of the client's personal experience and understanding of the social world, including the client–clinician relationship itself. PCT holds that if therapists are to play a significant part in the exploration of another person's construct system there must be trust, emphatic understanding and genuine respect between client and clinician. Effective help only occurs when the therapist is able to see events *through the eyes* of her client. This understanding will in turn lead to changes in the way the client construes his therapist. We feel that this level of mutual understanding is a prerequisite for effective therapy.

PCT Principles

Kelly formulated a logical basis for the theory of personal constructs which necessarily involved the introduction of new terms and concepts. The theory is based on the *fundamental postulate* of *constructive alternativism* which is expressed as follows:

> A person's processes are psychologically chanellised by the ways in which he anticipates events . . . (Kelly, 1955b, p. 561)

The fundamental postulate was elaborated by eleven corollaries, the first of which states 'We anticipate events by construing their replications'. We view the world and ourselves through our own unique construct systems that have been built up through past experience. We use construct systems to predict what will happen in the future. We are able to anticipate the future because we have built up 'theories' about people, settings and situations. We construe replications when we try to build a model of some anticipated social encounter. Using this model of 'how it will be' allows us to 'try out' various ways of coping with the encounter in advance. If our construct system is adequate we will find that reality conforms to our expectations. If our construct system is in some way faulty, under-developed or out of date, then we are likely to feel both uncomfortable in the encounter and perplexed by the experience.

PCT argues that we do not have to stick with our past experience. If we anticipate events differently in the future (e.g., through becoming convinced that our interpretation of past events was incorrect) then there is a chance that we may revise our construct system and achieve outcomes that were not previously possible. PCT says we have a choice: 'all of our present interpretations of the universe are subject to revision and replacement', (Kelly, 1955) and so we are not simply victims of our biography; we do not always have to play the role that we grew up with; we can change and evolve our ideas about ourselves and other people *for our own benefit*.

Personal constructs vary in their breadth of application. The *range corollary* of the theory states: 'A (personal) construct is convenient for the anticipation of a finite range of events'. Few constructs have general utility over all the events confronting us. Perhaps 'good–bad' is an example of a very broad construct that can be applied in many settings but 'plain–purl' is a construct that is primarily concerned with knitting! So, constructs have a range of convenience and become meaningless to the individual if they are stretched too far. The verbal labels we assign to particular constructs do not necessarily imply any agreed definitions. A therapist's understanding of the construct 'success–failure' may be very different from that employed by a fourteen-year-old male stutterer. These differences in interpretation are the very essence of constructive alternativism. We can only begin to understand the meaning of another person's construct by knowing something of what it is not (i.e., its bipolarity). In order to understand 'day' we must have some understanding of 'night'. Three different individuals might see the contrast of 'independent' as 'dependent', 'tied up', or 'part of a group'. Only by coming to understand these nuances can the therapist begin to build up an accurate understanding of her client.

PCT stresses individuality: 'Persons differ from each other in their construction of events'. We each see social events in our own way because we employ our unique construct systems. We each wear a set of 'goggles' through which we view events; our interpretations are idiosyncratic. But PCT also recognises commonality: 'To the extent that one person employs a construction of experience which is similar to that employed by another his psychological processes are similar to those of the other person'. In addition the sociality corollary states: 'To the extent that one person construes the construction processes of another he may play a role in a social process involving the other person'. People do share commonly agreed perceptions of experience with cultural identities being a case in point. From the therapist's point of view it is essential to gain a thorough understanding of the construct systems employed by clients in order to characterize and anticipate their problems. This understanding allows much more detailed treatment planning than any categorical approach to fluency problems (e.g., mild, moderate, severe) would allow.

As mentioned above our personal construct systems *should* be in a constant state of change and adaptation. If we have built up a construct system about 'Joe' as a mean and miserly person we are forced to make changes when we hear Joe has made a very generous charitable donation. We accept that we have got the wrong impression of Joe, and we must make adjustments to our constructs about Joe to accommodate this new information. But not always! Sometimes we simply refuse to make radical changes to our construct system even in the face of overwhelming contrary evidence. We seem to prefer to believe that the 'evidence' in question was a temporary aberration rather than a genuine facet of Joe's make up. Much of the psychological distress that people suffer in their lives can be traced through PCT to faulty or static construct systems. Change and adaptation result in healthy construct systems (and hence healthy people); denial and guilt are the products of an inflexible and impermeable construct system.

One final principle is central to a full appreciation of the value of the PCT approach to treatment. Construct systems exist to make sense of two entities: the social world 'out there' and our experience of 'self'. Our *Core Role Constructs* form a system of beliefs about *ourselves*. We develop personal ethics and pinpoint our strengths and weaknesses. We can predict how we will react in a moral dilemma by analyzing our core role constructs. Of course, we can *choose* to act in accordance with these core constructs or we can *choose* to act 'out of character'. Often people are surprised at their own reactions to various situations. They may dread some particularly formal social gathering and find afterwards that it was thoroughly enjoyable. If we are healthy we profit from such positive experiences. If we are negative we see them as no more than a chance occurrence devoid of implications for change in our construct system.

Summary

In summary, PCT characterises people as *scientists* who are constantly setting up predictions about the future based on a 'working model' of how people, institutions and life operate (construct systems). These predictions are then tested against reality. Like a good scientist the individual must be prepared to discard any discredited hypotheses in the face of contradictory evidence. As we noted above not everyone can do this, particularly with longstanding and firmly held beliefs. Applying the PCT model to speech dysfluency Fransella (1972) observed that dysfluent people inevitably end up *choosing* to stutter because that is the most familiar and predictable role to play. Making the psychological transition from dysfluency to fluency is considerably more difficult than bringing the overt speech behaviours under control.

In the effective treatment of stuttering we would suggest that two main strategies need to be pursued. Initially, technical motor therapy may provide immediate and effective control over speech fluency in the clinical setting. This may well transfer in the short term to other particular situations. Whilst such improvement is to be welcomed it may remain the case that the *universal* generalisation of these gains is still some way off. The second treatment strategy involves a psychological appraisal of the client's difficulties and the pathways through which he may resolve these to his own satisfaction.

Exploring Personal Construct Systems

Personal Construct Theory is perhaps best known for its associated *Repertory Grid Technique* which allows an objective evaluation of the interrelationships in a personal construct system. Grids provide a structured framework for exploring the nature of personal construct systems where both client and therapist seek to reach an understanding of the reasons for the client's inability to make the changes he desires.

A repertory grid usually contains a number of personal constructs that have been elicited in relation to a number of relevant *elements*. Grid elements can be significant people, institutions, relationships or situations that are personally meaningful to the client and are suspected by the therapist of having a bearing on the problem. When a suitable set of elements has been established and a set of personal constructs has been elicited the process of grid construction can begin. A typical grid (see Figure 1) has the elements arranged along the top axis and the constructs down the vertical axis. The client is then asked to construe each element in turn in relation to each construct. This process may involve the client *ranking* each element on the construct in question or it may involve the client making *ratings* on a 9 point scale in relation to the construct. For example 'Father' may be rated as 9 on the construct 'good–bad' where the ratings run from 'good' = 9 to 'bad' = 1.

When every cell in the grid has been ranked or rated the resulting data matrix is analysed using a computer program (Higginbotham and Bannister, 1983) which reveals the relative significance of each element and each construct in terms of their contribution to the overall variance in the scores. These statistical associations are indicators of the psychological significance of constructs and elements. The program then undertakes a cluster analysis of the elements and constructs. Here clusters of elements and constructs which 'go together' are formed using rules which prevent significant overlap. This analysis portrays the complexity of the associations between the various components of the grid. It becomes possible to see 'hidden' associations between elements and between constructs. We will discuss the process of analyzing repertory grids in more detail later; at this stage we only wish to demonstrate that objective methods of grid analysis are available. The correlations between the constructs indicate the extent to which an individual is employing a 'tight' versus 'loose' construct system (Bannister and Fransella, 1986). The clusters are indicative of the relative psychological significance of the individual constructs.

The first step in PCT, as in many other types of therapy, is to gather information about the person, his history, his view of himself and of his problem. It is possible, even at this early stage, to begin to discern the themes and the constructs which recur in the client's description of himself and his social world. Once the basic details of the case have been established the process of eliciting personal constructs begins. Below we outline some of the most popular methods of eliciting constructs for use in a repertory grid.

Self characterisation

This technique is a particularly useful way of eliciting personal constructs from clients who are in the very early stages of treatment. It involves asking the client to provide a written character sketch of himself. The instructions are carefully worded to encourage the client to draw a sympathetic picture of himself with as few restrictions as possible:

> I want you to write a character sketch of (client's name) just as if he were the principal character in a play. Write it as it might be written by a friend who knew him *intimately* and *sympathetically*, perhaps better than anyone ever really could know him. Be sure to write it in the third person. For example, start out by saying (client name) is . . . (Kelly, 155a, p. 323).

The client, of course, substitutes his own name in the sketch. The idea of the 'sketch' is used in order to suggest a general outline, while the use of the third person helps the client to convey both his good and bad points. The resulting self-characterisations vary as much as clients themselves do. Some may only offer the essential biographical details whilst others contain extensive lists of personal strengths and weaknesses. For some stutterers speech is the predominant theme whilst others hardly mention it at all.

Whilst it may not be possible to evaluate a self characterisation in any scientific way it does provide a rich source of hypotheses about the significant core constructs that the author employs. The task of the therapist is to learn more about the client's construct system and begin to see the world through the client's eyes. We seek to build up an overall impression of the way the client sees himself and his current situation. We pay particular attention to the first and last statements in a self characterisation. These are often amongst the most revealing about the person. Then, the range of constructs and any recurring themes in the sketch are studied.

The issues that emerge are noted for further discussion with the client, not as truths or falsehoods, but simply in the pursuit of greater understanding. Constructs about change are particularly important and help the therapist learn more about the client's goals, and how realistic these are.

Eliciting constructs through triads

The most usual method of eliciting significant personal constructs depends on the prior establishment of a group of relevant *elements* as outlined in the section above. The choice of elements is determined initially by the kinds of questions the therapist wishes to pose about an individual's construct system. At later stages in the treatment process the client's questions determine the grid components. In the early stages the therapist may simply want to explore general issues about personal relationships but as therapy proceeds it is likely that more specific questions will emerge. This is a very important point about repertory grids. We use grids to answer questions. Without a question in mind it is meaningless to draw up a grid.

If we wanted to look at current interpersonal relationships, attitudes to self, and the way constructs cluster together we would choose elements from amongst the significant people in the client's life. We would also need to include the client himself as one of these elements. Therapists usually employ a range of 'role titles' (Father, mother, best friend, disliked teacher, self, etc.) to ensure that a wide range of elements are represented in the grid. One might otherwise find that the client simply chooses elements from amongst his well-liked friends. We find the role titles in Table 1 useful for this exploratory type of grid.

Table 1: Role Titles for Repertory Grid Construction

1. Father
2. Mother
3. Sister
4. Brother
5. Close female friend
6. Close male friend
7. Someone in authority
8. Someone who makes you feel uncomfortable
9. Someone you envy
10. Someone you feel sorry for
11. Someone you would like to be like
12. Self
13. Self without a stammer
14. Stammering self
15. Self in 5 years time

Of course there are many other relevant role titles available to the PCT therapist (see Fransella and Bannister, 1977). Selecting 10 elements for the early exploratory grids is guided by the prior analysis of interview information and the self characterisation. Having chosen appropriate role titles we ask the client to enter on the grid the actual names of the people that fit the role titles. Next we write the names and the roles on cards which we use during triadic construct elicitation.

Three grid elements are chosen at random and the client is asked to consider these three individuals and specify 'some important way in which two of them are alike and thereby different from the third'. The therapist records whatever the client says, be it one word or a phrase, and then asks how this similarity makes the two people different from the third. The latter provides the contrast pole for the similarity construct elicited in the former procedure. This exercise then progresses using new triads until the desired number of personal constructs has been elicited.

The process may take some time before client and therapist are satisfied with their efforts. The client gradually becomes aware of what is meant by 'personal constructs'. In the beginning there may be a tendency to cite rather concrete reasons for the similarities and differences between elements. The client may say that 'mother' and 'best friend' both have red hair or that they are 'both tall'. Whilst it is conceivable that these are significant personal constructs for a particular client it is more likely that these are statements of fact, i.e., they are non-evaluative. Personal constructs by definition are personally meaningful ways of evaluating elements. Thus 'mother' and 'best friend' may both be *caring, helpful* and *warm hearted*. The third element in the triad may in contrast be *ruthless, self-centred* and *cold*. These evaluations are personal constructs.

In this process of guiding the client to a better understanding of the nature of personal constructs the therapist must be careful not to influence the individual's construing. There is the danger that she might unwittingly 'shape' the client's responses in the direction of her own expectations. Grids must be made up of the client's constructs rather than the therapist's. The contrast pole is particularly prone to this type of contamination; the client may offer a simple semantic opposite for the contrast pole rather than exploring what he really means by the contrast pole of a particular construct.

A further pitfall lies in the hierarchical nature of personal constructs. Some constructs are superordinate to others. Thus 'good–bad' may be a superordinate construct of 'honest–devious'. We may find that there is a very high (.98) correlation between 'good' and 'honest' in the construct analysis because honesty implies goodness for a particular client. Where the therapist suspects that subordinate constructs are being offered she can ask for clarification and point out the hierarchical nature of constructs. In the grid we want to try to include a range of distinct constructs which will provide greater discimination in the final analysis.

Hinkle (1965) introduced the term 'laddering' to describe the process of exploring the hierarchical nature of a person's construct system. In laddering further questions are asked about each construct which helps the client to develop a more abstract superordinate idea. It provides a way of clarifying the meaning of a construct as well as understanding the implications of the subordinate idea. For example, if the client offered the construct 'tidy–untidy' in relation to particular elements the therapist would probe further by asking why 'being tidy' is an important quality. The client may respond by saying that people who are 'tidy' are 'well-organised'. The therapist may then ask why it is important to the client to be well-organised in life, to which the client may respond that it earns the 'respect' of others. Therapist and client may conclude that 'respect' is really the most important construct here rather than its subordinate construct 'tidy'.

Summary

In this section we have outlined the main stages in repertory grid construction. We would emphasise again that grids are created in order to answer particular questions about an individual's construct system. The process of constructing a grid begins with the initial interview and self characterisation. As hypotheses emerge the therapist formulates questions which can be 'tested' using the grid technique. Constructs may be elicited via the triadic method and further refined through laddering. Experience is required in the design of efficient grids and we move on to illustrate this process in more detail in the next section by citing a specific clinical case.

Personal Construct Psychology in Practice — A Case Study

In order to demonstrate the process of gathering the information necessary for a grid and the ways in which grids are analysed it is helpful to follow a client through the various stages. We have selected one of the older adolescents from our caseload whom we shall call 'Keith' to illustrate the process.

Keith was 17 years old when he referred himself to our department. He had been stuttering for as long as he could remember. A decade of speech therapy had taught him a variety of speech techniques which he had found 'very helpful' and which had indeed enabled him to be fluent, albeit with great effort and for relatively short periods of time. He asked us for intensive help with his stuttering in order to build up his confidence in using a speech fluency technique. He felt that if he could exercise more control over his stuttering this would improve his social life and make it easier for him to participate in the discussions and debates he would become involved in when he entered higher education.

Formal fluency assessments revealed a speech rate of around 104 words per minute with a stuttering frequency of 37% of his output. We began by asking Keith to draw up a self characterisation which is reproduced below.

Me Old Mate Keith

He's a good bloke really — quite honest, can take criticism and can bounce back. He seems quite flexible, being able to adapt to various people: enthusiastically agreeing with a loud chatterbox, tactfully guiding a sympathy-attracting person, or manipulating a rebellious junior at school. Quite shy with strangers though, takes a while for confidence to emerge, but with friends he is quite lively and humourous and eager to exchange ideas.

He is not blunt though, even with blatantly wrong people; he tries to guide people to his way of thinking rather than bludgeoning through his partner's argument. His temper, when it comes, is more directed towards himself and situations, although sometimes he embarks on a controlled outburst against someone near to him. He gets frustrated trying to put over his ideas to those whom he feels don't understand, but his inexperience at speaking has made him a good listener — although probably playing a less prominent role in the outside world than he feels he deserves. He has a latent potential possibly kept down by his own self-consciousness rather than by circumstance.

If we look at Keith's self characterisation and examine the first statement we can see that he feels good about himself and there is some indication that he will be able to make constructive use of therapy. The last statement tells us that he sees himself as someone who has, potentially, a capacity to change and therefore is optimistic about his future. Themes that we would want to address further would be those of frustration, temper, outbursts, 'bludgeoning' as well as the notions about inexperience, self-consciousness, shyness and confidence.

Even at this stage we have elicited a wide range of personal constructs from Keith that appear to be relevant to his view of himself. The next task was to create a repertory grid where these constructs could be seen in relation to significant elements. We wanted to explore Keith's views about himself and his interpersonal relationships further and so we selected specific elements from the role titles for inclusion in the grid. The resultant grid complete with ratings is displayed in Figure 1.

The elements in Keith's grid were rated on each construct using a 9 point scale. The analysis revealed that the most psychologically significant construct in the grid was 'WARM-COLDER'. Several other constructs were related both positively and negatively to this focus (see Figure 2).

When we look at the raw grid and compare elements 6 (me now), 9 (me I'd like to be) and 11 (me fluent) with the constructs 1 (warm), 2 (assertive) and 4 (open) we can see that Keith rates himself consistently as a fairly warm and open person. Looking at assertiveness we see that he currently sees himself as more 'easy going' than assertive, but he would ideally like to be more assertive, and if he were fluent he *would be* much more assertive.

Figure 2 shows us that 'warmth' and 'assertiveness' are negatively correlated. Assertive people are therefore 'not warm', and warm people are 'not assertive'. We set up the hypothesis that perhaps Keith cannot afford to be fluent because of these implications. Fluency will either require an increase in 'assertiveness' or it will inexorably

Repertory Grid Form

ELEMENTS

CONSTRUCTS

#	Construct		MOTHER	FATHER	SISTER	SISTER	CLOSE FRIEND	ME NOW	GRANDFATHER (Uncom.)	Admired Person	Me I'd like to be	Friend	Me Fluent	12
1.	WARM	COLDER	3	7	2	4	5	4	6	4	4	6	4	
2.	ASSERTIVE	EASY GOING	7	2	6	6	4	7	2	6	4	3	4	
3.	ADAPTABLE	INFLEXIBLE	4	6	4	4	6	3	8	4	5	8	4	
4.	OPEN	DEFENSIVE	3	6	2	4	8	4	7	3	4	7	3	
5.	IMPULSIVE	ANALYTIC	3	8	2	7	4	6	2	7	6	4	4	
6.	SHY	CONFIDENT	7	7	7	4	4	2	4	7	8	7	6	
7.	WORLDLY	HOMELY	8	3	6	6	4	4	7	5	3	3	3	
8.	DIRECT & FIRM	UNAGGRESSIVE	6	2	6	6	4	7	2	6	5	3	6	
9.	SOCIALLY RESTRAINED	GOOD COMMUNIC.	6	8	8	4	3	3	3	8	8	7	6	
10.	FRANK	SECRETIVE	4	7	3	6	6	5	2	3	4	6	4	
11.	TEMPER	CONTROLLED FEELINGS	3	7	2	6	3	6	2	4	6	4	4	
12.			1	2	3	4	5	6	7	8	9	10	11	12

Figure 1: Keith's Repertory Grid

lead to an increase in assertiveness. This would then be incompatible with being a warm open person. Earlier in the process of laddering these constructs Keith supplied us with the following implications:

Construct Implications

WARM	COLDER
You'd be more in touch with people, humane.	You would be unemotional
It would be more rewarding You would have deeper contact	Contact with people would be limited. You would not get to know them.
You would feel more genuine You would have genuine relationships.	People would not be certain of how you feel. You would have uncertain relationships.
You would have some existence, some identity.	You would be unfulfilled in relationships.

ASSERTIVE	ACCEPTING/EASY GOING
You would not always be prepared to accept the ideas of others or see their viewpoint.	You would be open to new ideas and flexible.
Your own views could be wrong and this could lead to unhappiness in the long term.	Having different views would help you form your own attitude to the world
Your own attitudes might be blinkered and inflexible.	You would have a broader view
You would have a very limited viewpoint.	You would have greater understanding of the people and things around you. You would get greater satisfaction from this understanding. You would be able to adapt to new situations.

The second most significant component in the construct analysis centred on 'temper'. Looking again at elements 6, 9 and 11 in the grid we see that both Keith now and as he would like to be are rated nearer the 'controlled feelings' pole of the construct. When we look at what might happen were he to become fluent we see that he would shift towards becoming more prone to 'temper'. Here again we see an implication of fluency that may be preventing Keith from developing greater fluency. The transition might threaten his core role constructs about himself.

We discussed the above points with Keith to obtain his reactions. Did these ideas make sense to him? Keith wrote down the following observations based on our analysis of the grid:

Figure 2 Keith's Construct Analysis using GAB

	1	2	3	4	5	6	7	8	9	10	11
1	1	− .83	.76	.82	.30	− .10	− .41	− .86	− .13	.45	.31
2		1	− .84	− .71	.03	− .17	.42	.92	− .07	− .16	− .03
3			1	.83	− .28	.10	− .12	− .92	− .08	.09	− .25
4				1	− .04	− .29	− .25	− .80	− .43	.42	− .03
5					1	.01	− .47	.07	.21	.55	.90
6						1	− .14	− .13	.93	− .11	− .04
7							1	.17	− .27	− .51	− .55
8								1	− .01	− .21	.05
9									1	− .06	.15
10										1	.64
11											1

Constructs in order of contribution to variance:
1 8 4 3 2 11 5 10 7 9 6

Component 1 — Principal construct is: 1
Included in order of importance are constructs: 8 4 3 2

Component 2 — Principal construct is: 11
Included in order of importance are constructs: 5 10

Component 3 — Principal construct is: 7
No related constructs

Component 4 — Principal construct is: 9
Included in order of importance are constructs: 6

1 I seem to be afraid of impulsive temper, a characteristic I see embodied in my Grandfather and which repels me.

2 I'm stuck between two options: do I want to be warm and adaptable and open — or assertive, direct and firm? The grid shows that people cannot be both. I tend to admire the warmth of some people but I do not identify with the assertive characteristics of others. I want to be more assertive whilst retaining my warmth.

3 There are differences between 'me as I'd like to be' and 'me fluent'. Perhaps I'm not so sure what the 'me I'd like to be' entails.

Warm	Direct
Adaptable Vs	Assertive
Open	Firm

Ideally I want to have all these characteristics but do not want to strive for one side for fear of losing the other.

The process of change (reconstruction) may begin with self characterisations, eliciting constructs from triads and laddering but the discussion of the grid analysis is the most important stage in diagnosis and planning therapy. At the end of the discussion Keith went away to write a further self characterisation this time about Keith in five years time.

My new mate Keith well old mate really except he seems to have changed

This guy seems quite easy going with people; he's sure of himself, handles people very well although at times he can be a bit too open, too frank about his feelings, yet has the tact and wit to stay on the right side of people.

He's no pushover though; he'll tell you why you're wrong and isn't afraid to put forward his views strongly and guides rather than bulldozes people towards a different viewpoint.

Although he is seen as being very much in control of his life he still feels an uncertainty about himself which he can express to people he is close to, for he isn't defensive about himself; perhaps he is too aware of his openness. He sometimes feels he should have more contact with people; maybe he feels insecure about controlling and limiting his contacts with people; sometimes he feels that he is too friendly to strangers and too frank and assertive with friends.

He seems to adapt and mould himself to people and, that achieved, exerts his own pressure on the relationship. A warm and humourous person though; gets on well with all styles of personality, charming his way with some and enjoying some friction with firmer characters. He does have a temper though and can be quite scathing about things which are illogical or 'bad' in his view.

Above we see many of his original themes recurring, but this time Keith is struggling with how these same constructs might act for him in the future. The purpose of this second sketch is to see what notions the client has about change following the grid analysis and how that change may come about. For some clients the picture is highly idealized and unrealistic. For others such as Keith it sheds further light on the uncertainty in his constructs and the implications of change. Most significantly it demonstrates that these are possibilities worth exploring.

PCT with Younger Clients

The case above was chosen in order to illustrate the sequence of grid construction and the basics of grid analysis. It features an intelligent older adolescent who is both articulate and interested in the procedure under discussion. Construct elicitation and grid construction are however easily adapted to the individual and it is possible to devise alternative ways of eliciting constructs in relation to elements for younger clients. Perhaps a great deal of the appeal of PCT lies in the fact that it allows us to explore areas of cognitive and emotional functioning where words often fail. It can be very difficult indeed for any client to explain their mixed emotions about particular situations or people. Grid technique allows the therapist and the client to move from fairly basic and concrete constructs to much deeper and more personally significant ways of construing people and problems without resort to confrontational exchanges.

There are no compelling reasons why PCT should be restricted to the adult and adolescent populations. A number of workers have applied the principles of PCT in the treatment of very young children. For example, Ravenette (1980) devised an interesting technique for self-evaluation with young children. They were invited to select a person who knew them well and were asked 'What three things might that person say about you?'. Another example from Ravenette involved employing simple line drawings of happy and sad faces. The children were asked to give three reasons why the faces were happy/sad. Further drawings were used to elicit a much wider range of constructs. These approaches are discussed in more detail by Butler (1985).

Our experience with younger adolescents over the past several years suggests that many of them initially limit their construing to issues concerned with speech and the reactions of others to their speech. This indicates to us that the adolescent is developing and becoming preoccupied with construct systems about the stuttering self. The most common category of construing that we uncover about other people is concerned with whether they are 'easy to talk to', 'hard to talk to', 'patient with me', 'impatient with me', etc. We feel this is indicative of a constriction in the development of the adolescent's construct system. We see them reducing their perceptual and evaluative systems down to a few interrelated meaningful constructs that enable them to operate under conditions of maximum control. We see our role as helping the adolescent stutterer to 'broaden his perceptual field' (Kelly, 1955b) in order to learn more about the constructs of (fluent) others. We aim to help these clients to become more objective about themselves in relation to others. We hope that they can begin to realise that dysfluency is only part of their make-up and that it is certainly not the core.

Personal Construct Therapy

Kelly's notions about personal change and reconstruction have become a central theme in our approach to intensive therapy for dysfluency. Therapy should be a creative process both for client and therapist. Emphasis is placed upon the client actively elaborating his own construct system by releasing his imagination and discovering novel ways of helping himself to deal with the issues that confront him. This also involves the client in action to 'test out' the validity of older hypotheses and gain confidence in the validity of new alternative hypotheses. Kelly (1955a) states 'Creativity always arises out of preposterous thinking' and we make a start on this process by asking clients at the beginning of therapy to *brainstorm* ideas about stuttering.

The 'brainstorm' technique is employed widely in the social skills training area (e.g., Priestly *et al.*, 1978) and demands free unbridled thinking from participants. We encourage our clients not to rationalise their ideas but to present 'the first thing that comes into your head no matter how crazy it may seem'. When we use this technique in group therapy with adolescents we begin by asking them to brainstorm on a topic quite unrelated to their fluency. For example we have asked for as many novel uses as possible for an empty baked bean can! Once we feel the group has mastered the technique we gradually introduce more relevant topics related to communication. The aim is to break away from well rehearsed notions about a theme and to recreate that theme in the group context. We select topics like: 'What is stuttering?', 'What is fluency?', 'What is technique?'. The typical responses we get to the 'stuttering' topic cover ideas like repeating words and sounds, getting stuck, staying too long on one sound, speaking too fast/too slow, hesitating, ums and ers, fillers, pauses and so on. Having elicited these ideas we go on to encourage the group or individual to discuss whether these notions only apply to stutterers and if indeed all of them apply to all stutterers. In the course of this kind of exercise we expect our adolescent clients to become less inhibited about talking frankly about their problem and as a consequence to become more involved in the process of treatment.

Another key concept in PCT therapy is the role of the *CPC cycle* in the process of change. This is a consequence of construing which involves, in succession, *Circumspection, Pre-emption and Control*. The CPC cycle leads to a *choice* which precipitates the individual into a particular set of actions in a given situation. In other words this relates to the client's ability to see the alternatives in situations and to arrive at a choice of action from amongst these alternatives which is aimed at bringing the situation under control. We provide opportunities to experience the CPC cycle through an activity we term *Problem Solving* on our treatment courses. The exercise begins by simply asking clients to describe a current situation that is causing them a problem, such as coping with buying a bus ticket. We next ask them to brainstorm as many alternative solutions to this problem as they can imagine (circumspection). We then encourage them to think through the consequences of these various alternatives and then finally select from the alternatives the one which offers the maximum chance of success (pre-emption). We encourage 'testing out' the chosen strategy in reality to see how comfortable it feels and how successful it is in practice (control). The level of success or failure the chosen strategy achieves is less important here than the elaboration of the construct system which produced it. Either outcome is likely to lead on to further elaboration and development of the individual's construct system which will in turn lead to the development of further more adaptive strategies.

Role play is another technique which is central to the process of PCT therapy. Many clients are naturally apprehensive about testing out new strategies in public and indeed Kelly argued that anxiety was a prerequisite for change. In treatment we find that a *supportive* role play environment can provide a valuable bridge between theory and practice. In particular the use of 'role reversal' exercises within the treatment setting is an important adjunct to teaching the client to 'construe the construction processes of others'. Role reversal results in a much clearer appreciation of how to play social roles in relation to other (fluent) people. When the client plays the role of the bus conductor he has an opportunity to elaborate his constructs about the impact of stuttering which leads to the development of a more realistic view of the 'ticket problem' employed above.

We can gauge the impact of such experimental exercises through group discussion, written assignments, further grid construction and analysis as well as through behavioural assignments in the real world. If we came up against specific obstacles to progress with an individual client we can design a grid that may reveal the conflicts and apprehensions that lie behind such obstacles to progress. The essential point here is the importance of *client initiated change* in both construction and action, a goal that is further realised in the *fixed role therapy* described below.

When our clients are reaching the stage where they are becoming aware of the extent to which their actions are limited by their construct systems we encourage them to *imagine they have changed*. The essence of fixed role therapy is to experiment with alternative ways of behaving and to cope with the uncertainties and pitfalls as well as the positive benefits that this brings in its wake. Even when things go wrong it is not a signal to return to the safety of the 'old self' but rather an opportunity to learn and profit from the experience. If a client feels he should be more assertive and actively tries to be more assertive in everyday life there is always the danger that inexperience will lead him to be simply objectionable and his worst fears of humiliation may be realised. Fixed role therapy provides opportunities to make mistakes and to discuss these mistakes with a supervisor. The client returns to his new role with an elaborated construct system which should ensure he does not repeat the previous errors.

Fixed role therapy involves the drawing up of an explicit contract between client and therapist. Together they plan how the 'new self' will operate in practice and set specific goals for the 'new self' to achieve. The worst that can happen is that the client will fail to achieve particular goals, or fail to achieve them with adequate success; but this does not mean that the client himself is a failure.

This supervised treatment may be carried out over a period of several months but the sessions are spaced increasingly further apart. The emphasis throughout is upon a shift to self-supervision where the therapist is no longer the primary source of change-inducing constructs (Fransella, 1983).

Conclusion

We hope that this discussion has conveyed to the reader the flavour of the psychology of personal constructs. We each employ construct systems to guide our life choices and we inevitably develop particularly significant systems around our personal difficulties. It is our role as therapists to help clients explore their construct systems and appreciate how construct systems provide both the basis of current functioning and the vehicle for future change. We try to assist our clients in elaborating their construct systems where we feel this would be helpful. In the process we get to know our clients well; they share with us their strengths and weaknesses and we in turn try to provide learning opportunities which will allow them to revise and reconstrue their problems. For many clients the chance to reconstrue themselves and their communication difficulties can at the very least make the problem more acceptable. For others such basic reconstruction is the prelude to more comprehensive change in many areas of social functioning including speech fluency.

We do not suggest that all there is to the treatment of stuttering is a period of personal reconstruction; but equally we are convinced that it takes more than motor speech training to achieve lasting change in the treatment of dysfluency. Therapists trained in the 'scientific approach' to the treatment of speech disorders may be rather too ready to see the personal dimension of handicap as being the domain of other professionals in the caring services. We may be reluctant to switch the focus of our treatment from the objective and the scientific to the subjective and emotional dimensions of the problem. We hope that in this brief account of PCT we have been able to demonstrate that this is a false dichotomy. Scientists do not have the exclusive rights to scientific reasoning. We believe the problem of dysfluency can benefit from a more psychological approach to treatment.

9 The Treatment of Childhood Dysfluency Through Active Parental Involvement

Lena Rustin

Introduction

Research into the nature of stuttering has taken many paths. The problem has been studied at virtually every level of analysis from genetics to social learning theory. Perhaps part of the reason for this plethora of research perspectives lies in the popularity of speech dysfluency as a problem ripe for theoretical development. Human communication in general and motor speech production in particular is of considerable interest to theoreticians and model builders from diverse disciplinary backgrounds. Stuttering is a fascinating academic problem. It is also a very considerable human problem and treatment programmes which alleviate the condition are our first priority. The task for the clinician is to grasp the significance of new developments in fluency theory and translate them into applied action in the clinical context.

Currently, a general consensus is emerging that stuttering is best characterised as a developmental disorder where multiple etiological factors are likely to play a role in determining onset. For example, Adams (1982) discusses the enormous psychological and physiological changes that occur in children during the period between 2 and 7 years of age when stuttering is most commonly detected. Conture (1982a) and Conture and Caruso (this volume) start from the position that stuttering is the result of a particular *interaction* between the neuropsychology and the social psychology of fluency. For clinicians this implies opportunities for intervention at two levels of analysis: at the neuromotor level and at the social/environmental level.

Further, we have abandoned the notion that stuttering will simply go away if we ignore its development in young children. After a 'hands off' policy towards fluency development in young children (Johnson, 1961a) we are now seeing valuable opportunities to practice *prevention* through early intervention. Of course, to offer therapy at this age we need to be able to discriminate between children who are at risk for developing the chronic dysfluency syndrome and those who are within the acceptable limits of developmental dysfluency. Although research has been carried out on this problem there can be little doubt that a finer assessment grain (e.g., Conture and Caruso, this volume) is needed here. However, criteria do exist to identify the young stutterer and this chapter sets out to describe a programme of intensive and consecutive therapy which has been geared to the needs of young stutterers.

Early Intervention

As knowledge of the dynamics of developmental dysfluency has grown so therapists have seen the importance of preventative work. Whilst it may be unrealistic to eliminate the development of stuttering in very young children it may be possible to carry out useful secondary prevention work through early identification of the problem. If we can examine the child's neuromotor, cognitive and linguistic skills together with the prevailing social context of the problem, then we can begin to offer help which might arrest and reverse this particular course of development.

In this chapter I shall focus on the social and family context of early stuttering rather than on the cognitive factors which play a role in its development. After many years of work with stutterers of all ages it seems to me that special attention needs to be given to the *context of stuttering* in the course of clinical treatment. Stuttering is a highly context-sensitive problem. Perhaps the most graphic example of this fact is seen in the levels of fluency that clients can achieve in clinical treatment settings; many of them do become perfectly fluent in the clinic. For the young child the most significant context is the family, with school becoming a further consideration amongst older children. Of course 'the family' has received careful scrutiny in the search for the causation of stuttering, and often with mixed reviews. Less attention has been paid however to the influence of the family on the *maintenance* of fluency.

As therapists enter the arena of early intervention they quickly become aware of the need to develop effective treatment programmes and appropriate service delivery models. If the problem of speech dysfluency is the result of an interaction between child and environment then intervention must be targeted at both; too often we 'treat' the problem from only one perspective. To include any contextual intervention it is vital to involve the family. Indeed, recent reviews of the field of early intervention in child development have consistently pointed to the family as the key factor in the success or otherwise of early intervention schemes:

> The involvement of the child's parents as active participants is critical to the success of any intervention programme. Without such family involvement any effect of intervention, at least in the cognitive sphere, appears to erode fairly rapidly once the programme ends (Bronfenbrenner, 1976).

We came to believe that the informal education that families provide for their children makes more of an impact on a child's total educational development than the formal education system. If the family does its job well the professional can then provide effective training. If not, there may be little the professional can do to save the child from mediocrity. This grim assessment is the direct conclusion from the findings of thousands of programmes in remedial education (White, 1984).

In the work described below the family is seen as the main focus for early intervention with the young dysfluent child. At the simplest level family participation involves parental training in the techniques of improving motor speech fluency. At the social level it means studying family dynamics with a view to promoting changes in the family systems which are likely to lead to further fluency development.

Early Intervention for the Young Stuttering Child

Detailed consideration of the process of assessing young stuttering children is given in the earlier chapter by Conture and Caruso in this volume. Here I briefly outline several mainstream approaches to the management of the young stuttering child which can be incorporated into early intervention programmes.

Personalised Fluency Control Therapy (Cooper, 1976; Cooper and Cooper, 1985c) is an established treatment programme for young stutterers and Cooper discusses the theoretical and practical basis of PFCT elsewhere in this volume. In contrast to the Monterey programme (Ryan, 1978) Cooper's approach provides a much broader front for intervention. The therapy tackles the social and emotional dimension of speech dysfluency directly. The treatment process is akin to the cognitive–behavioural therapies that have made such an impact in clinical psychology in recent years. Therapists are able to help both the child and his parents to develop more accurate perceptions of the problem whilst training the child to employ a variety of specific fluency initiating gestures (FIGs) to control episodes of dysfluent speech. Parents are encouraged to participate in the treatment process by supervising the child's use of FIGs and actively supporting the child throughout the course of therapy.

Gregory's Therapy (Gregory, 1984a; 1985) is not available as a formal manual-guided therapy but a number of papers set out the basic approach to treatment. Here too there is an emphasis on the interaction between intrinsic characteristics of the child and multiple environmental variables in the causation of stuttering. The treatment process is preceded by a period of systematic evaluation of the problem which ranges from a detailed developmental history to a careful analysis of the child's overt stuttering behaviour, level of linguistic development and general learning capacity. Attention is also given to typical patterns of parent–child interaction.

Gregory offers several criteria for selecting the most appropriate intervention strategy for young dysfluent children. In each case Gregory stresses the need for active parental involvement in the treatment process. This may range from participation in individual and group counselling sessions to direct instruction in the fluency techniques they are expected to reinforce in their children.

Systematic Fluency Training for Young Children (Shine, 1980a) begins from the premise that most stuttering is the result of underlying constitutional factors which lead on to particular neurolinguistic/motor programming deficits. Stuttering is not therefore *learned* but is rather maintained by a fundamental lack of coordination between respiratory, articulatory and phonatory mechanisms. Shine argues that there is no conclusive evidence that parents *cause* stuttering but they do however have a central role in creating the conditions necessary for inducing a remission in their child's stuttering behaviour. Shine therefore advocates involving parents extensively throughout the treatment process.

From the outset parents are requested to make systematic observations of their child's stuttering behaviour on two separate occasions during the day. This data is used throughout the therapy process to gauge progress. Once a reliable base line has been established over a reasonable period of time the stuttering is targeted for specific forms of intervention. The child is taught to use an 'easy speaking voice' where both rate and intensity are significantly reduced. In addition, both length and complexity of utterances are controlled and manipulated to decrease the likelihood of stuttering. The aim here is to create a set of speech habits that are incompatible with dysfluency. Whilst there are a number of parallels here with the Monterey programme (e.g., the use of a token reinforcement system for fluent speech) Shine's spproach is less highly structured and there is greater explicit parental involvement in the treatment process.

The Component Model for the Treatment of Stuttering (Riley and Riley, 1979) is derived from a more interactionist view of dysfluency where both constitutional and environmental variables are seen as playing a significant role in the development of stuttering. Several neuropsychological processes may be involved in the development of stuttering such as disorders of attention, auditory processing disorders, sentence formulation disorders and oral motor deficits. The environmental factors that play a part involve the existence of a disruptive communicative environment, unrealistic parental expectations, high self-expectations by the child, and manipulative gains that may be achieved through stuttering.

Intervention in this approach is divided into three distinct levels. Level one is suitable for the non-chronic stutterer and involves the parents in counselling sessions aimed at modifying the child's speaking environment. Level two aims to help the child outgrow the problem through appropriate management of the 'underlying and main-taining factors', but without direct symptomatic treatment. Level three follows on from level two and here direct fluency training strategies are employed with the child to modify the motoric aspects of stuttering.

The treatment programmes outlined above have influenced the thinking of many clinicians about the treatment of the young stutterer. We have evolved our own methods of working with the families of young stutterers which we believe are both effective and efficient.

Rustin's Approach

The heart of this approach to early intervention in the treatment of stuttering lies in a detailed series of child and family assessments which provide both an adequate case history and a picture of the current context of the stuttering.

The parental interview schedule

Both parents are required to attend the interview (excepting one-parent families). The aim of this interview is to gather relevant information about the child's difficulties, the reactions of other siblings and parental attitudes to the problem. However the interview covers many more issues and places particular emphasis on gaining a picture of the family structure and its operating system. Specific questions are posed about the child's developmental history. Here we look for any evidence of uneven development and related concerns. We question the parents about the child's current behaviour in different contexts and look for variability in reported fluency. A considerable part of the interview is spent gathering information about family dynamics and social contacts. We enquire about other developmental and psycho-logical problems in the family history as well as trying to build up a picture of the current circumstances of the family unit.

We begin by asking parents to present their child's problems in their own words. For some families their child's dysfluency is the only problem mentioned at this stage whereas for others it is only one in a long list of behavioural, social and emotional concerns. Even at this early descriptive stage we learn a great deal about the family system from the ways in which the parents express their concerns and the examples they offer of their child's difficulties. Following the initial parental description the interviewer probes for specific developmental information that may have a bearing on the emergence of stuttering. The obvious questions about the onset of stuttering and the events surrounding onset are often met with non-committal responses and few clear recollections of what was happening within the family at that time. In many such cases as the interview progresses it becomes clear that several major events did take place in the family around the time of onset. We learn of bereavements in or close to the family, moving house and/or schools and illnesses that required hospitalisation. In other cases the events are less dramatic, such as a playmate moving away from the area, a frightening or painful experience or a series of unconnected and minor upsets. Whilst we cannot be sure to what extent these events are associated with the onset of dysfluency we do feel there may be a cumulative effect on the child which may trigger the emergence of stuttering.

The interview naturally focuses on the child's general health and developmental progress, on current behaviour and emotions, and upon relationships with other children and the family members themselves. For research purposes we note any significant developmental difficulties experienced by grandparents and parents as well as the other siblings in the family. We enquire about the physical environment, the type of housing, whether the family likes the area and whether there are any additional pressures (e.g., social, financial, etc.) on the family at this time. If the child is at school we ask about his progress and attitudes towards school. Towards the end of the interview we ask the parents to tell us in more detail about any other problems the child may have and specifically about the temperamental characteristics of their stuttering child.

Although this interview procedure is time consuming (it typically takes 2 hours to administer) we find the information it generates of very great value in planning rational intervention. An example may help illustrate these benefits. An 8-year-old boy was referred to our department with stuttering as the sole problem. During the parental interview procedure it emerged that around the time of onset a favourite grandfather had died suddenly, the family had moved house three times in the space of six months, a new baby had arrived and the boy had witnessed an uncle being arrested and charged with murder. In addition to his speech problem the child had developed enuresis and both he and his sister had developed marked behavioural problems at school. The general level of family disturbance here was very high indeed and we were able to arrange further specialist help immediately. We undertook further detailed appraisals of the child's behavioural difficulties at home and at school before we attempted to tackle the dysfluency.

Under normal intake procedures where the parents are simply asked to describe matters which they consider relevant to the child's problem the events above might never have been uncovered. Again, whilst we cannot attribute any causal role to the events that surrounded the onset of dysfluency we were at least able to take them into account when we prepared treatment programmes for the child within the family context.

The parental interview is structured in such a way that the basic and noncontentious case details are gathered in the early stages of the process. As time moves by so more sensitive and emotional material is probed. The interview procedure highlights

further problem areas and ensures that we do not treat stuttering as an isolated phenomenon (Rustin and Cook, 1983).

The child assessment schedule

This assessment is carried out whilst the parents are being interviewed. A standard
speech sample is obtained (frequency/rate of dysfluency and overall rate of speech). We
also note the type of stuttering behaviours that are present (whole/part word repetitions, prolongations, struggle, blocks and other concomitant behaviour, Ryan and
Van Kirk, 1978). If during the course of these assessments we suspect the child of
having any further linguistic, cognitive or temperamental problems we employ a
further range of standard assessments to define these deficits in more detail. We assess
basic neuropsychological functions and note laterality as well as constructional skills
and motor coordination of speech. With the very young child it is of course essential to
make the differential diagnosis between normal non-fluency and the dysfluency that is
characteristic of the young stutterer. The core of this discrimination depends on the
occurrence of audible prolongations and double unit repetitions together with the
overall frequency of repetitions and prolongations (Bjerkan, 1980; Floyd and Perkins,
1974).

The therapist tries to explore through conversation and play with the child how
he feels about his dysfluency and whether there are any further concerns currently
troubling the child. Specific questions may be asked about home and school life with
attention focussing on the child's account of social and emotional relations with adults
and other children. We need to know whether the child has close relationships with
other children or siblings or whether the child is isolated from peer support.

When stuttering rather than normal dysfluency is apparent the therapist encourages the child to experiment immediately with several fluency techniques such as
slowing the rate of speech, reducing the complexity of utterances, making the words
'flow together', and so on. The aim here is to find a method of control that is close to
the child's own speech and which can be developed further in therapy. This device
quickly establishes confidence in the child that the problem is controllable and provides
the information necessary to determine the type of intervention that is likely to be
required.

The Treatment Formulation

Once the child and parental assessments are over the therapist is in a position to answer
some fundamental questions about the child, his family and this particular case of

speech dysfluency. A profile of strengths and weaknesses can be drawn up which covers the cognitive, linguistic, social and emotional components of the child's stuttering. On the basis of this individual profile we begin to formulate treatment goals which are tailored to individual needs.

At the end of the assessment phase we also ask the parents to undertake a simple task prior to their next session. The task is termed *talking time* and is designed to test out whether the parents are able to make the kind of commitment we feel is necessary for therapy to be successful. The therapist negotiates with each parent to agree to spend 3, 4 or 5 minutes with their child 4, 5, 6, or 7 times per week. The child must agree to help his parents with their task and he will choose what he would like to do during this time, e.g., drawing, toys, plasticine, etc., but excluding reading and television (Rustin, 1987).

Taking the findings from the child assessment and the parental interview together we begin to build up an overall picture of the problem within the family context. A number of therapy options may be recommended in the light of this evidence. These might include:

1   Counselling sessions for the parents.

2   Sessions aimed at training the parents and the child in ways of enhancing fluency.

3   A direct structured therapy programme for the child.

4   Participation in the intensive treatment courses with active parental involvement.

The parental counselling sessions

A series of parental counselling sessions will be advocated if it emerges from the intake assessment that a. the child's 'dysfluency' falls within the normal range of non-fluency taking the child's age into account (Gregory, 1985a) and b. if there are no further phonological and/or language problems associated with the 'dysfluency'.

Parental counselling is also undertaken where it is clear dysfluency is established but in addition there are issues in the family which are not conducive to further fluency development. If there are marked relationship problems between the parents or if there are difficulties with other children in the family we try to ensure that the identified dysfluency problem does not divert attention away from these fundamental issues. We try to get the parents to face coexisting difficulties before embarking on any direct therapy with the child.

The aim in these counselling sessions is to address parental anxieties about the quality of their child's speech and if appropriate to extend the discussion to other concerns within the family. We spend time giving the parents a thumbnail sketch of the process of speech and language development and the nature of normal non-fluency. The parents are seen on a regular basis until we feel that their anxieties have been allayed or they have agreed to tackle other issues prior to commencing direct therapy. After a period of time we follow up these families to ensure that the situation is improving.

Often the counselling approach also involves the child. We were recently referred a 4-year-old with part-word repetitions, prolongations and a significant amount of struggle behaviour. In addition this child was developing moderate behavioural problems in the home. The family were seen together in the counselling sessions where it emerged the parents had previously separated on two occasions and the current situation was one of serious marital discord and physical violence. The child's speech was the central problem for these parents yet they were able to fulfill their 'talking-time' agreements. Shortly afterwards the mother left the family home and was later granted custody of the child. She was supported by the speech therapist during these upheavals and was able to carry out homework tasks designed to stabilise the child's behaviour. Gradually an acceptable level of fluency was achieved without the need for a direct intervention programme with the child.

Parents and children working together

We undertake this model of working where it emerges from the intake assessment that although the child's speech falls within the range of normal non-fluency there are enough signs to indicate incipient stuttering. Typically this child is beginning to develop prolongations and other struggle behaviours and there is some evidence of a steady increase in part- and whole-word repetitions. The child is usually quite unconcerned about his speech and the parental interview usually uncovers a number of areas of further concern such as sibling rivalry, additional behavioural problems, a highly competitive family environment and poor speech models within the family.

Children falling into this category are invited to attend for treatment sessions accompanied by their parents. Many features of the parental counselling model above are included here but the general discussion includes an emphasis on the nature of stuttering and its remediation. We try to avoid any implication that the parents are responsible for their child's speech difficulties but we do encourage them to experiment with alternative ways of managing the child at home. One of the commonest strategies here is to divert parental attention away from the instances of dysfluency and redirect attention to periods of normal fluent speech. In the same way we encourage them to attend to examples of 'good' behaviour rather than focussing on instances of less acceptable behaviour.

We base our treatment recommendations on the outcome of the talking-time assessment. We ask the parents to undertake talking-time sessions in the clinic and we video-record these sessions for further analysis and discussion with the family (Rustin and Cook, 1983). A wide range of fluency disrupting behaviours has been documented and regularly appear in the videos (Gregory, 1985a; Gregory and Hill, 1980; Starkweather, 1984). Such behaviours include rapid speech rate, interruptions, asking too many questions without waiting for a reply, parental overdirection in play and conversation, parental passivity, poor listening skills, ambiguous non-verbal communication, and conversation that is unrelated to current activity. Where parents have difficulty in grasping these issues the therapist will model both good and bad examples of each behaviour. Further role play rehearsal may be necessary before the parents demonstrate an adequate grasp of the problem and its effect on their child's speech.

One case graphically illustrates the value of these teaching sessions. Three years ago we saw a 4-and-a-half-year-old boy who was living with his mother and grandmother following the sudden death of his father eighteen months previously. The boy was clearly developing the stuttering syndrome with prolongations and struggle but without any apparent accompanying anxiety. His mother had a very rapid rate of speech herself and in addition she was very anxious and over-protective towards the child. After viewing her talk-time session on the video she was immediately able to identify many points which were contributing to her child's dysfluencies. From that moment on her handling of the child changed dramatically and was matched with a corresponding decrease in her child's dysfluency. We recently reviewed this case and happily the child no longer exhibits any speech dysfluency.

Direct intervention

We advocate a programme of direct intervention with the child when it is clear to us that stuttering is well established, the child is concerned about the problem and the child is either too young for our intensive therapy programmes or there are factors in the family's lifestyle that preclude attendance on the courses. We draw on other treatment approaches as indicated previously in much of our direct work with individual children and their families and tailor the treatment components to the specific needs of each individual child and family (Rustin, 1982; Rustin and Cook, 1983).

Intensive Treatment with Active Parental Involvement

The treatments offered on these courses have evolved over the years through a process of evaluation of the effects of intensive therapy and experimentation with new treatment components. It had become obvious that speech control attained in therapy was seldom achieved in any consistent way in the child's normal social world. Intensive treatment courses offer adequate time to establish a consistent level of speech control and the opportunity to carry out treatment in a social context.

Our earliest experience of intensive therapy courses concerned adolescents and older children (Rustin, 1978, 1982, 1984; Rustin and Purser, 1984). The importance of involving parents in the treatment of the 7 to 11 year old group had already been highlighted by several clinicians (Conture, 1982a; Cooper, 1976; Gregory and Hill, 1980; Riley and Riley, 1979; Starkweather, 1984). Initially, parents attended courses on an ad hoc basis for information about their child's progress. We gradually had to increase the parental time as we began to appreciate the crucial role that parents played in the therapy process. Currently, children are only accepted on the course if both parents agree to attend each day with their children.

We see this level of parental involvement not only helping in the process of establishing fluency but also in the transfer and maintenance components of therapy. Our initial evaluations of active parental involvement in the intensive courses have convinced us that treatment gains do now persist in the majority of cases beyond twelve months from the end of the therapy (Botterill and Rustin, 1987). Further comparative research is planned to replicate these findings with larger samples. The treatment components of the intensive courses are outlined below.

Child Programme

The children's programme is made up of several types of activity which are considered prerequisites for the development of normal fluency in social settings. There are three principal components.

Social and relaxation skills training

Social skills training (Trower *et al.* 1978) is an integral part of the intensive course. We have found (Rustin, 1984) that deficits do exist in the social skills repertoires of many adolescent stutterers. The problems range from inappropriate eye contact during conversation to a serious lack of specific skills (making friends, assertive behaviours, negotiating skills, etc.). We employ skills training exercises both to assess the level of social competence a child has developed to date and to identify particular areas where further training could be usefully carried out (see Rustin and Cook, 1983). The specific areas with which we are concerned are observation, listening, turn-taking, reinforcing and problem-solving skills. Role play exercises afford us the opportunity to teach individual skills which may be missing or poorly developed in the individual's repertoire (Cartledge and Fellowes-Millburn, 1980).

There are of course difficulties in trying to establish developmental norms for particular social behaviours in young children. Our approach here is therefore much more focused on specific social situations which cause particular problems for the child. A very common source of difficulty for the young child is coping with teasing from other children. This problem-oriented approach to skills training captures the child's imagination and coupled with the use of role play and problem solving exercises provides opportunities to practice and explore alternative coping strategies in the controlled intensive course setting.

Relaxation training is also a feature of our work on the intensive courses. Many children do become very tense indeed when anticipating some speech act. High levels of muscle tension do contribute to stuttering behaviours and we therefore try to get the children to appreciate the difference between relaxation and tension through games (Rustin, 1987). As the children become more proficient at the relaxation process we encourage them to use the techniques as a coping mechanism when stuttering becomes particularly marked.

Fluency control techniques

The aim of many treatment programmes is to facilitate the acquisition of specific motor speech skills which allow stutterers to speak at a slower rate, with an 'easy relaxed' onset and more continuous airflow whilst blending sequential sounds smoothly together (e.g., Cooper, 1979a; Gregory and Hill, 1980; Prins and Ingham, 1983; Rustin and Cook, 1983).

Prior to any specific speech control training we hold group discussions with the children on such topics as normal speech production, what can go wrong with speech and fluency facilitators. The latter topic might include the following examples which would be modelled by the therapist:

1 A slow controlled speech rate
2 Blending the words together
3 Using 'soft sounds'
4 Easy breathing with appropriate phrasing
5 Normal intonation

In teaching speech control to the children we place emphasis on the various factors which facilitate fluent speech rather than on any rigid adherence to a particular technique. The advantage here over more prescriptive approaches is greater flexibility which allows the individual child to concentrate on those features of control which genuinely aid his fluency. A therapist works with each child individually to devise specific fluency goals for the rest of the course (Rustin, 1987). The speech control is introduced to the child using cognitive problem-solving skills. The child examines what goes wrong with his speech and what he can do to help himself.

Cognitive techniques

One of the strategies we employ to get the child using fluency techniques comfortably in social settings is termed *problem-solving*. Here we draw on the *Think Aloud* programmes developed in the USA to prepare the child to use motor control techniques in the establishment phase of the course. There are four steps in the problem-solving component:

1   My problem is . . .
2   What am I going to do about it?
3   How am I getting on?
4   What am I going to do about it now?

The first step involves encouraging the child to describe what goes wrong with his speech and to illustrate this in a diagram. In the second step the fluency technique training is then practised and the child is tape recorded using the technique to solve his speech problem. The third step emphasises the need for the child to evaluate his own performance by completing individual progress charts. These charts can be discussed with the therapist and provide a launchpad for the child to take greater responsibility for his progess. The final step encourages the child to set new goals for fluency control and lead on to the setting of 'homework' tasks to be completed outside of the course. Parents are of course involved in these tasks.

Spivack and Shure (1974) discuss the use of such cognitive problem-solving skills amongst young children and conclude that children who are good problem-solvers show higher levels of social adjustment when dealing with conflict situations. In our experience direct training in problem-solving skills is extremely useful to stuttering children and may account for a great deal of their continuing fluency outside the therapy context.

The Parental Programme

During the first week the parent group sessions are taken up with a carefully prepared series of discussion topics and exercises (Rustin, 1987). We give parents experience of the games and exercises we routinely use in treatment, including direct instruction in speech modification techniques, systematic muscle relaxation (Mitchell, 1977), and cognitive problem-solving techniques. Each day homework tasks are set which are discussed at the group meeting the following day. It is our intention that the parental groups should generate a variety of viewpoints about the problem of stuttering and its management within the family setting. This exchange of ideas may initiate productive changes within each family without the need for explicit professional intervention. At certain points the group discusses topics without professionals being involved as we feel this is an important step towards utilising the power of the group to create informal contacts between parents which can last well beyond the courses themselves.

During the second week of the course family sessions are conducted which provide an opportunity to tackle issues that are specific to that family unit. Every family member over 4 years of age is invited to the session including the grandparents where appropriate (especially where they have a role in the running of the household). The purpose of this meeting is to set up systems of communication between the family members which acknowledge the roles they play in the maintenance of the stuttering problem.

The child is encouraged to state his preferences for the way he would like family members to deal with his problem. Further, we try to explore the situations that arise within families which exacerbate the problem. One child objected to the way his older sister was constantly coming up to his room and 'messing with my models'. The sister was asked how she thought her brother should deal with this problem and in this way was given the opportunity to see this conflict in a different light. Together they were able to find a mutually acceptable way of dealing with this problem. Although this may seem a trivial example of negotiation it represents an important shift in the balance of power within families.

The family sessions are also conducted by the family in the home each week where progress and further grievances can be aired and further solutions reached. In this way the family acquires new skills in negotiating conflicts which we hope persist beyond the timescale of the intensive courses.

Maintenance

I hope that it will be apparent from the outline above that we do not employ active family involvement merely as an adjunct to the treatment of dysfluent children. The implicit aim of this method of working is to shift the responsibility for treatment from the professional therapist to the family unit. In this process we try to transfer the traditional clinical skills of fluency control to the parents and their child in order that they can continue the treatment process on an intensive basis for as long as may be necessary.

In order to ensure that the treatment gains are being maintained a regular post-course commitment is vital. Parents need support to implement changes they have decided to make in their management of the child within the family unit. To facilitate this we set the parents tasks which have been agreed during the course. They are required to record the outcomes on a homework sheet and return this to their supervising therapist. The therapist then replies to the family praising their efforts and advising on specific management points where necessary. The original group meets after the conclusion of the course at 3 and 6 weeks, 3 months and 6 months with further follow up sessions every 6 months for two years. These sessions last around 2 hours and problems of management are discussed, homework assignments are renegotiated and further family sessions arranged where necessary. The children attend these follow up occasions in order that we can reassess and monitor both their fluency and their social interaction. Instruction and advice is offered where necessary. Some children also require continuing weekly treatment and therapists are able to offer distinct levels of help depending on the stage the fluency has reached.

Conclusion

We do not claim that parental involvement is by any means a panacea for the successful treatment of a complex problem. There may well be instances where parental involvement works against progress rather than promoting it. These are however empirical questions and it is our hope that we will be able to distinguish between families who are likely to be able to help their dysfluent child and those who cannot. In the meantime we feel that in the majority of cases active family involvement is likely to promote a far more enduring response to treatment than the traditional clinical model of intervention for speech dysfluency.

10 Paradoxical Therapy in the Treatment of Stuttering

Armin Kuhr

Introduction

Psychotherapists are constantly faced with the problem of formulating feasible and economical therapeutic programs for a heterogeneous population of clients. Therefore a constant search is going on for the specific and general factors facilitating change. One of the main elements seems to be a good therapist–patient relationship (Goldfried, 1980), which should be characterised by trust, mutual respect and positive feelings. Sloane *et al.* (1975), comparing the effectiveness of different therapeutic approaches, asked successful patients undergoing psychoanalysis or behaviour therapy: 'What were the most important factors in your treatment?' The following items were each termed 'important' or 'extremely important' by at least 70 per cent:

1 the personality of your doctor
2 his helping you to understand your problem
3 encouraging you gradually to practise facing the things that bother you
4 being able to talk to an understanding person
5 helping you to understand yourself
6 encouraging you to shoulder your own responsibilities by restoring confidence in yourself
7 the skill of the therapist
8 the confidence that you would improve (pp. 206–207)

The main factors cited are encouragement, advice or reassurance.

Similar results were reported by Silverman and Zimmer (1982). Stutterers saw warmth, empathy, good listening skills, and patience as the most important attributes of their therapist. However, Mitchell, Bozarth and Krauft (1977, p. 483) state that it is

...increasingly clear that the mass of data neither supports nor rejects the overriding influence of such variables as empathy, warmth, and genuineness in all cases . . . The recent evidence, although equivocal, does seem to suggest that empathy, warmth, and genuineness are related in some ways to clients' 'change', but that their potency and generalizability are not as great as once thought.

When I trained as a psychotherapist, warmth, acceptance and unconditional regard for the client used to be of prime concern. Over the years I have become impressed with the importance of the therapist being able to demonstrate that it *is* possible to help the client with specific problems. Relationship variables obviously are very important, often crucial, but generally they are insufficient to effect long-lasting positive treatment outcome. In order to make clients more effective in handling certain situations or in overcoming maladaptive fears therapists have to be good problem solvers. The objective in therapy, fluent speech, may be reached in many different ways; the therapist has to find the right one. No single technique or set of techniques is useful to all patients. What a particular patient can do is highly idiosyncratic and therapy must therefore be tailored to the needs of the individual. Sheehan (1970a, p. 262):

> Stuttering is not a unitary disorder, but a cluster of disorders of varying degrees of complexity and relatedness . . . Varying treatment is indicated for varied stutterers, yet certain underlying principles must apply to all.

Describing his own 'career' as a stutterer Murray, (1980, p. 163) states that:

> Many stutterers who say they want to get better are actually deeply resistant to the exposure that stuttering therapy entails, to the threat of having to confront a part of themselves that they have tried for many years to sweep out of consciousness . . .

And this view is supported by Van Riper (1973, p. 284–285):

> Most advanced stutterers have made avoidance almost a career, developing very elaborate rituals to escape the revealing of their stuttering.

There are powerful forces against change, the most important ones being the fear of the unknown, continued failure in therapy and primary or secondary reinforcement for stuttering. To overcome these obstacles, the therapist needs to cope creatively with resistance: avoid it altogether, meet it head-on, or use it as a means for change. In short, the therapist has to be able to use paradoxical techniques.

Very often clients have a deep-seated need to maintain the status quo and if the therapist is not skilful, therapy might degenerate into a fight for control: clients want to retain it, therapists want to gain it (Haley, 1976). Therapists should avoid power struggles that they are bound to lose. They should therefore refrain from placing themselves in the untenable position of trying to 'force' the client to do what needs to be done.

Clinical experience teaches us that those stutterers who 'spontaneously' recovered from their disorder without therapy, did so because they were able to overcome their fears by repeatedly and consistently being exposed to anxiety-inducing communicative situations (Van Riper, 1973, p. 296). From this experience therapists are tempted to 'make' clients do what is good for them. But the clients must take responsibility for their own treatment and the therapist's duty is to put them in a position where change must occur, without the need to cajole.

To summarize: the main feature of an effective therapist is the ability to react flexibly to the client's needs. Treatment should be matched to personality and aptitude variables. To help the client to discard the symptomatology the therapist might be required to look for new methods of therapy including non-commonsensical paradoxical approaches.

Paradoxical Approaches — History

Paradoxes have a long history in human thought. In the sixth century B.C. the Cretan Epimenides of Megara developed the famous paradox of 'all Cretans being liars'. At that time paradoxes were of great interest to philosophers and logicians, in the West as well as in the East. Zen philosophy is a centuries' old tradition in Japan that conceptualizes change paradoxically. In Europe paradoxes seemingly dropped from sight for several centuries. Neither philosophers nor scientists seemed to be interested in it. The pioneering research project on human communication (1952–1962) led by the anthropologist Gregory Bateson changed this attitude. From this came the well-known double-bind theory of schizophrenia, a formulation emphasising the interpersonal and reciprocal dynamics underlying schizophrenic development. The Palo Alto group and the scientists at the Mental Research Institute (including Jackson, Haley, Weakland, and Watzlawick) not only worked on the nature of the pathological double-bind but looked at the 'mirror opposite' cure for it: the 'therapeutic double-bind'. In the course of this work it was realised that other approaches used techniques that could be construed as paradoxical.

Morita developed his 'Morita Therapy' in Japan in the 1920s using basic ideas of Zen philosophy. In Europe Alfred Adler (1914) probably was the first psychotherapist to use and write about paradoxical strategies (Mozdzierz, Macchitelli and Lisiecki, 1976). One of Adler's non-specific preliminary paradoxical strategies was to avoid power struggles with the client. He viewed neurotic symptoms as uncooperative in principle, and as an inadequate way of dealing with the demands of life. As the therapist would lose direct power struggles with the client, he would try to shift resistance towards co-operative behaviour by accepting it.

Mozdzierz *et al.* (1976) described some of the specific Adlerian-based techniques:

1   permission — giving the client permission to have a symptom
2   prediction — predicting the client's symptoms would return, or that he would have a relapse
3   pro-social redefinition — redefining or reinterpreting symptomatic behaviour in a positive instead of a negative way
4   prescription — directing the client to engage in a symptomatic behaviour
5   practice — asking the client to refine and improve symptomatic behaviour

Dunlap (1928) developed the technique 'practice' further. He called it 'negative practice' and used it for stuttering as well as for other symptoms. He would direct a client to practise stuttering under prescribed conditions with the expectation of losing the habit. Dunlap (1946) failed to develop an adequate rationale for the technique of negative practice. However, theoretically, it rests on the learning theory developed by Hull who stated that every time a certain act is performed, the power inhibiting this act is strengthened — he called it reactive inhibition — the inhibition resulting from fatigue and negative reinforcement (Foppa, 1968).

In his major work on negative practice Dunlap (1972) further discusses several causes of stuttering including malnutrition, but comes to the conclusion that:

> ...the stuttering habit is actually induced by psychological caus-
> es...(p. 198).

He reasons that in many cases the original causes of stuttering have ceased to operate, thereby the task is 'simply' to break the habit. After reviewing various systems designed to cure stuttering he comes to the conclusion that there is a 'desperate lack of better methods' for 'the majority of cases' (p. 202). Introducing his approach he writes (p. 202):

> There is, however, one thing the stutterer can do, and which has been strangely overlooked in the past. He can stutter! This is a performance which obviously should be considered as the possible basis for an adequate system of practice.

The basic (and paradoxical) idea is that the stutterer does voluntarily what so far was done involuntarily. Therapy is started by making the stutterer practise the stutter. This should be done 'eagerly and enthusiastically' (Dunlap, p. 204). The client is required to practise stuttering for about three to four weeks and try to perfect it, i.e., make the so-called fake stuttering as similar as possible to the usual stutter. Gradually the practice of stuttering will be interspersed with periods of fluent speech. If the client fails to speak fluently, stuttering practice should be immediately reinstated. Dunlap advises the therapist strongly to avoid the situation where the client tries to speak correctly and fails.

The most explicit use of paradoxical techniques was made by Frankl with his 'paradoxical intention'. He focused on the client's fear of the abnormal and desire for the normal. He tried to persuade the client to desire the abnormal. The client might be concerned about the frequency of a 'spontaneous' behaviour, so if the client wants to reduce this, paradoxical intention would require an attempt to increase its frequency. Thus, the therapist apparently promotes the worsening of problems rather than their removal.

The basic idea of paradoxical intention is to fight anticipatory anxiety. Every therapist knows that avoidance strengthens phobias. Frankl (1959, p. 130) states:

> A given symptom is responded to by a phobia, the phobia triggers the symptom, and the symptom, in turn, reinforces the phobia.

Paradoxical intention is designed to interrupt the vicious cycle of avoiding and re-inforcing anxiety by asking the client to actively strive for what is feared. Frankl emphasised that he was not merely treating the symptom, but endeavouring to change the patients' attitude towards their neurosis. He called this change 'in attitude an existential reorientation' and saw humour as an essential ingredient in the patients' ability to detach themselves from their neurotic condition.

Looking at these different approaches they seem to have one basic element in common, i.e., that symptoms are not being construed as enemies, but as friends. They should not be fought at any cost but be 'invited' to enable the client to study them closely, learn from them, and then, maybe, change them.

Definition of Paradox

Up to now a great deal has been written about paradoxical approaches in therapy, but it seems to be very difficult to define what makes a treatment method paradoxical in the first place. Dell (1981b) believed that 'the meaning of the term has been blurred and corrupted almost beyond usefulness'. Even if this is an overstatement, what is the essence of a paradox? In one basic definition (The Pocket Oxford Dictionary, p. 638) a paradox is a

> . . . statement or proposition seemingly self-contradictory or absurd, and yet as explicable as expressing the truth.

The core of a paradox obviously relates to the defeat of one's own or the other person's 'common sensical' expectation. The possible reactions to paradoxes might be confusion and surprise. They seem to be a prerequisite for perceiving something as paradoxical. A standard definition was developed by Watzlawick, Beavin and Jackson (1967) who saw a paradox as 'a contradiction that follows correct deduction from consistent premises'. In psychological terms this definition is too simple to be true. What is correct? What is consistent? Using the Palo Alto group's term 'pragmatic paradox' we move closer towards its psychological nature. Andolfi (1974, p. 222) wrote:

> . . . if the message is an injunction, it must be disobeyed to be obeyed . . .

The example often used for this kind of pragmatic paradox is if we instruct someone to 'be spontaneous'. They would be unable to succeed. Only when the command is not obeyed can one behave spontaneously.

Looking at a paradox from a psychological standpoint its interactional aspect comes into view. Within the therapeutic setting the therapist defies the client's assumptions and expectations in a premeditated way. Haley (1963), discussing Frankl's paradoxical intention, notes that it would be inaccurate to designate the client deliberately performing the feared event as paradoxical *per se*. What makes a client's act appear paradoxical derives from incongruities in the therapeutic procedure. The therapist offers to help a client overcome a problem and within that framework proceeds to encourage it. This constitutes formal paradox of an interactional nature. The message at one level of communication directly conflicts with another message on a different level.

Dell (1981a) remarks on the subjective, relativistic aspect of paradox that 'all 'Paradox' exists only in the mind of the beholder' (p. 127). Anything that is alien to one's common sense could correctly be identified as 'paradoxical'. Mozdzierz *et al.* (1976, p. 169) have a dialectical view of paradoxes:

> A paradox is dialectics as applied to psychotherapy. It consists of seemingly self-contradictory and sometimes even absurd therapeutic interventions which are always constructively rationalizable, although sometimes very challenging, and which join rather than oppose symptomatic behaviour.

Seltzer (1986, p. 10) tries to give an adequately integrative definition of the concept:

> A paradoxical strategy refers to a therapist's directive or attitude that is perceived by the client, at least initially, as contrary to therapeutic goals, but which is yet rationally understandable and specifically devised by the therapist to achieve these goals.

Paradox and Behaviour Therapy

During the last two decades paradoxical techniques have become increasingly popular with psychotherapists of different theoretical orientation. Many (e.g., Lazarus, 1971) incorporate these techniques into their repertoire of treatment procedures in an eclectic manner. Others operate within a more organized framework and try to conceptualize the method to achieve consistency with their own system (e.g., Haley, 1963). Irrespective of the underlying rationale, there is a great deal of similarity in the manner in which paradoxical methods are employed.

Behaviour therapy, being directive in nature, lends itself very well to paradoxical techniques as it has an action-oriented way of dealing with problems. Little time is spent finding out about the origin of the complaint as this is very often difficult to detect, but a great deal of time is focused on how the complaint is maintained. Both paradoxical and behavioural approaches are not necessarily concerned with insight because it does not change a person. These approaches are more concerned with making clients aware of what they can do. On a theoretical level Hudson (1980) maintains that he cannot see any real differences in the thought concepts of behavioural therapy and paradoxical therapy. If behavioural therapists were just to retain a linear causal model they certainly would not be able to use or benefit from structural or paradoxical thinking. But there is nothing to prevent behaviour therapists considering circular patterns of stimuli and response.

Any one event can be seen as both a response to a stimulus and stimulus for a further response. Having this circular model in mind the therapist is able to test the hypothesis if the problem is maintained by the attempted solutions. Several behavioural techniques that have been developed seem to be transferring paradoxical techniques into learning terms, for example, negative practice (Dunlap) or the closely related technique of massed practice (stressing the almost unremitting diligence in the repeated performance of unwanted behaviours); stimulus satiation (repeated presentation of a positive stimulus to the point of satiety, Ayllon, 1963); implosion and flooding (Stampfl and Levis, 1967) which require the exposure of clients to the anxiety contingent upon contact with phobic or contaminated stimuli — all include more than just the behavioural rationale. In these procedures the paradoxical component is quite evident.

How does paradoxical intention work? Attempts by the client to control the stuttering symptom generate performance anxiety. This anxiety either strengthens avoidance behaviour or leads to increased stuttering because of the resulting tension. Ascher (1979) thinks that this performance anxiety component which arises from attempts at symptom control by the client, sometimes poses a problem for the clinician attempting to administer the behavioural treatment of choice. Ascher suggests the use of paradoxical approaches in these cases which would obviate the goal that served to generate and maintain performance anxiety. The basic ideas would be outlined to the client as follows:

— avoidance strengthens phobia
— to experience anxiety is not necessarily bad and should not be avoided at any cost

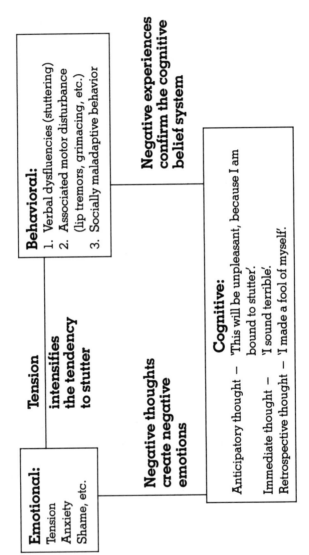

Figure 1 Stuttering cycle: The stutterer finds himself in a self-perpetuating cycle in which cognitive, emotional, and behavioral components continually interact in a closed system. (Burns and Brady, 1980 p. 718).

— trying to control anxiety might lead to a worsening of the problems

— instead of trying to control anxiety one should try to concentrate, e.g. on the physiological concomitants of anxiety and reinforce them to experience the anticipated catastrophic reaction

— if it is possible to switch the anxiety on, eventually it will be possible to switch it off (control it).

The stuttering cycle as described by Burns and Brady (1980) illustrates the process very well (Fig. 1).

Another aspect of paradoxical approaches relates to the fact that trying to control 'spontaneous' behaviour makes it difficult to perform. The symptom, by definition, is an involuntary act. If someone is asked to perform it deliberately then the symptom is, by definition, no longer a symptom. The client gets at least a modicum of control over it. In the therapy process this feeling of control gradually amplifies until the 'involuntary' symptom is under voluntary control. The client is placed in a double-bind by being told to change by staying the same. If the client complies, then by doing it actively (Watzlawick *et al.*, 1967) the client demonstrates control over the symptom. If the client resists the therapist by not behaving symptomatically, the purpose of therapy is achieved as well. The pathogenic double-bind places the person in a no-win predicament; a therapeutic double-bind moves the client towards a no-lose situation.

When should paradoxical approaches be used in behaviour therapy? Naturally they would be considered if the linear treatment of choice unpredictably fails to produce the desired results. This might happen in cases where performance anxiety is the presenting symptom. It might not be possible to break the vicious cycle of anticipatory anxiety leading to the feared result in any other way. Paradoxical techniques might be employed to good effect in behaviour therapy as strategies to enhance the client's cooperation, especially in difficult or resistant cases. Sometimes it might be useful to introduce a paradoxical statement as a 'door opener' suspending the normal frame of reference for the client and enabling exploration of new experiences with the old behaviour. This could be seen as a seed; straight behavioural techniques would have to be used to let the seed develop and grow.

The basic stages in therapy using paradoxical techniques will now be presented. It should be reiterated, however, that therapists should adapt their methods to the client, not vice versa. Flexibility and creativity on the part of the therapist are of utmost importance.

The first steps are:

— establishing a positive client–therapist relationship

— defining the problem clearly

— listing the goals that are to be achieved in therapy.

The therapist then develops a strategy. If the therapist decides to use a paradoxical approach the symptom would be related in a positive way and given a different frame or connotation. In the case of stuttering the therapist might say:

— thinking about it fills time, avoids emptiness
— something to blame for failures in life
— gives a great deal of anxiety but adds weight to your words
— anxiety is very useful for human beings, you have to keep your stutter to have your barometer of anxiety.

These rationales have to be adapted very carefully to a specific case, otherwise the patient will have the feeling of not being taken seriously.

Rohrbaugh, Tennen, Press and White (1981) divided paradoxical intervention into two categories, depending on whether the purpose of the intervention was to have the client carry out the paradox or reject it. The compliance-based paradox would bring about change if the client tried to obey the paradoxical prescription. A defiance-based strategy would be used on the assumption that the client will defy or oppose carrying out the paradoxical directives and thus allowing the client to change (e.g., predicting something will happen that the therapist does not want to happen).

The symptom is prescribed, the client is required to stutter, possibly in a different way. The therapist might decide to change the stutter in some way so that it is, e.g., divided up into subparts, interrupted, or linked to another behaviour. The basic idea is to modify the experience of the problem for the client. The delivery of relabelling and prescribing is absolutely essential. If the presentation is done in the correct way, the client might be surprised, even angry, but after repeated unsuccessful attempts of solving the problem might think 'why not try something stupid?'. The advantages of this would be:

— to enable the client to take the first step towards therapeutic change
— to give the client responsibility for the problem
— to help the client make the uncontrollable controllable
— to add an element of unpredictability and creativity to a therapy.

As soon as change occurs the therapist should consider restraining the client by telling him about the negative consequences of change — maybe even inhibiting or forbidding it. The client is advised — when the therapist inhibits change — to go at a slower pace. Change should come cautiously, as problems might arise if the client changes too quickly. The next stage would be to forbid change. The client might be told to give in to the symptom: 'I want you to give in to stuttering, however often it occurs next week.'

To deal with a client's extreme resistance, the therapist could declare that change is impossible and that the situation is hopeless. This strategy should only be used as a last resort when the client has failed to respond to any other strategy, and the harder the therapist works, the less the client does to promote change. It is rarely necessary to go to these lengths but this tactic might be useful for the 'yes, . . . but' client. If the therapist is being actively fought by the client the therapist should declare his or her impotence. If the timing and the delivery are right the client is bound to spring into action. Now the client will be the one to work and the therapist has to be convinced or prodded that continuing therapy is of use.

A dangerous point in therapy is when paradoxical techniques lead to the sudden disappearance of the symptom. The therapist is not allowed to take any credit for the change, but has to wonder, out loud, if it will last, or even predict a relapse. By doing so the therapist places the client in a therapeutic double-bind. If the symptom occurs again, the therapist predicted it. Therefore it is under the therapist's control. If it does not come back, it is under the client's control. The symptom is being defined in such a way that it can no longer be perceived as being uncontrolled or spontaneous. If it reappears, it is no longer as threatening since it was predicted. Very often clients will view a relapse prediction on the part of the therapist as a challenge. The only way to prove the therapist wrong and to win the power struggle would be by avoiding a relapse. If there is none the therapist should go one step further and prescribe it. Erickson had a very elegant way of prescribing relapse. He instructed his patients to go back, to experience the symptom again, and see if there was anything worth retaining in the future (Haley, 1963).

To use a paradoxical approach, the therapist must be experienced, skilful, and needs a great deal of practice. It is also necessary to be able to think about problems in a gamelike or playful way, even while realising that these are real problems causing serious distress.

Paradoxical Techniques in the Treatment of Stuttering

There are occasional reports in the literature of stutterers who were not able to stutter when they badly wanted to do so. Frankl (1961) reports a case of a severe stutterer who, when caught without a ticket on a tram, tried to arouse the conductor's pity by stuttering as badly as possible, but found that he was unable to do so. Murray (1980) was shocked when he received an order to report for an army physical examination. He had been rejected once because of his stutter, but during his second checkup when he desparately wanted to stutter, he talked fluently and had to join the Army. Experiences like these no doubt led to the introduction of paradoxical techniques into the treatment of stuttering. They will be reviewed here briefly.

Darwin (1796, cited in Rieber and Wollock, 1977a, p. 11) who used logopedic exercises for his clients, advised them to interact as much as possible with others. He writes:

> To this (speech practice) should be added much commerce with mankind in
> order to acquire a carelessness about the opinions of others.

This is not a paradoxical prescription in the true sense of the word, but it has a paradoxical flavour about it. It is suggested that the clients speak as much as possible and
obviously not care too much about their speech. This relaxed attitude would
counteract stutter-generating tension.

Frankl (1961) described his treatment of stuttering using certain speech techniques
and de-reflection which is a quasi-paradoxical technique. Clients are advised to train
themselves not to concentrate on their speech but on something else. Every time they
think about speech it will disturb the proper performance. The next step (as with
Darwin) is to have as much contact with others as possible. Clients are told to talk to
themselves — 'It is not illegal to speak with anxiety'. Clients are asked to risk failures;
if they cannot do this, they will never achieve their goal. Eventually the reduction in
anxiety will lead to the first small successes.

Nystul and Muszyska (1976) report on the use of paradoxical intention and de-
reflection in the treatment of stuttering within Adlerian psychotherapy. They centre
their approach on the client's fear of failure in talking which results in a 'hyper-
intention' to speak fluently, which leads to the above mentioned anticipatory anxiety.
This mental anxiety and the concomitant physical symptoms are so distressing for the
stutterer that fluent speech is impossible. In therapy the symptom's direction is
reversed by asking the clients to stutter intentionally, e.g., by being asked to do
something that they can do very well. The clients will therefore not fear failure and
with 'the wind taken out of the sails' of this self-defeating cycle they can stutter in a
more relaxed way. The therapy process is geared toward helping the clients to detach
themselves from the symptom.

In the inital phase the client is required only to stutter. If there are any difficulties
communicating, therapist and client should write notes to each other. During this
stage therapist and client work together on drawings confirming the client's
problems. These are discussed from a 'teleological' perspective. The therapist probes
into the goals the clients have in their lives and the role of their stuttering behaviour.
The clients will realise the purpose of their stutter, e.g. it could be to create a barrier
separating themselves from others. In the second phase of therapy, loosely following
the guidelines of Ellis (1977) basic mistaken ideas should be identified, e.g., in order to
establish a relationship with a girl one must be a 'good' talker. During the third phase
the clients are confronted with the irrationality and uselessness of their basic ideas. This
self-defeating cycle is explained to the clients and their resulting frustration is used as a
source of motivation for further therapy. Three main techniques have been used:

— paradoxical intention; instructing the client to try to stutter in social
   situations

— de-reflection; changing the client's own focus from negative to positive aspects of self

— 'open communication'; using non-verbal communication when the client feels too tense to talk.

During the last part of therapy the client is advised to put the techniques into practice. Eventually this will lead to a dramatic reduction in stuttering. In the usual paradoxical session the client is warned against letting the fluency level increase too dramaticaly for fear of a return to the self-defeating cycle of wanting to be such a good talker that fear would cause failure, etc.

Dunlap's negative practice spawned some basic and applied research. As mentioned previously it rests on the premise that every time a specific behaviour is performed, inhibition develops in the central nervous system. In negative practice the stuttering client would have one or two sessions per week, possibly more. The first five sessions last approximately 30 minutes, later the sessions might be extended to an hour. Every 10 or 15 minutes there is a brief break as negative practice is very exhausting for the client. Every time the symptom occurs the client is interrupted and is required to imitate the stutter as precisely as possible. This is important, as otherwise further stuttering behaviour would be added to the client's repertoire. It is not therefore advisable to use negative practice outside the therapy session. Dunlap (1942, p. 127) stressed:

> The essential point is to bring under voluntary control the behaviour pattern which has been involuntary. It is a very difficult task to teach a stutterer voluntarily to reproduce his involuntary pattern, but unless this is done, the method of negative practice is not applied.

As there is no detailed description of the techniques, negative practice procedures used in later studies differed. Dunlap, for example, did not specify the amount of phrase repetition or stuttering practice that should follow a dysfluency. Fishman, (1937) provided the first use of negative practice used with stutterers. Stuttering decreased for the patients who mainly showed repetition; it increased for those whose speech mainly showed blocks. Fahmy (1950) used negative practice to treat adult stutterers who were described mainly as tonoclonic or tonic. The tonoclonic subjects improved, the pure tonic subjects tended to regress. Case (1960) used Dunlop's technique with a larger group of stutterers; in his study no beneficial effects were found.

Looking at the results of research over all it seems that negative practice is not useful for clients who suffer from tonic stuttering (speech blocking). Nevertheless, variations of negative practice are still being used. The main reason for this is that it was employed by therapists from the 'Iowa School' in the management of stuttering. Bryngelson (1943, 1950) used 'voluntary stuttering' among other techniques. His rationale was to bring the problem behaviour under voluntary control and also reduce the stutterer's concern about displaying the problem. During his first stage of therapy clients practise the technique before a mirror until they are able to mimic their stuttering behaviour. Having mastered the technique they use it outside the clinic in speech situations. If attempts at stuttering voluntarily on a difficult word result in an involuntary reaction, they have to repeat the attempt until the block is completely under their control. Bryngelson realized that their approach had its limitations in that it was impossible to eliminate all fear of stuttering in the majority of cases. There frequently remained a considerable amount of stuttering. Therefore, even when fear was reduced modifications of the stuttering behaviour were undertaken.

Johnson (1948) also used voluntary stuttering. His main thrust was to encourage the stutterer to stutter openly in order to remove any attempts at avoiding non-fluency. The approach differs from negative practice as clients are encouraged not to repeat the exact pattern, but use effortless repetitions of stressfree prolongation of sounds to produce 'easy stuttering'.

In a more recent study by Ingham, Andrews, and Winkler (1972) four different treatment procedures were tested, among them a variation on negative practice termed 'increased stuttering'. In this group the clients were required to double their stuttering above base rate. The technique was introduced as a method of reinforcing the use of syllable-timed speech. The rationale was that the acceptance of ST speech might be enhanced if its facilitative effects were contrasted with the debilitative effects of increased stuttering. This type of negative practice did not show any impressive results as compared with the other techniques.

Sheehan (1970a), using voluntary stuttering, stresses the role acceptance of the stutterer:

> The acquisition of fluency in stuttering should come about indirectly, through the reduction of avoidance, through being open, through accepting the role of a stutterer. (p. 25).

> For adults, a paradoxical feature of the problem is that role acceptance as a stutterer leads to being able to perform the role of a normal speaker, and the attempt to become completely normal speaker leads back to the role of a stutterer. (p. 30).

Sheehan believed that a stutterer could learn to succeed by stuttering openly and easily, resisting time pressures and pausing whenever necessary. Increased fluency would be a by-product of these activities. Another prominent researcher and therapist, Bloodstein (1975) also uses a paradoxical element. As quick cures are normally not durable the most

> reliable way to achieve a lasting reduction of stuttering is to do it slowly and gradually (p. 79).

He asks clients to accept their role as a stutterer and analyzed very carefully what they do when they stutter. Only through this intensive analysis might they understand their stuttering behaviour and thus how it could be altered.

Van Riper (1973), who was a very severe stutterer in his youth and who later developed a popular aproach to therapy, incorporated several paradoxical techniques. Van Riper makes ample use of 'pseudo-stuttering', which is basically the same as voluntary stuttering. He uses these techniques to reduce anxiety, lessen word and situation fears, as the means of teaching the stutterer a fluent form of stuttering, and as a tool to vivify the cues which lead to error.

> To eliminate the seemingly uncontrollable responses, the person must become aware of the stimuli that trigger them. (Van Riper, 1973, p. 284)

In pseudo-stuttering the client is supposed to do this 'faking' on non-feared words, and should start with fakes that are not too severe or unduly traumatic. Van Riper claims that an important added advantage of pseudo-stuttering is the experience that most listeners react fairly indifferently.

> One of his (the stutterer's) worst experiences has been the loss of control over his behaviour, the feeling that he has suddenly been seized by mysterious forces that manipulate him and render him helpless. By deliberately assuming stuttering behaviours and resisting their automaticity, he directly attacks this vital feature of his problem (Van Riper, 1973, p. 286).

A further paradoxical technique is Van Riper's 'response prevention'. He instructs the stutterer to commence blocking and to continue until the therapist signals that it is time to cease. The client is not to attempt to interrupt the block, nor adopt any of the behaviour patterns which usually accompany a block. The duration of the core stuttering behaviour is gradually increased and the stutterer learns that it can be tolerated more easily.

In striking similarity to Frankl, Van Riper (1973, p. 290) writes about the effects of his paradoxical techniques:

> It's hard to fear something you very much desire.

Indication and Contraindication of Paradoxical Approaches

Paradoxical techniques are very flexible and can be used with a wide variety of clients. However, they certainly are more appropriate for certain types of cases, and there are also clear contraindications.

There is a group of adult stutterers that might be called therapy-addicts. They a long history of treatment failures. They do not seem to be really motivated to change, rather, they seem to derive some pleasure from defeating therapists. The therapist might start in a linear fashion, but soon discovers that the client's willingness to change is very small, because the client forgets to do homework and refuses to do assignments, etc. Bona fide paradoxical techniques might also be indicated, if the therapist realizes that the family or partner of the client starts to sabotage treatment. In general, paradoxical approaches should be considered for resistant and chronic clients. As in other therapeutical approaches, the will to change, responsibility and effort on the part of the client are the basic success criteria.

Paradoxical techniques are contraindicated when it is impossible to actively involve the client in the therapeutic process. Care should be taken with clients who are liable to distort reality in a paranoid way. They might become very suspicious, and the client–therapist relationship might deteriorate and break up. Paradoxical treatments are inappropriate in situations of crisis or instability (Rohrbaugh, Tennen, Press, White, Raskin and Pickering, 1977).

The therapist who uses paradoxes in therapy should be carefully trained and have sufficient experience. Paradoxes should not be used as a gimmick or for their shock value. They should be used in a very discerning way. The treatment with the lowest risk should be implemented first. When using paradoxes in therapy, therapists should be very careful not to act out their own hostility towards clients. Therefore, it is advisable to do this type of treatment under supervision or discuss it with colleagues.

Discussion

The use of paradoxical techniques has raised the issue of professional ethics. Some see this approach as too manipulative or controlling, but these criticisms have been refuted by several writers. Watzlawick, Weakland and Fisch (1974) and Haley (1976) have pointed out that it is impossible not to manipulate in the therapeutic relationship. Despite the fact that the client gives his informed consent, it is impossible to discuss every therapeutic manoeuvre. The techniques, obviously, should be used responsibly.

The basic ethical problems are amplified by the fact that the practical and theoretical aspects of paradoxical intervention are not well developed. Frankl failed to give an unambiguous didactic definition of paradoxical intention. He vividly described case histories that give the reader ideas but are of little help in determining treatment strategies in specific cases. Most literature still consists of anecdotal case descriptions without giving data. We might pose the following questions:

Did clients try to follow the therapeutic directives?
Did they really work on increasing their anxiety?
Did the paradoxical techniques lead to increased anxiety at all?

Were there any panic attacks?

What did the clients think?

However, over the last five or six years a greater number of empirical studies have appeared that try to identify the main effects of paradoxical techniques (Ascher, Schotte and Grayson, 1986; Mavissakalian, Michelson, Greenwald, Kornblith and Greenwald, 1983; Ascher, 1981; Ascher and Turner, 1980). Paradoxical psychotherapy does not have a theoretical structure or basis that links its diverse techniques and approaches. Only Watzlawick *et al.*, (1967; 1974) attempted to provide a kind of theoretical explanation. There is an urgent need to develop the theoretical basis further as paradoxical methods can no longer be viewed as a fringe development. Dell (1981b, p. 41) observed:

> . . . paradoxical therapy, much like Pirandello's play, remains a set of techniques in search of a theory.

To illustrate the proverb 'one man's meat is another man's poison' we end this review with a case vignette by Murray (1980, p. 162):

> Charles Van Riper spent several months in therapy, often under Dr. Bryngelson, who had him work through voluntary stuttering to gain control over his involuntary blocks. During this time he made remarkable progress. Within a year he had learned to talk well enough to start teaching. Johnson was at Iowa at the time, his stutter had decreased somehow, but it was still a serious problem for him. As he saw Charles Van Riper's success, he decided to put himself on a similar programme. Immediately his stuttering became so much worse that he was told to stop speaking altogether and to go off on a week-long fishing trip, during which he was to continue his silence.

11   Self-Help for Stutterers — Experience in Britain

Bryan Hunt

Introduction

Not very much is known about the utility of self-help groups in the treatment of stuttering and no systematic study of the subject appears to have been carried out. An Association for Stammerers was established in Britain in the 1960s, when the self-help movement was going through its period of most active development. This chapter attempts to set the Association for Stammerers (AFS) within the context of the self-help movement in the UK in general, goes on to describe the results of an ad hoc survey of self-help groups affiliated to the AFS and concludes with some personal reflections on the contribution of self-help groups to the management of stuttering.

The self-help movement

In many developed countries today a more critical attitude on the part of certain sections of the public towards the professional care offered to them has become evident. This has two components: the introduction to the medical field of the 'consumerism' which is evident in so many other fields already; and the development of doubts amongst a small but articulate section of the public about the efficiency and benefits of so-called 'technological' medicine. The result has been an upsurge of diverse, confusing and often contradictory opinions and activities of which the most useful summary is still the introduction of Ilona Kickbusch and Steven Hatch to the WHO publication 'Self Help and Health in Europe' (1983). They mention a range of activities including traditional self care, lay care (i.e., the informal, unorganised forms of care provided by members of a recognisable community such as a church, a voluntary association or charity) and self-help, often referred to somewhat self-consciously as the 'self-help movement'. The last of these seems to represent a significant new development and appears to have at least the following distinguishable attributes:

1 Mutual aid and support including emotional support by groups of people with common problems. This is the major part of the self-help movement and may include groups of people who are themselves suffering from chronic complaints, e.g., diabetes, or subject to social stigma, e.g., Alcoholics Anonymous, or the families and others caring for those suffering chronic, disabling conditions such as schizophrenia. Such organisations may engage in a very wide range of social activities.

2 Provision of information and advice.

3 Direct provision of services, often on a charitable basis, e.g., in mental handicap.

4 An interest in 'alternative' therapies — this may be an expression of dissatisfaction with the health professions or with the official, established health care system.

5 Fund raising and pressure group activity, working through the political system to press for the special interests of the group concerned.

The scale of the self-help movement is remarkable, as can be seen from the Directory entitled *Self-help and the Patient* published by the Patients' Association (1984) which lists in the region of 250 separate organisations, each catering for a different disease or handicap.

The Americans Katz and Bender (1976) provided what has come to be regarded as the classical definition of self-help groups:

> . . . voluntary small-group structures for mutual aid and the accomplishment of a special purpose. They are usually formed by peers who have come together for mutual assistance in satisfying a common need, overcoming a common handicap or life-disrupting problem and bringing about desired social and/or personal change. The initiators and members of such groups perceive that their needs are not or cannot be met by or through existing social institutions. Self-help groups emphasise face-to-face social interactions and the assumption of personal responsibility by members. (p. 9)

Richardson and Goodman (1983) define self-help groups more succinctly as 'groups of people who feel they have a common problem and have joined together to do something about it.'

History of the Association for Stammerers

The AFS began in 1968 as part of the self-help movement which was developing rapidly at that time. It originated largely due to the efforts of one man, Robin Harrison, and was at first a single group, essentially concerned to explore the possibilities of group therapy of various kinds without professional input. The comments of Richardson and Goodman (1983) on the initiation of self-help groups in general, apply very aptly to the early development of the Association:

> Whatever the considerable rhetoric to the contrary, self-help groups do not generally spring up wholly spontaneously, like Venus from the waves. They come into being because someone wants them to do so and, typically, puts a great deal of effort into their cause . . . behind such developments there are usually one or more individuals who are keen to see something happen;
> . . . Launching a local self-help group successfully is a challenging activity for which few people are in any way prepared. The founder, often already burdened by his or her own problems, suddenly has to deal with the problems of a whole new set of people plus those of running an organisation. The latter requires some administrative skills (keeping membership lists, setting up meetings, etc.), some public relations skills (getting publicity, informing local professionals) and a great deal of time and energy. (pps. 33–34)

The Association took more defined shape as a nationally organised support group ten years later in 1978, when a number of enthusiasts in co-operation with a handful of interested speech therapists set up a more formal constitution under which the Association obtained charitable status and expanded its activities substantially. The Association now provides an important focus for information and advice for stutterers and their families but still retains its essential self-help element, for its core is a network of self-help groups up and down the country. It has been most successful in a few areas such as London, Scotland, Birmingham and elsewhere, where a support group structure linking speech therapists with a few stutterers and dedicated helpers has provided the continuity which is required in order to sustain self-help groups as they come and go, and to provide an information service on an on-going basis.

How Does AFS Fit into the Self-Help Movement?

As a voluntary organisation in support of an identified group of handicapped people the Association aims to act as a source of information and advice and a focus of activity in its chosen field. In practice, however, its ability to operate effectively in this way has been severely circumscribed by shortage of funds and the difficulty it has encountered in engaging in fund-raising activity amongst the general public. What the Association has been able to do, however, is to function effectively as a self-help group, and at the same time link together other self-help groups throughout the country.

If we refer back to the five types of activity mentioned earlier as being character-istic of the self-help movement in general, we find that the bulk of the activity of stut-terers' self-help groups falls into the first two of these. More will be said on this topic later, but broadly speaking it seems to be the case that the mutual advice and support obtainable within the group setting represents their most valued feature. They are able to provide a substitute for more normal social intercourse, which is often barred to stutterers, or difficult or stressful for them to participate in. In addition the groups act as an 'information exchange and mart' regarding what treatments are available, where they can be obtained and what benefit others have obtained; all subjects on which many stutterers are surprisingly ill-informed.

It is generally recognised that effective treatment of stuttering in the adult requires at the least active participation by the patient. In this context the shared experience of the disorder and its treatment provided by self-help groups can be helpful. Many stut-terers find themselves socially isolated to a greater or lesser extent; learning what difficulties others have experienced and how they have coped can be revealing and beneficial.

By contrast, stutterers' groups tend to be less active in the field of public cam-paigning. Although successful in using the media to disseminate information about their existence, they have not, in general, taken a prominent or active role in improving treatment facilities, complaining to the authorities about deficiencies in services, finding alternative therapy, providing a counselling service, etc.

The Present Survey

As the Association for Stammerers has expanded it has developed a network of area representatives throughout the country. In the majority of cases these are stutterers who have themselves undergone intensive therapy courses and have subsequently undertaken to organise groups. In others, they simply agree to act as focal points for the dissemination of information and literature.

For the purpose of the present survey 30 area representatives and group organisers were written to and asked for particular information about groups in their area: their size, membership, duration and activities. In addition, they were asked open-ended questions about their views on the benefits of self-help groups for those who par-ticipated in them. 20 replies were received.

Additionally, specific enquiries were made about their views on self-help groups to five speech therapists known to have taken a special interest in this field of activity. The respondents covered all parts of the country, including all regions of England, together with Wales and Scotland. There were no systematic divergences between the responses received from area representatives and speech therapists and the two sets of replies have not been analysed separately.

The scientific limitations of data collected in this way will be evident to the reader and must be considered when assessing the results. The Association for Stammerers is in no way representative of the population of sufferers from this disorder. Epidemiological evidence suggests that between 0.5 and 0.9 per cent of the adult population shows some evidence of dysfluency (Van Riper 1982) but only a tiny proportion of those persons belong to the Association. The findings have therefore not been presented in tabular, numerical form which might appear to lend them a spurious statistical validity. It seems reasonable to assume, however, that the active and interested group of people who constitute the Association's area representatives are in touch with a substantial proportion of the self-help groups in the country, through their contacts not only with other Association members but also with interested speech therapists in their locality. Given the two-thirds response rate achieved, it is suggested that, in the absence of more systematic data, the results of this survey may provide some pointers to the role of self-help groups for stutterers and may prove useful as a basis for formulating hypotheses or planning more definitive enquiries.

Results

Reports were received on 15 self-help groups being attended at the time of reporting by around 120 people. The information provided was multiplied perhaps three or four-fold by the accounts, some of them extensive and detailed, that many of the respondents were able to give of personal experience of participating in self-help groups over a number of years. In addition, respondents noted the existence of 17 additional groups attended and usually led by speech therapists.

Age range

The majority of members fall within the young adult range, from 25 to 40. There is a substantial sprinkling of older people, however, whilst relatively few teenagers seem to attend groups regularly. The average age of those attending self-help groups seems to be rather higher than those attending therapy groups, few clients over 50 probably being found in the latter. One speech therapist who maintained a knowledge of clients attending both kinds of group quoted an age range of 20 to 53 for the treatment group and 29 to 63 for the self-help group.

Form of groups

A consistent pattern emerged with regard to the form taken by self-help groups. They tend to be small, even as small as two or three, while four to six is common, and they rarely exceed 12. Groups meet weekly as a rule but sometimes fortnightly or even monthly if this seems to suit the membership best.

Origin

Almost without exception self-help groups have taken origin as an offshoot of therapy groups managed by speech therapists. They sometimes describe themselves as 'follow-up' groups and may have titles such as 'Transfer and Maintenance Groups', i.e. they have the specific aim of transferring to everyday life the speech control methods taught in therapy sessions or the maintenance over time of the techniques taught.

A common pattern is for a speech therapist actively to suggest their continuation as a self-help group to a group of stutterers who have come together over a period of time in a therapy setting. More rarely, the groups of friends who have been established in this way spontaneously decide themselves to continue meeting after the therapist has declared the therapeutic sessions to be at an end.

Activities

The activities of groups can be extremely variable depending on the needs of the participants, including personal testimony, practice interviews for jobs and, very importantly, simple social gossip. But most self-help groups begin with a programme of speech-related activities and many continue in this form throughout. More will be said later about the importance of leadership in the survival of groups but the following quote from one very successful group organiser illustrates the kind of activities which many groups undertake:

> I must be perfectly honest and state that I lead the group and I provide the majority of the activities that we practise. These range from practising speech therapy techniques, speaking to a metronome beat, having a dummy stage phone on which any member can 'ring' any other member at any time through the meeting and hold a conversation (I do most of the ringing), role

playing where we have ongoing interviews for a shoe-shop salesman, and lately video cameras with instant playback.

Other respondents refer to practising slowed speech, reading aloud, quiz games, giving talks and group discussion.

Special interest attaches to those groups whose activities move on from the direct pursuit of fluency through speech exercises to a deeper consideration of the personal, psychological concomitants of the specific situational difficulties which most stutterers encounter, as in the following report:

> . . . Broadly speaking we spend far less time on speech techniques as such, i.e. slow, prolonged speech, breathing, fluency, etc., than on discussing the 'hidden agenda' — the fears, anxieties, feelings of inferiority, powerlessness, frustration, and ways of overcoming these through changing the image of 'myself as a stammerer' into 'myself as a fluent person', building up an individual's self-image by drawing attention to the positive gifts and qualities he/she may have which he/she may have underestimated, discussing ways in which the so-called 'fluent speakers' may also have their anxiety problems under different manifestations, concentrating on the 'gifts' of the stammerer, e.g., empathy, understanding of people with disadvantages, conscientious-ness . . .

In spite of this report, the responses to the survey as a whole show quite clearly that it is true only in a minority of groups. It seems that it is those groups consisting of the more mature members and those who have done relatively well in speech therapy, who are likely to feel, therefore, that for them, control of their speech pattern is possible. Consequently they devote more time to discussion of personal experiences with exchange of opinions about the psychological aspects of stuttering, responses to different situations and so on, with the high degree of mutual support which springs from such personal testimony.

Duration

By far the most striking and consistent feature of self-help groups to emerge from the reports is their tendency to come and go. They are characteristically short-lived, few lasting more than one to two years. Groups form, dissolve, and re-form as members come and go; there is little evidence of continuity. Even if a group persists its member-ship fluctuates. As one member put it, the group

> fulfils different needs for different people at different times — they join, gain something from it, then go. People with employment problems are common recruits at the present time. These people rarely feel any personal loyalty to

the group or the organisation as such, although they may develop on-going personal relationships with the group leader or other member.

Factors making for permanence of groups

A self-help group may be judged 'successful' if it attracts sufficient loyalty from its members to ensure its continuity as a group for a substantial period of time. By this criterion the following factors seem important:

1   Determined and energetic leadership seems to be essential if the group is to have any continuity. There is almost universal agreement on this point. 'Someone must be responsible for hosting and developing the group — listening to the individual needs and making sure that they are met . . . '. When a group develops continuity it often reflects the efforts of one dedicated person, commonly a stutterer with drive and personal experience of hardship, coupled with a conviction of the possibility of change which he wishes to share with others and therefore with a commitment to keeping the group going.

2   Support from local speech therapists is also commonly mentioned. Many respondents said that they found it necessary to be able to refer problems to a speech therapist from time to time, although the speech therapist did not attend the meetings of the group itself.

3   The support of a speech therapist is also helpful in maintaining the size of the group, i.e., as older members drift away, the membership can be recruited by a speech therapist referring people whom the therapist thinks may benefit.

4   It was interesting to note that 'Self-discipline' was mentioned by several respondents. The following comments go beyond the issue of group continuity as such and reflect the importance of motivation and the need for a persistent effort to achieve self-control which many stutterers perceive as a key factor in achieving fluency:

> It needs three or four people to confidently arrange and organise the meetings along progressive lines. I found that just meeting in a pub lends itself to loss of discipline quickly, so a meeting place needs to be carefully researched. Discipline is the key word. You, I and anyone else who attempts to modify his natural speech pattern with a technique knows the importance of self-discipline. A self-help class needs to utilise its time with a well-structured programme of practises. Use of one's technique is the number one priority, aiming to bring it very gradually up to an acceptable quality for use in the outside world.

Another respondent commented along similar lines:

> A self-help group can easily fall into the trap of being a friendship group
> rather than a speech therapy group. The first rule we all must learn is to tell
> the truth, however bitter, about each other's speech. A certain amount of
> self-discipline is required by all members of the group. Speech is the primary
> consideration: friendship afterwards.

Comments like this demonstrate the personality features and motivation responsible
for the success of some group organisers in ensuring the survival of their groups over
time. They do not necessarily reflect the areas in which positive benefits are most
commonly felt to occur.

Reports by respondents of benefits received

It is generally agreed that stutterers are deficient in social skills, presumably as a result
of disuse, avoidance or dependency. Positive social skills training is the optimal solution
but this is hard to obtain. Experience of the self-help group may itself constitute a
worthwhile social experience and therefore be helpful in this respect. This point is
illustrated in the following comment:

> We all get tremendous benefit from our meetings, I know — support,
> friendship and encouragement certainly rate high on the list for us as we are
> mainly single stammerers who perhaps have not found our niche socially but
> can really relax in the group atmosphere. Several of us had spent many lone
> years of stammering, not meeting anyone else with the same problem, and
> tending to bury the problem and not talk about it.

Another respondent commented:

> I have found being a member of a group helpful in a number of ways. It has
> helped me to get into fluent speech and convinced me that it is at least possible
> under some circumstances for me to speak without stammering. I feel that I
> have benefited a great deal from the atmosphere of support that groups
> provide, particularly when things are not going well. I have also learned a bit
> about speaking situations which perhaps are more difficult for stammerers to
> pick up in the normal course of events than it is for non-stammerers.

Several respondents made the point that the absence of speech therapists encourages
honesty. The most valuable elements in a self-help group, according to one report, are
'those that allow people to talk about their problems and difficulties freely — they then
realise that they are not alone, others have coped successfully, so they are encouraged
and motivated to do the same'.

Role of self-help groups

Stuttering in the type of adult client group which is the concern of this study is a chronic and intractable disorder, often showing periods of improvement followed by recrudescence. The only way to determine the benefits of any form of intervention in such a condition is by long-term follow-up of comparable groups who have followed different career pathways. This has not been done, and that there is an urgent need for such a study is demonstrated by the marked differences of opinion of the most appropriate role for self-help groups noted in the course of even this small survey.

Several self-help groups, particularly those led by energetic organisers, see themselves as 'therapy groups without the therapist'. It is in fact from just such a group that the AFS itself has emerged, and the approach fits well with one of the basic themes of the self-help movement as a whole, namely the active rejection of the 'medicalisation' of disability. This is an approach supported by one progressive group of speech therapists whose declared aim is to 'wean stammerers off speech therapists'. After considerable experience with therapist-led group therapy they concluded that 'it encouraged members to be far too dependent on speech therapists and thus minimised the effort which they put into their progress. We also considered that the meetings were looked upon as 'treatment' which we really did not feel was an accurate or desirable concept . . . Our policy now with new referrals is to give them a short course of individual therapy and encourage them to join the self-help group as soon as possible.' It may be significant that, having been given this greater degree of autonomy and responsibility by the speech therapists, this group has re-styled itself 'a self-help fluency group.'

Another, equally experienced speech therapist takes a very different view. Major progress, for those capable of achieving it, is most likely to come, she feels, through therapist-led work. Self-help groups may even be counter-productive from a fluency-gaining standpoint. She writes:

> The main value of the self-help group is social. To that extent the group serves to *maintain* the problem of stammering in order to continue with this social interaction. It is primarily useful for people who have found it difficult to come to terms with their problem and who are unable to change their attitudes and behaviour in therapy. It is a valuable support group.

Before drawing far-reaching conclusions from such an expresssion of opinion it is important to remember the dominant position of the therapist, who often has the power to allocate clients to one form of group or another and so, by selection of the membership, determine the outcome.

This survey could not, by its nature, obtain the views of persons who had ceased to participate in a group because they felt it provided little benefit. Some evidence suggested, however, that it is those stutterers most strongly motivated to gain fluency who move on most readily from a self-help group to some wider social arena.

The Survey: Conclusions and Summary

Of the 20 respondents to the present enquiry, few reported knowledge of more than 20 persons actively participating in self-help groups, strictly defined. This would suggest that at any given point in time, participation in a self-help group is a significant component in the life experience of not more than 400 to 500 stutterers in the UK.

Considering the frequency of the disorder amongst adults, its often intractable and chronic nature and the dissatisfaction with professional help so often expressed by sufferers, the overwhelming conclusion from the present survey, therefore, must be concern at the paucity of self-help groups, their small size, transitory nature, dependence on enthusiastic individuals and the relatively minor impact they make on the lives of the large majority of stutterers. And this in spite of almost universal reports from those who have participated, of at least some benefit received. Of course, it might be the case that there exists a large pool of flourishing self-help groups, actively conferring benefits on their members, totally unreached by the present survey but this seems improbable.

The responses to the questionnaire shows that it is difficult, and may not always be helpful, to draw a clear-cut distinction between self-help and other types of stutterers' groups. The present survey provides positive evidence of benefit from self-help groups for only a minority of stutterers, but there is a suggestion that many more obtain much needed support at critical stages in their lives from the group experience.

On a short-to-medium term basis, the self-help group seems able to provide:

1   social contact,
2   new insights for the individual into the nature of his condition,
3   a way of helping others. The business of maintaining the group provides useful experience of constructive activity without the necessity of competition with fluent speakers.

If effectively maintained over the longer term their provision includes:

1   a link with professionals. The collective voice of the clients may provide professionals with valuable insights,
2   an information service — useful for those who have had no treatment and may help to make expectations more realistic.

On the other hand, these groups generally seem to be less helpful for teenagers and immature adults, perhaps because many of them have only recently become aware of the social consequences of their handicap and quite often are disillusioned following relapse after therapy. Without adequate personal counselling they find it hard to come to terms with this situation and look to 'the group' as yet another possible external 'cure', expecting attendance and participation to have almost magical curative properties. The groups are least successful, not surprisingly, in the case of very severe stutterers whose need is for more effective therapy.

Self Help Groups: What Have We Learned?

Few writers on stuttering, particularly if they suffer from the complaint themselves, can lay claim to scientific objectivity in dealing with the subject. Their conclusions will be biased by the views they hold regarding the nature of the disorder, the importance they attach to the stutterer's self-perception of his disorder and the social stigma surrounding it. Before concluding this chapter with some positive proposals regarding the kind of organisational arrangements which might best meet the needs of stutterers, it will be appropriate to clarify the author's own position on these points.

Positive rejection of the suggestion that they are suffering from any kind of 'abnormality', whether of mind or body, is a significant component of many stutterers' self-concept. And they are probably correct. So far as psychological features are concerned no studies have ever demonstrated any consistent personality differences between stutterers as a group and the remainder of the population. Stuttering is not the province of the psychiatrist. The essential nature of the underlying speech dysfunction which triggers the development of the stuttering behaviour pattern is still unknown; although probably neurological it may well not be structural in nature. Whatever it is, it has secondary consequences in terms of emotional reactions which can be disturbing and learned responses which, paradoxically, are frequently maladaptive. It is the overt manifestations of these secondary effects which constitute the symptomatology called 'stuttering'.

Those with mental handicap, many spastics, and some physically handicapped persons often have to struggle, both personally and through the organisations which speak for them, against pressures tending to exclude them from society. Stutterers, by contrast, are freely admitted to society to which they can contribute in many ways; indeed their contribution is positively welcomed, always provided their aspirations do not go beyond a supporting or subordinate role. Contemporary social attitudes in this respect can be unclear and ambivalent so it is not surprising that the social consequences of stuttering are not always immediately apparent to the young sufferer; hence much of the unreality of his attitude and consequent difficulties of adjustment.

This chapter discussed previously the major factors producing the overt manifestation of stuttering, namely emotional reactions and maladaptive learned responses. Given appropriate motivation, these are susceptible to control, treatment, counselling and support. It might therefore be assumed that self-help would play a more prominent and significantly beneficial part in the management of stuttering than appears to be the case. Is it possible to develop a hypothesis explaining why its role appears to be so limited?

Experience gained within the Association, not only from the present survey, strongly suggests that an important influence militating *against* the success of self-help groups in this disorder is the unwillingness of many stutterers to be categorised as speech-defective. Linked with this is the fact that many stutterers do not wish to associate regularly with others similarly affected. A point to note is the paradoxical effect which the stigma attached to stuttering may have. In some cases it will drive sufferers to associate with others like themselves, a feature which is common in self-help groups for other forms of handicap. In other cases, however, it will have the reverse effect and cause them to try even harder to dissociate themselves mentally from their own handicap and to 'pass' as successfully as they can in normal society. Interestingly, this feature appears also in the case of some physical handicaps to which no social stigma of any kind is attached. A recent book by a diabetic (McLean, 1985) describing her own experiences of the disease, includes this perceptive and relevant comment:

> Diabetes must be almost as old as humanity itself but it has only been an English institution for fifty years. It is now an official subculture. Besides the natural camaraderie of its doctors and patients, there is a British Diabetic Association, complete with newspaper, clubs, dieticians, medical and legal advice, video cassettes, and even diabetic tea-towels. I ought to belong to the BDA, which is obviously a marvellous organisation, but I do not. I ought also to think of myself as a diabetic but I do not. Instead, I think of myself as someone who happens to have diabetes and I would rather not belong to an association in which diabetes is the sine qua non; there are better ways to be counted. (p. 158).

It is clear, however, that numerous benefits for stutterers can and do accrue from the group experience, but under appropriate circumstances the same can apply to many kinds of group, not just self-help groups. Is it possible to learn any general lessons about the management of stuttering from the experience of self-help groups? And since some stutterers do report benefit, is it possible to identify particular features either of the groups themselves or the individuals concerned, which might suggest the persons for whom participation in a group might be recommended?

We find that activities reported as useful take place in either self-help or therapist-led groups, or both. One respondent, quoted above in the section on 'Activities', made special reference to the value of the self-help group in promoting exploration by the participants of the psychological 'hidden agenda'. But one of the speech therapists included in the survey saw this aspect as precisely the one where the therapist's role was needed. Having explained that the self-help group in her district spent its time mainly on speech exercises of various kinds, 'the therapist-led group', whe went on to say, 'concentrated largely on Personal Construct Therapy including elaborating the members' construction of fluency, understanding the construction processes of listeners, dealing with avoidance and self-assertion, and using video and bio-feedback to monitor behaviour and relaxation'. So it is not the specific activities undertaken by the group which account for all the benefits.

The greatest specific virtue of self-help groups we have been able to identify is the relief from the sense of isolation they can provide, giving the stutterer someone to talk to who can understand the distress, frustration and isolation endured. It may be vital for some people to pass through this phase of communicating and sharing a troubling experience, and to come to terms with it, before they become able to devote the necessary personal effort to the practical aspects of dealing with their own unique speech problem. For some this can only happen in a group of fellow stutterers. An observation made during the course of the survey by one perceptive and experienced group organiser may be relevant here: 'Life histories of many adult stammerers show it is often only in middle age that the true extent of their speech difficulty dawns on them and they realise the profound influence it has had on their career prospects and life experience'. Results can be very varied, depending on personality features: depression, resignation, renewed determination for self-change and a fresh start; all the elements, in fact, of the so-called 'mid-life crisis'. The life history of the chronic stutterer includes phases of exerting greater control, others of asserting greater self-expression, yet others of acquiring greater understanding of his or her personal problem. Depending on numerous individual factors, joining a group for a period of time may assist any or all of these phases. We have found that successful self-help groups tend to be those whose members are somewhat older and more self-aware, who have succeeded in establishing some degree of control of their speech and are therefore able to communicate effectively and gain benefit from the insights which come from the exchange of personal testimony about coping strategies. This often leads to a more realistic awareness of the attitudes of others towards stuttering which in turn can lead to either a greater determination to develop better speech patterns or to adopt a more challenging and assertive attitude towards communicating with others; often both. Our experience is that a self-help group 'works':

1   when the leader acts as therapist,
2   when the leader acts as counsellor,
3   more rarely, when the group dynamics enable a member to perceive the possibility of change — either in his speech as such, or in attitude or in communication performance.

What is needed to achieve better results in adult stuttering and what existing services fail to provide is a combination of *counselling* with *continuity of follow-up* so that stutterers can be directed to appropriate treatment and also helped towards a fuller understanding of their disorder and a better adjustment to it. Counselling may come from a fellow-sufferer or an older, more experienced speech therapist with a special interest. It is necessary for those who counsel stutterers, whether they be speech therapists or others, to tread a very narrow dividing line, supporting and confirming the stutterer in the sense of his own normalcy and using this to build self-confidence, whilst at the same time promoting greater realism by enhancing the stutterer's awareness of others' perceptions of his speech patterns and coming to accept these responses too, as 'normal'. Stutterers themselves must assume control, both of their speech and their situation, and assume responsibility for promoting communication.

The self-help movement, properly organised and funded, could make a major contribution to both counselling and follow-up by providing a focus for maintaining contacts over time, but in practice would often need the institutional support of speech therapy clinics. In Britain, the National Health Service alone is a long way from being able to provide this kind of service. Continued voluntary endeavour, perhaps in closer collaboration with the speech therapy profession, will certainly be needed.

Acknowledgment

Many friends and colleagues have contributed to this chapter by recounting their experiences and offering much helpful information and advice. I am most grateful to them all and particularly to the area representatives of the Association for Stammerers without whose collaboration the survey could not have been carried out.

12 Informing Stutterers About Treatment

Gavin Andrews, Megan Neilson and Mary Cassar

Introduction

Successful treatment of stuttering depends on many hours of speech retraining with an appropriate technique (Andrews, Guitar and Howie, 1980). In the treatment programme for adult stutterers which is the focus of this article, the technique used is referred to as smooth speech, and involves emphasis on the gentle onset of each utterance and on continuous phonation from one phrase juncture to another. At slow rates this eliminates stuttering. Gradually, this abnormal but stutter-free speech is systematically shaped to become normal speech in terms of both rate and prosody. Each subject then undertakes a series of graded assignments outside the clinic so that the new fluent speech skill is generalized to the outside world. The treatment programme was developed from that of Andrews and Harris (1964), with the original fluency-producing agent of syllable-timed speech being superseded in 1970 by the prolonged or smooth speech technique. The present treatment programme has been conducted as a service programme since 1971 and some 50 new patients are treated in this clinic each year. It has been the topic of many research reports and was most recently described by Andrews and Feyer (1985).

The smooth speech technique has been shown to fulfill criteria for a satisfactory treatment. Data on more than 300 subjects have been reported since the prototype treatment was introduced by Curlee and Perkins (1969). Subjects, both adolescents and adults, have had their speech assessed by reliable and objective techniques on a number of occasions from the end of treatment to 18 months later. Speech attitudes have also been measured. Both speech and speech attitudes have been shown to improve significantly with treatment. Evidence has been presented that neither regression to the mean nor response to placebo could account for these changes (Andrews and Harvey, 1981). Since comparable reports have come from clinics in different countries and since this treatment is in routine service use throughout Australia, it is unlikely that the later reports of benefit are due to the halo that surrounds a new treatment, or to the charisma associated with a particular clinician.

The principal goal of therapy has always been to produce stutter-free, natural-sounding speech and thus the focus of the treatment process has been the elimination of stuttering. In recent years it has been realized that the acquisition of normal communication attitudes and an internalized locus of control are other important determinants of long-term fluency (Guitar and Bass, 1978; Craig, Franklin and Andrews, 1984). After treatment the majority of subjects speak without stuttering, and for most these gains are permanent. However, one year after treatment one in six will be stuttering on more than 3 percent of their syllables, the criterion for entry to the programme. The one-sixth of patients at risk of relapse can be identified at the end of therapy because they will not have attained the goals of absolutely fluent speech, normal speech attitudes and internalized locus of control. In the latest revision to the programme the subjects who remain at risk undertake remedial programmes during week three of the course to hasten achievement of these goals.

This paper addresses a further strategy that we use to maximize improvement. We inform stutterers in considerable detail about the entire treatment programme before treatment commences by means of a detailed patient's manual which is reprinted herein. We also inform them about stuttering by providing a summary of the review of stuttering we published in 1983 (Andrews *et al.*, 1983) and that summary is also reprinted as the introduction to this volume. Those who are interested to read further are referred to that review and to the meta-analysis of treatment outcomes (Andrews *et al.*, 1980). Becoming fluent is hard work. We consider that if our subjects are fully informed about the nature and treatment of stuttering before they begin then they are more likely to persevere with the practice that is essential for continued fluency.

THE UNIVERSITY OF NEW SOUTH WALES
PROFESSORIAL UNIT IN PSYCHIATRY
and
DIVISION OF PSYCHIATRY
ST. VINCENT'S HOSPITAL
SYDNEY, N.S.W. 2010

PATIENTS MANUAL
for the
STUTTERING TREATMENT PROGRAM

This manual is for use by patients
during treatment under the direction
of an appropriately trained therapist.
It is not a treatment in itself.

PROGRAM SUMMARY

WEEK 1

SUNDAY:

Introduction to the program commences at 10 a.m. Please have someone from home attend with you for the first hour. You will then stay on for your pre-treatment assessment. This is usually finished about 1 p.m. Please bring with you a blank C-60 cassette tape and, if possible, your own cassette recorder (see below).

MONDAY–FRIDAY:

Group treatment begins at 8 a.m. each day. On Monday you will be taught 'smooth speech', a technique for controlling stuttering. Initially you will have to speak very slowly but, as the week progresses and your new speech skills improve, you'll gradually be allowed to speed up. By Friday you should be speaking fluently at normal rates and not stuttering at all. Such rapid changes can only be achieved by many hours of intensive work. Your progress will be paced and your departure time each evening will depend on how efficiently you have achieved the goal for that day. Earliest departure time is 6 p.m., 8 p.m. is more usual, and people sometimes have to stay on far into the night before reaching their goal.

WEEK 2

MONDAY–FRIDAY:

From 8 a.m. to 10 a.m. you will practise your smooth speech skills in the clinic. If your progress is satisfactory you'll spend the remainder of the day doing assignments that effectively transfer your new fluent speech from the clinic into the outside world. There are set assignments to be completed by 6 p.m. each day and if this is not accomplished you will be required to stay for up to two hours longer for extra practice.

WEEK 3

MONDAY:

Your arrival time on Monday morning will be by appointment and we will assess your achievement up to that time. If your progress has been consistent and all your expected tasks are complete, you will be invited to continue with an extra four days of advanced, individually based therapy for which there is no charge. Those who do not qualify for the advanced course will leave the program at the end of the Friends and Relatives meeting on Monday evening. This starts at 6 p.m. and lasts about two hours. You should arrange to bring at least one family member or close friend.

TUESDAY–FRIDAY (ADVANCED COURSE):

Your day will begin at 8 a.m. with a series of individually designed tasks. These will be aimed at minimizing your chance of relapse and will allow you to consolidate your fluency in even the most challenging real life situations. Departure time will vary but will usually be no later than 6 p.m.

IMPORTANT

(1) Please clear yourself of any external commitments for the duration of the course. Your days will be full and since assignments often take up part of the evenings and weekends, you will welcome spare time to do nothing.

(2) You will be using a compact hand-held cassette recorder throughout the course. The clinic can lend you one if necessary but it's far better if you have your own as you'll need to continue working with it after the course finishes. The newer pocket-size recorders which take a standard cassette are ideal e.g., Tandy Model 14-1047. Larger recorders or recorders without a pause button are not suitable.

INTRODUCTION

Stuttering is basically a physical disorder, not a psychological one. The part of the brain which controls a stutterer's speech does not work as efficiently as it should. The result is the malfunction we call stuttering.

The aim of this program is to enable adults who stutter to speak fluently and well. Unfortunately it is not possible to change an inefficient part of the brain simply by plugging in a new component, as you would with a car or a computer. Nevertheless stutterers can become reliably fluent by mastering a special technique called 'smooth speech'. The smooth speech technique simplifies certain aspects of speaking and focusses the stutterer's attention where it is most needed. This allows the inefficient speech system to operate safely within its own limitations.

It is important to realise right from the start that this course is not a miracle cure for stuttering. Learning smooth speech is like learning to drive your car a whole new way. Relearning an existing skill takes time and hard work and you constantly have to guard against returning to your old methods. But once you've mastered it thoroughly you'll be able to use it easily and well. If you use it all the time, it will continue to prevent you from stuttering. If you don't use it consistently, your old way of speaking will gradually take over and your stuttering will return. You should therefore regard your weeks at the clinic as the beginning of an ongoing commitment to practise and maintain a new form of speech. If you stick to that commitment, you need never stutter again.

WEEK 1

FLUENCY INSTATEMENT PHASE

WORK SCHEDULE

On Sunday there will be an introductory session lasting approximately three hours. For the first hour of this session we ask you to bring along someone from home so that we can explain to you both what is going to be happening to you over the next weeks. There will be some forms for you to fill out and your speech will be assessed. You will also get to meet the other members of your group. Each of you will take home a cassette tape which will introduce you to 'smooth speech', the new way of speaking that you will learn during the course. You must listen to the tape carefully overnight.

Monday to Friday you will arrive at the clinic at 8 a.m. sharp. The group will work intensively throughout the day with only brief breaks for refreshment. There will be a one hour break for lunch which will be eaten together at the clinic. Before going home each evening you are expected to reach a set goal. How quickly you reach this goal will depend on your performance during the day. If you have performed constantly well you may get away as early as 6 p.m. and will eat at home. If you have had lots of difficulty you may have to stay on at the clinic for several hours so you will eat there. You will also have some homework to complete each night.

TREATMENT PROCEDURES

Treatment is conducted by means of group conversations which are called rating sessions. As well as giving you lots of practice at smooth speech, rating sessions enable you to learn and practise many aspects of conversational skill. For example, knowing when and how to interrupt or lead a conversation can be very difficult for a stutterer, so the program has been designed so that these interactions will occur. The competitive nature of the course means that unless you speak up in each session you will fall behind. In this way your speaking confidence will increase as you become more able to be active in a conversation.

In each rating session you must complete a minimum number of syllables, this number depending on your stage in the program. Syllables rather than words are used as the basic units of speech. During each rating session the therapist will use a computer to record the number of syllables spoken, the number of errors and the elapsed time. The computer monitors the rate at which each person speaks. Speech rate is measured as the numnber of syllables spoken per minute. We refer to this measure as your SPM (Syllables Per Minute). At the end of each rating session you will record your SPM, the number of syllables spoken and any errors on a progress sheet.

Early Monday morning you will begin learning the techniques of smooth speech. This will be described by the therapist and a demonstration of each sound will be followed by each patient practising both individually and with the group. To start with you will be speaking very slowly, at 50 syllables per minute, which is about one quarter of normal speech rate. You will be shown how to breathe into the words and use your airflow properly.

Before lunch a practice rating session will be held at 50 SPM. To help you concentrate on your speech and not on what you are saying, you will play a simple game such as 'I Spy' or 'Animal, Vegetable, Mineral'. After lunch you'll start your first proper rating session. You will need to complete six successful rating sessions at 50 SPM and the last one must be free of any error in your smooth speech before you can move up to the next speed. During the week your target speech rate will increase in easy steps until you get up to 200 SPM (normal speech rate).

In this way your new smooth speech will be learned and established at a very slow speed and then practised and consolidated at gradually increasing speeds. By Friday you should be speaking fluently and at normal speed.

To pace your progress during the week we set speech rate goals which you must reach before you leave each evening. You will see these in the rating session schedule which follows.

RATING SESSION SCHEDULE

	MON	TUE	WED	THU	FRI
8:00	Introduction	50/5	90	160	Weekend briefing
9:00	to smooth	50/NE	100	165	200/1
10:00	speech and	55	110	170	200/2
11:00	practice rating	60	120	175	200/3
12:00	session	65	130	180	200/4
1:00	**LUNCH**				
2:00	50/1	70	140	185	200/C
3:00	50/2	75	145	190	Assignment briefing
4:00	50/3	80	150	195	
5:00	50/4	85	155	200	
	EVENING BRIEFING				
	Extra sessions until goal for the day is achieved				
GOAL	50/4	85	155	200	200/C

HOW A RATING SESSION WORKS

As mentioned earlier, rating sessions consist of group conversations. These conversations last a set time of 45 minutes. Each of the six group members is expected to contribute to the conversation for a total of seven minutes ($6 \times 7 = 42$) leaving only three minutes spare. The amount of information (i.e. the number of syllables) you are able to communicate during the conversation will depend on your speech rate. For instance, if you speak at 50 SPM you will only be able to contribute $7 \times 50 = 350$ syllables, whereas at 120 SPM you will contribute $7 \times 120 = 840$ syllables and at 200 SPM you will contribute $7 \times 200 = 1400$ syllables.

In the first rating session everyone has a target speech rate of 50 SPM and a target information output of 350 syllables. You must continue contributing to the conversation until you have reached your 350 syllables. If you speak at exactly 50 SPM this will take exactly 7 minutes. If you speak too fast it will take less than 7 minutes and if you speak too slowly it will take more. With the help of the computer to monitor your speech you will learn to keep your rate close to the target SPM. This is very important because if you speak faster than you should your new smooth speech skills may break down. Likewise, if you speak slower than you should you will not consolidate your smooth speech skills at the required target rate and you will also use up more than your allotted seven minutes in the rating session. Because sessions have a time limit this means that you may not be able to reach your required number of syllables before the session ends or if you do, you may leave another group member without enough time to finish.

To complete a rating session successfully you must:

1. Achieve your required number of syllables without stuttering.
2. Achieve your required number of syllables within the session time limit.
3. Maintain your speech rate close to the target SPM throughout the session. Your overall rate for the session must be within + or − 20 SPM of your target.

If you miss on any of these points you'll have to repeat the session.

The above three conditions must always be satisfied in every rating session. For some sessions there will be other requirements as well; for example, the final session at 50 SPM must not only be stutter free but it must also be free of any errors in your production of smooth speech. The therapist will tell you when extra conditions must be satisfied.

During the first day or so, because of the slow speeds, it's often difficult to have very meaningful conversations. As the speed increases, a more natural type of discussion will be possible and we expect you to start tackling interesting and challenging topics. At this stage you may find the therapist will refuse to rate speech which is not relevant to the general conversation of the moment or which is just a monologue. Remember that the program is designed to help you CONVERSE fluently, not just to talk! This is also the reason we set a time limit for each rating session. Not only do you have to be fluent at your target SPM, but you also have to be able to organise what you want to say quickly enough to get into the conversation. Otherwise you'll run the risk of not having reached your required number of syllables by the time the session ends.

As mentioned earlier, there are only three spare minutes in a 45 minute rating session. This time remains spare only if all six people keep exactly to target rate and speak promptly and efficiently without undue hesitations. If you make an error in your smooth speech the therapist may stop you and show you how to correct the error. Normally the clock is left running while this happens, so any spare time will get used up quite quickly if lots of errors are being made.

Sometimes though, the therapist may decide to interrupt the session to give special revision or to make an important point. In this case the clock will be turned off so that the time used is additional to the 45 minutes for the session.

As you will see from the rating session schedule, sessions are timed to start each hour, so additional time is not plentiful. The remainder of the hour, after the actual rating session has finished, is used for recording your performance on your rating session record, collecting any payment (see below) and, if there's time, a quick break.

Your rating session record sheets detail your progress throughout the fluency instatement phase of the program. Please fill them in promptly and accurately; they will be collected from you at the end of the course.

REWARDS SYSTEM

The busy schedule of rating sessions is designed to give you lots and lots of practice so that you can develop your new smooth speech skills. Learning a new skill requires concentration and effort and you'll often feel you're working very hard. To help you learn quickly and efficiently we give you a reward each time you perform well.

Whenever you complete a rating session successfully you will be allowed to move on one step in the schedule, which usually means moving to a slightly faster speech rate. Each successful rating session therefore takes you one step closer to your goal for the day. As mentioned earlier, the quicker you reach your goal the earlier you'll be able to go home, so a successful run of rating sessions rewards you with an 'early mark'.

At the end of each successful rating session we also pay you a small amount of money. Payment is 5¢ for the first successful session of the day. If you follow this with another successful session you earn 10¢, then 15¢ and so on.

If you don't achieve your required number of syllables before a session runs out, or if your speech rate is more than + or − 20 SPM off target, you'll have to do the next session at that same target rate. You won't be paid for the unsuccessful session and your next payment will be set back to 5¢.

If you stutter during a session, your syllable count will be zeroed. If this happens well into the session you'll have to sit out for the remainder and do the next session at the same rate. If it happens early, you may be allowed to start again. If you manage to complete the session successfully after the restart you'll move on to the next rate. But you won't be paid in either case and your next payment will be reset to 5¢.

The program is self-limiting, in that when you need consolidation of earlier steps your skills break down and an additional session is necessary. Stuttering is an indicator that your skill at that stage of the program is not robust enough. Repeating any session should not be viewed as a failure but rather, as revision of earlier learning. A stutter is therefore not a 'failure', it's just an indicator that your skill level, or the degree to which you are applying the skill, is inadequate.

If you stutter outside a rating session, or if you use speech which is too fast or not smooth, you'll have to pay a fine. Fines are 5¢ Monday afternoon and Tuesday, 10¢ Wednesday and Thursday and 20¢ from Friday to the end of the course. You are expected to use the new speech AT ALL TIMES after Monday lunch. At this stage you must be specially wary of making spontaneous remarks. If you speak without first paying attention to your smooth speech technique, you run a high risk of stuttering. The prospect of a fine helps to emphasize the need to use smooth speech all the time.

VIDEO SESSIONS

To maintain your new fluency successfully you must learn to recognise when you are using the correct speaking skills and reward yourself accordingly. For this reason the treatment program trains you to assess your own speech accurately and objectively. It is important to develop a realistic attitude to your speech rather than an emotional one. If you can be objectively critical about specific aspects of your speech skill, you are in a better position to correct problems.

From Tuesday of the first week, two sessions daily will be concerned with teaching you to evaluate your speech. Payment for these sessions depends on your correct evaluation of your own speech and the speech of the others in the group.

In these sessions each person speaks for one minute on a topic selected by the therapist. This is video taped and played back immediately. Everyone assesses the quality of the speech according to the criteria listed below.

The criteria for video assessment are:

1. Breathing
2. Gentle onsets and offsets
3. Joining/continuity (all syllables in a phrase must be joined up — there must be continuous airflow, continuous movement and continuous sound)
4. Phrasing and pausing
5. Intonation (appropriate pitch and emphasis; no sing-song or monotone)
6. Presentation (facial expression, eye contact)
7. Correct speech rate (within $+/-20$ of the target)

If there are two or fewer errors in a particular category you award a tick for that category; if there are more than two errors you award a cross. Your rating of each group member's speech is then compared with those of the therapist. Since the aim of the video session is to train you in assessing the quality of smooth speech, your payment for the session will be based on how frequently your ratings are in agreement with the therapist, rather than on how well you spoke during your video. Payment is usually 5¢ per agreement with the therapist's assessment of your own speech during the video, plus an additional 20¢ if you agree on at least two thirds of the assessments on the rest of the group. However, irrespective of your assessment skill and payment, if you stutter during your video or if your speech rate is too far from your target, you will have to repeat that rate in the next normal session in order to consolidate your skill at that level.

GOING HOME AT NIGHT

When you go home each night it is very important that you continue to practise the new speech that you've been using during the day. Before you leave the clinic each evening we'll ask you to leave an amount of money as a 'bond'. It's up to you how much you choose to leave, but it should be an amount you'd be reluctant to lose. Each morning you'll be asked about your speech at home and, based on this, how much of your bond you think you deserve back. The most important person to be honest with is yourself. Each night you'll also be given a homework assignment. This will usually involve recording three minutes of smooth speech at your correct target rate. On Monday night you'll record yourself reading aloud and on Tuesday, Wednesday and Thursday you'll tape your side of a conversation at home. The therapist will assess your assignment and you'll be paid 25¢ if it's satisfactory. You should only consider your homework finished when you've listened to the tape and have completely satisfied yourself that it contains good quality, stutter-free smooth speech at the correct rate. If it doesn't, you should rewind the tape and do it again.

At the end of each day you should also make time to review your progress in your 'speech diary'. The blank paper at the back of your folder is there for that purpose. You should also use it for making notes on information and advice the therapist may give you. After you finish the intensive program and are back on your own, you'll find it useful to look back over your record of how you felt during your fluency instatement and to revise information you found meaningful and helpful.

WEEK 2

TRANSFER PHASE

The purpose of this phase of treatment is to enable you to transfer the skills you have learned in the treatment room into the outside world. You will do a series of assignments designed to give you practice at using smooth speech in a variety of everyday situations. This week is often considered to be much harder than the first week because there are more stresses on you in the outside world.

THE COPING TECHNIQUE

Before you start the outside assignments you will be taught a special smooth speech technique called 'coping'. The coping technique is designed to help you through difficult situations where you may feel unsure about remaining fluent. It involves using exaggeratedly slow smooth speech whenever you encounter a potential trouble spot. So that you will be able to use the technique efficiently in real life situations you need to practise slowing down and smoothing out your speech at will. After the teaching session, you will be asked to include examples of the coping technique in a variety of assignments, inside and outside the clinic.

Remember:
    1. You must increase your speed gradually. You must not increase from half speed to full speed over just one or two syllables.
    2. You must plan for the potential trouble spot to occur in the slow section. The technique will not be helpful if you're already up to full speed by the time you get to the difficult bit.

RATING SESSIONS

There will be a rating session from 8 a.m. to 10 a.m. each morning. In these sessions each person must complete three minutes of fluent speech at 100, 150, 180 and 200 SPM. During the three minutes at 200 you may be required to practise your coping technique. Rating sessions help make your new speech more automatic and allow you extra practice speaking at the faster rates needed for the outside world. After completing the morning session, you will go out and start the assignments. If you successfully complete your required number of assignments before 6 p.m., you can go home right away. Otherwise you'll stay for extra rating session practice. Each rating session you complete during this week should be entered on your transfer phase rating session record; these sheets will be collected at the end of the course.

ASSIGNMENTS

There are 15 set assignments to be completed in Week 2. The daily goals are as follows: By 6 p.m. Monday evening you should have completed 3 successful assignments, by Tuesday evening 6, by Wednesday evening 9, by Thursday evening 12, and Friday evening 15. Most people attempt the assignments in the following order and thus do the easier ones first. If a particular assignment is likely to be especially difficult for you, then do it later in the series.

1. Conversation with a family member of close friend using coping.
2. Conversation with a family member or close friend.
3. Conversation with a stranger (male or female) using coping.
4. Conversation with a stranger (male 1).
5. Conversation with a stranger (male 2).
6. Conversation with a stranger (female 1).
7. Conversation with a stranger (female 2).
8. Telephone calls to strangers (1).
9. Telephone calls to strangers (2).
10. Shopping.
11. 20 enquiries.
12. 14 introductions and requests.
13. 10 deliberate stutters with coping recovery.
14. 5 telephone appointments and cancellations.
15. Identifying at least 6 important points from Van Riper's discussion of stabilization after therapy.

Assignments 1–14 must be taped and must satisfy the following criteria:

1. Fluent (i.e., no stutters or more than one re-start).
2. Correct rate (200 + / − 20).
3. Good quality smooth speech.
4. Correct length.

Assignments 1–10 must be at least 1400 syllables long.

Assignments 11–14 must contain the correct number of items.

The therapist will assess your work and if you haven't fulfilled these conditions, or if you haven't carried out the assignment as instructed, you'll be asked to do it again. Before you start an assignment make absolutely sure that you know what is expected of you. The following paragraphs give you a brief outline of how to do the assignments and the therapist will give you more details where necessary. If something isn't clear, ask about it.

Assignments 1–2 (conversations with family/friend) are done at home and can be attempted during the weekend. It's best to do these first assignments with people you feel completely comfortable with. Make sure you make frequent use of the coping technique in one of these assignments. If your coping technique is not correct, or if you don't use it often enough, you'll have to repeat the assignment even though it may be O.K. in other respects.

Assignments 3–7 (conversations with strangers) are usually done within a few blocks of the clinic. The therapist will suggest places where you're likely to find people who'll be willing to let you talk with them. On approaching a stranger you should explain that you are doing a speech course at St. Vincent's Hospital and that it would be helpful if you could sit down and talk for a few minutes. Demonstrate the pause on the tape recorder and explain that you will only be recording your side of the conversation. If you don't manage to record enough speech for the full assignment with your first stranger, listen back to what you've done so far and if it's o.k., continue on with another person. If it isn't, you should rewind and start over again with someone else. Continue doing this until you have enough for the whole assignment. Except for the coping assignment which can be done with either males or females or both, you should keep male and female conversations on separate tapes. As before, your coping assignment must contain frequent examples of good coping technique in order to pass.

Assignments 8–9 (telephone calls) are usually done at the clinic. By using yellow pages, classified ads, and some imagination, you'll find lots of things you can enquire about at length. Choose things that will allow you to do much of the talking, rather than the other person; e.g., enquiring about hiring equipment for camping, catering for a party, spare parts from motor wreckers, trekking holidays in the Himalayas, etc. Assess each phone call before going on to the next. If it's O.K., continue on, if it isn't, rewind to where that call began and continue from there. Because the clinic has very few phone lines, no more than two people should be doing phone assignments at the one time, so plan accordingly with other members of the group.

Assignments 10–13 are all done away from the clinic. For these assignments your tape recording must be done discreetly, without telling others what you are doing. This means either hiding your tape recorder in a pocket or bag, or disguising it as a 'Walkman' by wearing earphones around your neck. Test your recording quality and if the environment is too noisy go somewhere quieter. If your assignment can't be heard it can't be passed. As you complete each item in an assignment, review it before you go on, and if it isn't satisfactory, tape over it. If you don't do this you run the risk of finding that your tape is unsatisfactory after you've come all the way back to the clinic, in which case you'll have to have to go out again.

Assignment 10 (shopping) is best done by choosing an area where there is plenty of scope to make detailed enquiries about goods or services. Big shopping plazas, department stores, or back street speciality shops all offer the opportunity to record away from street noise.

Assignment 11 (enquiries) consists of approaching strangers with brief enquiries such as asking directions, conducting a 'survey', etc. Again, try to choose places without lots of street noise.

Assignment 12 (introductions and requests) requires you to invent situations where you will have to give your name at a counter or desk and then make a request likely to involve you in some negotiation; e.g., picking up photos, dry cleaning, repairs, etc. supposedly left in your name, reporting to the wrong place for an appointment, collecting a message that isn't there. Engage in as much conversation as you can, but don't put people to excessive trouble. Be ready with a plausible reason as to why you must have made a mistake.

For Assignment 13 (stutters and recovers) you should put yourself in a situation with a stranger where you previously would have been very likely to stutter. During the encounter you must pretend to stutter and then recover from it using the coping technique. The stutter that you simulate must be precisely the sort of stutter that you might really have done in that situation prior to treatment. Your recovery must be organized so that the slow section of the coping coincides with whatever you pretended to stutter on. Before you do this assignment ask the therapist to let you listen to your pretreatment tape so that the stutter you simulate will be just like your own. It's not acceptable to imitate some other sort of stutter in this assignment. You should demonstrate your pretended stutter and recovery to the therapist to make sure you are doing exactly what is required before trying it outside.

Assignment 14 (appointments and cancellations) is done at the clinic and requires you to give your name and other specific details on the phone; e.g., booking a table at a restaurant, or making an appointment for the dentist, a haircut, a car service, etc. Plan the assignment so that you do the cancellations after a considerable delay, preferably the next day. Make sure you keep a record of who you rang and what you told them, otherwise you won't be able to cancel!

Assignment 15 (Van Riper) is the only assignment which does not involve speaking. The therapist will lend you a copy of a chapter on stabilization after therapy from a book by Charles Van Riper, an expert on stuttering and himself a stutterer. Read the information and summarize at least six of the major points on ordinary writing paper (you don't need an assignment sheet). You will pass the assignment provided you have included what the therapist considers to be the most important things to be remembered.

SELF-ASSESSMENT OF ASSIGNMENTS

To help you learn to be an accurate judge of your speech, you must always listen to your tape of each assignment BEFORE submitting it to the therapist. When you've listened carefully to the whole assignment you should complete an assessment sheet which must be handed in clipped to your tape. As well as rating your tape, the therapist will read your assessment and give you feedback as to how accurately you've judged your performance. The ability to assess your own speech accurately is essential for long term survival.

The assignment assessment sheet lists the same criteria for good smooth speech as were used during your Week 1 video sessions; i.e., breathing, onsets and offsets, joining/continuity, phrasing and pausing, intonation, presentation, and speech rate. You should comment on each of these aspects of your speech performance during the assignment. You should also estimate the percentage of the assignment that you regard as good smooth speech. Write down examples of any things you recognize as problems. At the bottom of the sheet there is space for you to make overall comments about the circumstances of the assignment and how you felt about it.

There are two rules about handing in assignments which are there to ensure that the therapist does not have to waste time rating obviously unsatisfactory tapes.

Firstly, you must not hand in a tape which you know contains a stutter. If you happen to stutter during an assignment there is no point continuing. You must rewind your tape and begin the conversation again, if necessary with another person. Provided you are monitoring your speech properly you should be aware of a stutter right away. If one does slip past you should hear it when you assess the tape and you'll have to go back and re-do from the beginning of the conversation which contained the stutter. This means that for assignments consisting of several separate conversations or items (e.g., telephone conversations, shopping, enquiries) you should be sure to check your tape after completing each segment.

Secondly, you must make certain your assignment is long enough. Remember that pause time during the conversation does not count, so where 1400 syllables at 200 SPM are required, your recording should run for at least 8 minutes to be sure. If you're inclined to speak slowly, you should do more than 8 minutes.

If you apply yourself to the job and work consistently at your assignments, you should be able to reach the goals for each day without undue difficulty. Aim to hand in a tape at least every two hours. If you can't do this you should consult with the therapist. If you leave the clinic to do an assignment and then stay away because you're having trouble with it, the therapist is unable to help you. It's essential to report back regularly. If things are going well you'll be able to move on confidently to the next task, and if they're not, you'll get help in overcoming problems before they grow.

RECORDING YOUR PROGRESS

Each time you submit an assignment you should record the submission on your assignment work record. Each time you get an assignment back you should again fill in your work record with the details of how you fared. When you succeed in passing an assignment you should also fill in the details on your assignment completion record. The information on these sheets allows your progress to be monitored throughout the transfer phase of the program; they will be collected from you at the end of treatment.

You should also continue to use your speech diary to record your thoughts and feelings about what happens to you during this crucial period of transferring your new speech skills into the real world. This will be helpful to you when you are on your own again.

PAYMENT

Payment for Week 2 is $20, payable only if ALL assignments are successfully completed by 5 p.m. on the Friday of Week 2.

WEEK 3

ASSESSMENT AND ADVANCED TRANSFER PHASE

ASSESSMENT (MONDAY)

At this point in the program each person's progress is assessed in terms of whether or not they are likely to benefit from the advanced course which comprises the rest of Week 3.

Those who have completed all expected tasks by the end of Week 2 will automatically progress to the advanced course. They will arrive at the clinic around midday on Monday, having first been to their normal workplace to complete a work assignment. On arriving at the clinic they will complete a further assessment to help determine how best to organise their tasks for the remainder of the week.

Those who are unable to complete the Week 2 assignments within that week will arrive for assessment at an appointed time Monday morning. A decision about their suitability for the advanced course will be made at that time. In most cases people in this situation will have little to gain from the advanced course and are best advised to spend the rest of the week consolidating their fluency in their normal environment. The remainder of the day is spent on post-treatment assessment, planning of a maintenance program, and attending the Friends and Relatives meeting.

Friends and Relatives Evening for all group members runs from 6 p.m. to 8 p.m. on the Monday. Each person should bring at least one family member or friend for a discussion about fluency and the changes it may bring.

ADVANCED COURSE (TUESDAY–FRIDAY)

The advanced transfer phase of the course is designed to allow you to consolidate your fluency in a variety of challenging situations relevant to your individual needs and aspirations. You will be given some set tasks but you will also develop your own list of assignments in consultation with a therapist. These should include things that used to be a problem, even though they don't seem so now, and things which you perhaps never contemplated even attempting before. Although each person will have an individual program, everyone will be expected to include the following:

1. Work assignment. At least 1400 syllables to be taped at work if possible, usually on Monday morning.
2. Introductions. You will do formal introductions on Friends and Relatives night.
3. Public speech to a group of strangers. Your speech should be at least 1400 syllables long and can be on any subject you like. You may use notes, but must not read from a prepared text.
4. Talk Back Radio. At least 200 syllables of conversation on air. You must not talk about your speech or the course.
5. Debate. The group holds a formal debate, each member speaking for 3 minutes.

There is no charge for the advanced course and there is no formal payment for your assignments. For long-term survival, you need to learn to use self-motivation as an incentive to do your speech tasks. This is very important, as after you leave the course you will have to rely on your own initiative to do the daily speech practice needed to keep you fluent.

MAINTENANCE PHASE

After you've complete the treatment program it's essentially up to you to manage and maintain your fluency. You are now competent to take over as your own therapist.

During the program there were several crucial things your therapists provided for you; they observed and gave you feedback on your smooth speech skills, supplied you with structured objectives, and encouraged and reinforced your attempts to attain these objectives. You now have the skills to do all these things for yourself. The whole key to maintenance is self-management. You are capable of taking responsibility for your own fluency. That is what you should be striving for, FLUENCY THAT YOU ARE RESPONSIBLE FOR BY DESIGN, NOT BY ACCIDENT.

DAILY PRACTICE

Each day set aside at least ten minutes to go through a formal practice routine. If you have identified your difficult speech production areas you could refresh the relevant skills. Alternatively you could practise your total smooth speech techniques. This would consist of slowing down to a more obvious slurred level, say 100 SPM. If you have difficulty gauging your speed, recall that at 50 SPM you said two or three syllables on each breath and at 100 SPM you said five to six syllables on each breath.

The reason that you are slowing down is not to simply 'slow down' — you can still produce bad smooth speech at slow speeds — you should listen carefully to your technique. Check the breathing, gentle onsets and offsets, joining, phrasing and pausing, intonation and presentation. If you are being careful, you should take at least ten minutes.

You do not have to talk to someone. You can talk to yourself or your dog or the wall. The important thing is to produce speech out loud so that you can monitor and analyze your skills.

Try and get into a routine of formal practice; for example, get out of bed, brush your teeth, do your practice whilst dressing and so on. The excuse 'I don't have time to do it' is not a valid one. You can do your practice as a conjoint activity, that is, whilst doing something else, for example, having a shower, reading the paper, waiting for the water to boil for a cup of tea or coffee, during television commercials, doing the gardening — the list is really endless. If you cannot find ten minutes all at once, then divide the time — a few minutes in the morning then some more in the evening.

If your next excuse for not doing this revision is that you 'don't know what to talk about', then it's not really very original either. Talk about what you are going to do or have done that day, talk about the weather, talk about the spots on the wall — the point is to talk in smooth speech about ANYTHING.

You should also select real life situations for daily assignments. For example, a difficult phone call that you must make can be treated as an assignment. In fact ANY opportunity of speaking which you can PLAN, can be used as an assignment. Where possible you should tape record your speech and evaluate it critically.

To help remind yourself to practise during the day, use someone or something from your everyday surroundings to jog your memory. For example, you could ask a particular workmate/friend to help you; you could use morning and afternoon tea break as a reminder to practise, you could stick something on your phone at work to remind you and so on.

SELF-MANAGEMENT

This commences with the identification of trouble spots in your speech. Survey and analyze your speech skills. This is usually easier if you record your speech. Once you have identified what is wrong with your speech technique then you can structure your difficulties from easiest to hardest things to work on. For example: you think your voice sounds boring and choppy, also, that your breathing is poor. So work first on breathing; next on choppiness; last on melody of your speech. By improving your speech in that order you will make each thing you work on easier to resolve. You should design practice strategies. Pick the easiest level to work on for you, for example, Breathing: (i) breathing exercises; (ii) make sure that you do not start speaking without taking a breath; (iii) make sure that you do not stop suddenly and hold your breath — ensure that you are joining your speech. Set goals and rate your success. You may set a pass mark of 5/10 or 50%. When you can achieve that level of success you move on to expect more of your performance: 60%; 75%; 90%; 100%. Finally, reward yourself for your successes as you move through the work you have set for yourself. When you achieve a goal, give yourself something enjoyable. It doesn't have to be extravagant, a biscuit, beer or chocolate will do. You do not have to wait until you reach 100% — reward yourself as you go.

TROUBLE-SHOOTING

In order to 'not stutter' there are a number of things you need to remember. These things are all linked to the SMOOTH SPEECH TECHNIQUE.

If you are having difficulties it is not sufficient to say 'It doesn't work anymore' or a broad 'I'm having problems with my speech'. Saying that you are 'stuttering' does not help you stop, 'stuttering' is only a word, it is not a solution. You need to put some effort into working out what the difficulties are. In order to do this you should listen to your speech in the situations that you are noticing difficulty in. If possible record your speech in the situation/s.

Monitor your speech sample — what sounds wrong or what feels wrong? What seems to have preceded or surrounded your stuttered speech? A general comment about your speech first might help you to define what your difficulty is. For example, your speech might 'sound tight' so you would then work out why it sounds this way. Always analyze your speech in terms of the criteria you learned during your video sessions, namely, breathing, onsets and offsets, joining/continuity, phrasing and pausing, intonation, presentation, and speed. You can then focus on the specific areas to work on. Once you have analyzed your speech does simply correcting each error help to improve your overall fluency? If the answer is no there are a number of things you CAN do.

HIERARCHIES

The concept of a hierarchy is that you pass from one level of difficulty to another. The most logical way of working on a speech skill difficulty (and any possible problems that may have developed with those difficulties) is to commence at the easiest and most successful level and to move on to progressively more difficult tasks. This encourages you to be objective about what you are doing and how well you are working at getting rid of the difficulty.

To become your own therapist in the full sense you must acquire problem solving skills. When you encounter a problem you should try to write out what aspect of the situation presents difficulty for you speech-wise. For example, you may find it difficult to give precise information that you know will be called for, like giving your name at a counter. This situation can be imitated by making telephoned reservations at restaurants without volunteering any information. If you say only that you wish to make a reservation, it forces the other person to ask you the specific information with their own order and timing. You can therefore imitate the lack of control in the original name-at-the-counter situations. Sometimes just thinking about a particular speech situation may make you feel tense and unconfident. To cope with this, you need to learn to make up assignments which are easier approximations of the speaking situations in which you wish to succeed. This allows you to build up fluent 'mileage' and confidence. This is called constructing a hierarchy. For example, someone may find it difficult to make extended enquiries on the telephone. A possible hierarchy would be:

1. Speaking to a recorded message on the telephone (e.g. the time, weather etc).
2. Speaking to a group (or Speak Easy) member.
3. Speaking to someone who you feel relaxed with but who does not speak in smooth speech.
4. Making an enquiry of a stranger which is completely rehearsed before the call. (e.g., finding out the trading hours of all the large stores only requires you to say a single sentence which you can thoroughly rehearse beforehand).
5. Make an enquiry with some uncertainty. (e.g., Ring up about a car advertised for sale in the paper. The car may be sold in which case you finish the call, or it may still be available in which case you enquire about the price and other details).
6. Make an extended enquiry (e.g., travel agent).

Make sure that each step in the hierarchy is practised many times and that you feel completely confident about performing it before progressing to the next step. Remember, no step is too basic to be the first in a hierarchy, and the jump between steps can never be too small.

SELF-REINFORCEMENT

It is essential that you reinforce yourself for your fluency. Whilst you were in the program you had therapists, other group members and your clear progress to motivate and reward you for your efforts. Once you leave the program you may find that you miss the praise and the other signs of 'success'. It is most important to reward yourself for speaking well and even for 'just practising'. Praise yourself, give yourself something nice, perhaps have a break from what you are doing — do or give yourself something that makes you feel good! Other people may expect you to speak well and they may not be aware of the effort it costs you to do this. Remember to reward yourself when you know you have handled a difficult situation.

Make sure you keep on improving how you talk and how you FEEL about how you talk. If you begin to feel discouraged, look at how you are reinforcing yourself. If you begin to feel discouraged because you feel that your practice is not working well enough, contact the clinic to discuss with one of the therapists how you can improve this.

Do not be discouraged by speech difficulties. Having problems with your speech does not mean failure. However it is important that you do not ignore difficulties. Do not be embarrassed to approach your therapists about your speech — good therapists know when to seek help!

SPEECH DIARY

Continue to use the speech diary which you began during the course. The diary should include:

A review of the day's speech

Difficulties that you need to work on

Planned assignments

Evaluations of your recorded assignments

How you may have coped with problems so that stuttering did not occur

How often you felt your speech was good

Be sure to praise yourself when your speech has been good and when you have attempted to do the tasks you set yourself. Remember, other people may not realise what sort of effort you are putting into speaking fluently and so they won't be likely to praise you as much as you may deserve and need.

FOLLOW-UP CONTACT WITH THE CLINIC

You are required to attend five follow-up evenings at one, two, three, six and twelve months after treatment. These are your 'official' follow-up times and we expect to see you.

Follow-up evenings are held on the second Thursday of each month. You are welcome anytime between 5 p.m. and 8 p.m. These evenings help us evaluate your progress and provide assistance to you if necessary.

For official follow-ups you should bring with you a tape recording of at least five minutes of face to face or telephone conversation with a stranger. This is to be a sample of your speech in the real world. It is not an assignment to be made perfect. If you are making errors, we need to hear them to help you. You should also write an assessment to hand in with your tape, just as you did during the course.

If you live too far to come to follow-up, you should do your follow-up by mail. At each official follow-up time you should send us a tape. This tape should have (a) 5 mins phone to stranger (b) a 'rating session' (preferably done with someone rather than alone) consisting of:

3 minutes at 100 SPM
3 minutes at 150 SPM
3 minutes at 180 SPM
3 minutes at 200 SPM

Write an assessment of your tape just as you did during the course. Also let us know how things are going for you and whether you are having any problems. We will assess this tape and mail it back to you before the next tape is due. You are quite welcome to send us a tape anytime you feel you need some feedback. You are most welcome to come to follow-up even if it is not your official time.

PARTICIPATION IN GROUP SELF-HELP ACTIVITIES

The Australian Speak Easy Association is a national self-help group for stutterers. It has been proven to be effective in helping people stay fluent after they have completed treatment. Members meet at each others homes on a regular weekly basis to practise basic fluency skills in a supportive atmosphere. A Speak Easy Toastmasters group is also available for those who wish to develop their presentation and communications skills to a more formal level. We encourage you to attend your regional Speak Easy meeting or Toastmasters group each week for the first six months after you complete the program. After this you can decide how often you need to attend them. We will provide you with the details of the Speak Easy group nearest your home and work place.

SOME FINAL REMINDERS

After you have completed the treatment program you have a choice — you can stutter or you can be fluent. This does not mean that you are 'cured'. It means simply that you have the necessary skills to be fluent and take control of your speech. As your own therapist you must accept responsibility for your fluency.

You have had many years of practising your stuttering but only a few weeks of using your fluency. As with any new skill you must practise it — use it — in order to become better at it and eventually perfect it.

Be proud of the fluency you have achieved. Be realistic about your speech, acknowledge and praise your good speech, but don't pretend it's great when it's not.

Staying fluent requires your time, effort, and commitment from here on. In other words, you don't have to stutter anymore.

All the best!

MAINTENANCE IS DOING WHAT YOU KNOW HOW TO DO ALREADY; SO THE IMPORTANT QUESTION IS *not* 'WHAT SHOULD I DO?', *but* 'HOW CAN I ENCOURAGE MYSELF TO DO IT?'

III THE EFFECTS OF TREATMENT FOR STUTTERING

The treatment of any disorder requires several essential prerequisites. First we need a working understanding of the nature of the problem; next, derived therapeutic methods and techniques that have been demonstrated in experimental settings to have a reliable beneficial impact on the problem; finally, treatment requires evaluation. Without detailed objective evaluation of different treatment programmes there can be little prospect of further progress in the treatment enterprise.

Speech therapists, along with their colleagues in other health care professions, are increasingly being called upon to provide unequivocal evidence that their treatments benefit society. In times of economic stringency priorities have to be set by service managers and planners. There is no argument against the view that *all* services to patients should be scrutinised to gauge their capacity to deal effectively with the problems that confront them. Whilst effective human communication must be a major priority for any health care system it remains to be seen whether the methods currently being employed in this area do have significant and lasting impacts on the diverse problems that cluster under the broad heading of *human communication disorders*.

Although efficacy research continues to be carried out in this area there is no general consensus amongst clinicians on what constitutes an adequate treatment evaluation study. A variety of methodologies exist, but as yet there is no single paradigm that holds sway over all others. In this section of the book we have commissioned two papers that address the central issues in the evaluation of treatment for stuttering.

Ken St. Louis and Janice Westbrook have collaborated to review recent published studies concerning the effects of different treatments for stuttering. They concentrate on some thirty treatment outcome studies and highlight many examples of the kinds of limitations that currently confound much good research in this area. In addition they offer a number of suggestions for future clinical practice and research which would enhance work in this area. In the final chapter Harry Purser takes these methodological and conceptual problems further and outlines several distinct issues in the evaluation of treatment. This paper highlights the need for clarity in our conception of what *scientific evaluation* involves and how such principles translate into clinical practice.

The purpose of this concluding section of the book is to emphasise the need for objective evaluations of therapy for stuttering. We hope that the following discussions will highlight the importance of this topic for the profession and that further progress will be made in the coming years to elucidate the complex relationships between theory and practice that are to be found in this area.

. St. Louis and Janice B. Westbrook

ɔn

to be asked about stuttering by someone totally unfamiliar with
nguage pathology. After fumbling through the answer to 'What
we often find ourselves faced with questions about treatment.
volume have addressed the issue of cause and the questions about
ɔut it?'. Perhaps our goal in this chapter is to address this question
.

ious debate about whether or not we ought to treat stutterers as a
er, a great deal of contradictory information has been written
ss of our treatments. The purposes of this chapter are threefold;
ssues central to evaluating therapeutic effectiveness, review recent
it outcome, and suggest particular strategies which might assist
ng their treatment of stutterers. These are broad purposes, and
xpanded far beyond the detail covered here. Nevertheless, they are
inent to serious attempts by clinicians to improve their own effect-
tutterers.

ffecting Treatment Outcome

tcome of stuttering therapy is not a simple task. A multitude of
rs are involved in deciding whether or not a particular program of
is been effective (Andrews, 1984a; Shames, 1986). In what follows
f discussion of such parameters.

235

Definition of success

Obviously, the definition of success of treatment is an important variable in determining the effectiveness of stuttering therapy. Most current therapies utilize reductions in the frequency of stuttering as the primary criterion for success, measured in terms of stuttered words (or syllables) (e.g., Andrews, Craig, and Feyer, 1983; Ingham, 1980b; Shames and Florance, 1980; Ryan, 1974). Whatever else may be involved, the majority of serious clinical researchers expect their stutterers to achieve speech which is free of stuttering, or nearly so, in order to be considered successful in treatment. (It must be pointed out that this is not the same issue as whether or not any normal dysfluency is permitted (e.g., Boberg, 1986). Nevertheless, individuals such as Cooper (1986b) and Sheehan (1986) have argued that reductions in frequency of stuttering alone is neither a sufficient nor valid indicator of treatment success.

Achieving healthy client attitudes or feelings, or a reduction of avoidance or anxiety, are viewed as essential ingredients in many therapies and, thereby, are considered among the criteria for success (e.g., Cooper and Cooper, 1985b; Rubin, 1986; Sheehan, 1970a; Van Riper, 1973). Instruments such as the *Perceptions of Stuttering Inventory* (Woolf, 1967) and the Andrews and Cutler (1974) S-24 version of the *Erickson Scale of Communication Attitudes* (Erickson, 1969) have been used to assess or predict such internal variables and to gauge their relationship to therapeutic success (e.g., Guitar and Bass, 1978; Webster, 1980).

Recently, considerable research effort has been focused on the *quality* of fluency obtained in therapy, such as the notion of 'speech naturalness' as proposed by Martin, Haroldson and Triden (1984) and supported in a number of studies (Ingham, Gow, and Costello, 1985; Ingham and Onslow, 1985; Ingham *et al.* 1985). From these studies, it is clear that lack of stuttering *per se* may not constitute sufficient evidence to listeners that stuttering therapy was completely effective.

Other factors affecting clinical outcome

In addition to definitional issues, other variables must be taken into account in evaluating reports of clinical effectiveness with stutterers. Some are obvious and logical; others are subtle and troublesome.

Clinical Techniques: For a period of 20 years or so up to the early 1960s most 'mainline' treatments for stutterers in the USA focused either on anxiety-reduction or 'controlling stuttering' or both. During this era, psychotherapeutic approaches (e.g., Sheehan, 1953) and teaching 'controls' (e.g., Van Riper, 1958) were extremely popular. Most therapy efforts were directed at adults since Johnson's (1961a) hands-off policy toward stuttering children was widely accepted.

In the past two decades new stuttering treatments have been widely affected by empirical investigations of various techniques which were found to reduce stuttering very effectively (Beech and Fransella, 1968; Webster, 1977). Two new groups of therapies have emerged which have partly or totally replaced the earlier approaches. These are *contingency management approaches* utilizing operant technology, assumptions, and procedures (Ingham, 1975; Shames and Egolf, 1976) and *fluency shaping techniques* utilizing procedures such as breathstream management, vocalization training, prolonged speech, slowed speech, and delayed auditory feedback (Guitar and Peters, 1980; St. Louis, 1979). In general, although comparative data is limited, these latter approaches have resulted in more effective reductions in stuttering than earlier anxiety reduction or controlled stuttering approaches (Howie and Andrews, 1984; Ingham, 1984b).

Therapeutic model: In addition to consideration of therapeutic technique, the therapy delivery model is a further important factor in carrying out stuttering therapy. One aspect of this variable is the question of whether the stutterer is treated intensively (i.e., for at least several hours a day for a few weeks) as is typical of many stuttering clinics, or non-intensively (i.e., for only a few sessions or hours per week for months or years), as is often utilized in general speech–language clinics or public schools. Again, good comparative data are lacking; yet, it appears that most authorities agree that intensive models are more effective than non-intensive models (Gregory, 1983; Ingham, 1984b; Shames and Florance, 1980; Webster, 1986). Cooper (1986b) disagrees and has lobbied for the twice-a-week non-intensive model. Nevertheless, even Cooper (1979a) has stated that the intensive model may serve a useful purpose at the outset of therapy.

Another aspect of the model of therapy variable is the issue of whether or not maintenance strategies are included. The 1979 Banff conference in Canada on Maintenance of Fluency was a major effort directed at addressing this issue (Boberg, 1981). The clear consensus from experts at that conference was that stuttering therapy must include maintenance components, yet to be agreed on, if stutterers are to be expected to reduce the likelihood of relapse. This issue has become so important that it now appears likely that clinical reports of stuttering therapy without follow-up data for at least two years duration post-treatment will either not be taken seriously or, perhaps, will not even be publishable in journals serious about scientific rigour.

Client differences: Another important consideration in assessing the effectiveness of stuttering therapy lies in differences between clients. Age is extremely important. The current consensus is that stuttering therapy is more effective with children than with adults and that 'cures' are quite common among young and very young stutterers (Costello, 1984a; Gregory, 1979b; Ryan, 1986). It is important, however, to be aware that many of these treatment successes with young stutterers may have occurred without any direct treatment (Curlee, 1980). Spontaneous recovery data indicate that from 40 to 80 per cent of childhood stutterers will recover without any formal speech therapy (Andrews, 1984a,b; Ingham, 1983; Wingate, 1976) although certain authors (e.g., Cooper, 1979a; Ingham, 1983; Shine, 1984a,b) have written that many of these recoveries were likely due to direct parental and other influences. Given that a large percentage of young stutterers will recover without *professional* treatment, there is almost certainly a case to be made for the role of spontaneous recovery in the process of clinical treatment for young stutterers (Martin, 1981).

Severity: Severity is another important factor in evaluating stuttering treatments. In general, it is assumed that more severe stutterers do worse in therapy than less severe stutterers (Hinzman and St. Louis, 1983; Ryan, 1981; Sacco, 1986; Van Riper, 1973).

Etiology: It is possible that etiology may also play a role in treatment outcome. Certainly, neurogenic stutterers have different prognoses than developmental stutterers (Helm-Estabrooks, 1986; Rosenbek, 1984). Also, stutterers with various other atypical influences such as mental retardation (Cooper, 1986a), cultural differences (Leith, 1986), gender (i.e., female stutterers) (Silverman, 1986), cluttering (Daly, 1986), and psychological maladjustment (Cox, 1986) are likely to respond differently to treatment than the 'typical' stutterer.

Motivation: Motivation is another factor which significantly influences therapeutic effectiveness. Stutterers who have: the ability to self-reinforce (Cooper and Cooper, 1985b; Shames and Florance, 1980), an internal locus of control (Craig, Franklin, and Andrews, 1984), needs for fluent speech (Van Riper, 1973), and willingness to wait for and then complete a comprehensive therapy regimen (Ingham, 1981) do better than those who seem to require constant direction or reinforcement from others, have less natural penalty for stuttering, or do not complete therapy requirements consistently.

Summary

For all these client factors, with the possible exception of age, there is practically no comparative data available in the literature where clients with different attributes were systematically compared on the same treatments. All of the above statements are the result of *post-hoc* analyses of treatment outcomes, much the same as any careful clinician would do.

Clinician Characteristics

An area which has received very little research attention but which may well affect treatment outcome is that of clinician characteristics. Van Riper (1975) and Cooper and Cooper (1985a) have described the general characteristics of the effective clinician for stuttering, such as empathy, genuineness, and a willingness to 'mix it up' with the client. However, others within the behaviorist tradition have stressed the need for clinicians to be objective, unbiased, consistent, and rigorous in their clinical style (Ingham, 1981; Webster, 1986). The issue of training and experience is no doubt another important variable here as well, at least from the perspective of the clinician (Costello, 1984a; Leith, 1971; St. Louis and Lass, 1980). For example, clinicians have indicated in a number of surveys that skill in counseling techniques is an important ingredient within the clinician's repertoire (Cooper and Cooper, 1985a; Cooper and Rustin, 1985; St. Louis and Lass, 1981). In spite of the obvious importance of clinician training, orientation, experience and personal characteristics, there is no available systematic data which indicates clearly which clinicians are likely to treat stutterers effectively and which are not.

Recent Evidence

A review of the effectiveness of stuttering therapy is beneficial when it helps us refine our definition of success and when it challenges us to improve our skills. Several such reviews have appeared in the past few years. In 1979, Sommers *et al.*, examined 287 studies published from 1967 to 1977, and observed that many methodological faults which had been identified 10 to 20 years earlier remained prevalent in stuttering research. Many reports contained no information about sex, and sample sizes were usually small, i.e., less than five subjects. Studies involving children appeared irregularly with the average client being a young adult. Treatment studies comprised only 20 per cent of the total studies of stutterers in each of the 10 years. The authors did not survey the measures used (e.g., frequency of stuttering), but only 63 per cent of the studies (mostly non-treatment investigations) permitted formal hypothesis testing.

In 1980, Andrews, Guitar and Howie provided an ambitious meta-analysis of stuttering treatments spanning 31 years from 1948 to 1979. They examined a carefully selected sample of studies which had reported before and after measures of fluency, and from which *treatment effect sizes* could be calculated (see Smith and Glass, 1977 for details of the meta-analysis procedure). Forty-two studies, covering the treatment of 756 stutterers, were considered, and six common principal treatment models were identified and ranked in order of effectiveness:

1 Prolonged speech, 2 Gentle onset, 3 Rhythm, 4 Airflow, 5 Attitude therapies, 6 Systematic desensitisation

Overall the improvements from prolonged speech and gentle onset were reported to be more effective than the others and to be more stable over a 12-month period following therapy.

In 1981, Martin's review of research pertaining to the maintenance of fluency was published as part of the proceedings of the 1979 Banff Conference. In examining the efforts of thirteen clinicians and their clinical teams (from 1958 through 1977) Martin placed maintenance efforts in one of the two categories which seemed to be related to clinical effectiveness. The client's speech was either assessed at a predetermined date following the termination of therapy, or programmed maintenance activities were carried out after intensive treatment had been completed. Martin then stated that the data could not conclusively recommend either approach in regard to maintenance, but he did suggest that a review of the studies allowed a 'crude estimate' of clinical effectiveness to be made. The 'estimate' was that one-third of the clients achieved and maintained satisfactory fluency, one-third achieved fluency during therapy but regressed over time, and one-third either failed to complete treatment programs or were unavailable for follow-up assessment. He viewed this 'drop-out' factor as a crucial hindrance to the evaluation of therapy programs. He also observed that a higher quality of fluency improvement seemed to occur with children, and discussed the possible coincidence of treatment and 'spontaneous recovery'.

Adams (1984d) reviewed the research and therapy from 1977 to 1982 and noted a veering toward more psychological explanations of stuttering. He saw two major consequences of this shift. One was a renewed faith in prolonged speech as a tool of proven worth, especially for adults. The other was an increase in the use of more direct therapy techniques with children. Ingham and Costello (1985) compared effectiveness data from adults and children in 36 studies published from 1965 to 1981. They chose studies which permitted estimates of the treatment time required to decrease stuttering by at least 50 per cent. Their findings also supported the premise that children respond 'a shade more rapidly' than adults to most treatment procedures, especially the response contingent techniques.

Bloodstein (1981) reflected the profession's readiness for a new era of accountability and specificity when he provided criteria for judging client progress in stuttering therapy. He suggested that as clinicians we should provide objective measures of therapy results, with ample and representative groups of stutterers. He also stated that repeated and adequate samples of speech should be assessed in settings outside of therapy. Factors other than frequency of stuttering were recommended for speech assessment. Speech naturalness and spontaneity, as well as the client's 'sense of handicap' and 'need to monitor' should be documented. Estimates of effectiveness should be realistic, and the use of controls was recommended, as was consistent demonstration of success over time with various clinicians.

The Current Review

Bearing in mind these recent challenges, we reviewed the major journals and books published from 1980 to present, and using guidelines similar to those used by Andrews *et al.* (1980), we listed studies which were:

1 clearly intended to be therapeutic in nature
2 involved at least three subjects
3 reported data from which clinical effectiveness could be determined (Table 1).

The studies in Table 1 have been roughly divided according to the ages of clients receiving treatment. Eleven of the thirty reports pertained to therapy provided for children from 3 to 14 years of age. Three concerned therapy for children and adults, and sixteen outlined methods used with teenagers and adults.

The review of methods used with adults reinforces the observations of Andrew *et al.* (1980) and Adams (1984d) that prolonged speech (or some variant thereof) is currently the treatment of choice for adults who stutter. Rate control also figured significantly in these approaches. Modification of moments of stuttering was not a principal tool in any of the studies, although it was used indirectly by some. Many of the studies described provision for counseling clients, but few listed this as a significant part of therapy. Desensitization, which once played a major role in treatment of stuttering, was seldom mentioned. This is especially interesting when considered in the light of the fact that seven of the studies used attitudinal scales either as assessment tools or as efficacy measures.

Seven of the eleven methods used with children advocated direct manipulation of fluent speech patterns, in a manner similar to the prolonged speech and rate control used with adults. Six of the eleven methods mentioned parent counselling and even parental involvement in therapy. Delayed auditory feedback did not figure significantly in any of the methods used exclusively with adults, and it was the tool of change in only two approaches with children (Robb *et al.* 1985; Ryan, 1984). Overall, the programs for children were broader in nature than the adult programs. Desensitization and selective parental attention were used, along with language assessment and facilitation. Two clinical teams (Gregory and Hill, 1984; Riley and Riley, 1984) provided not only differential assessment, but distinctive therapy tracks for children who exhibited other communication deficits.

With Martin's (1981) 'drop-out' estimate in mind, we listed both the total clients who began treatment and the number of clients available for post assessment when this information was provided (11 of the 30 studies). Only two approaches with children utilized intensive scheduling, while 9 of the 16 programs for adults included a period of intensive therapy. Therapy durations ranged from two 90-minutes sessions (Ladoucer *et al.,* 1982) to two years (Runyan and Runyan, 1986). Interestingly, Runyan and Runyan were the only authors who reported empirical data collected specifically in the public schools.

Table 1.   Recent stuttering treatment studies.

Clinicians	Methods	Total Clients/ No. for Study and Client Ages	Therapy Schedule and Duration	Measures of Effectiveness and Averaged Results
		CHILDREN		
1 Craig and Cleary (1982)	Electromyographic feedback, self monitoring	/3 10–14 yrs. (range)	1 hr. sessions, 7–8 sessions (total)	Reductions (% change) in per cent syllables stuttered from baseline (after EMG feedback alone 25.83; after EMG and self-control 71.99; 2–9 mos. post 80.33)
2 Culp (1984)	Prolonged speech, language stimulation, parent counseling; desensitization	32/14 4.1 yrs. (mean)	1 hr./wk, 45 hrs. (mean)	% Stuttered words, average of 5 situations (pre 11.44; post 2.95; 3 mos. post to 2 yrs. post 2.85)
3 Gregory and Hill (1984)	Differential assessment and treatment depending on presence of concomitant communicative problems: parent counseling, modeling, desensitization, choral reading, modification of psychomotor speech responses	Children	2 1/2 hrs./wk., 9–18 mos. (total)	Clinicians's estimate of fluency (70% develop normal fluency)
4 Johnson (1984)	parental modeling of slow rate and continuous breathflow, and selective parental attention	/7 3.0 to 6.1 yrs. (range)	2 sessions/wk,	⁴% Stuttered syllables (pre 5.1; 2 mos. 3 wks. to 2 yrs. post 2.5, 6 subjects)

5	Riley and Riley (1983, 1984)	Differential assessment and treatment as needed in the following areas: attending disorders, articulatory or neurologic components, language disorders, parental counseling, and modification of remaining abnormal disfluencies	54/44 3-0 to 12-9 yrs. (range)	47.9 hrs. (mean)	Average ratings (0 to 5) of stuttering severity (pre, none reported; post 1.06; 12 to 23 mos. post; 24 to 48 mos. post .86)
6	Robb et al. (1985)	Delayed auditory feedback	/12 7-14 yrs. (mean)	5 days/wk., for 1 wk.	% Stuttered words (pre 15; post 3, 2 mos. post 5)
7	Runyan and Runyan (1986)	Fluency rules to modify rate, breathing, articulatory pressure, and secondary features	/9 3-8 to 7-1 yrs. (range)	20-30 mins./wk., 2-3 sessions/wk, 2 yrs. (total)	[4]Stuttered words/5 minute sample (pre 41.55; end of 1 yr. 2.22; end of 2 yrs. 2.0, 5 subjects)
8	Shenker et al. (1983)	Rate and breath control, easy articulation, peer-mediation, parent counseling	9/8 8-14 yrs. (range)	4 days/wk. for 3 wks., 5 hrs. at 3 mo. follow-up, 45 hrs. (total)	% Stuttered words (pre 20.7; post 9.5; 3 mos. post 7.7, 7 subjects)
9	Shine (1984a, 1984b)	Prolonged speech, modification of physiologic, prosodic and linguistic variables, parent counseling	18/14 2-9 to 8-0 yrs. (range)	40-50 mins./wk., 56.7 sessions (mean)	[4,5]Stuttered words/min. (pre 13.9; post 1.7; 14-64 mos. post 3.2)
10	[1]Stocker and Gerstman (1983)	Control of utterance length and linguistic complexity	28/24 6-11 yrs. (mean)	7.4 mos. (mean)	[6]Average ratings (1 to 6) of stuttering severity (pre 5.4; post 2.4)

Table 1. Recent stuttering treatment studies. (continued)

	Clinicians	Methods	Total Clients/ No. for Study and Client Ages	Therapy Schedule and Duration	Measures of Effectiveness and Averaged Results
			CHILDREN		
11	Wakaba (1983)	Group play therapy	5/3 4–6 to 5–3 yrs. (range)	1 hr./wk., 16.3 sessions (mean)	[6]Average ratings (0 to 7) of stuttering severity, clinician and parent (pre 2; post .6)
			CHILDREN AND ADULTS		
12	Cooper (1984)	Rate and breath control, easy articulation, loudness control, syllable stress, counseling	2–5 to 50 yrs. (range)	Dependent on age, severity, setting and other factors	Author's estimate of results (pre; post 60% had prolonged periods of fluency; 3 yrs. 20% had prolonged periods of fluency and 40% controlled their stuttering)
13	Ryan (1984)	Control of utterance length and linguistic complexity, delayed auditory feedback	/500 children and adults	19 hrs. for estab. and transfer, 2 1/2 hrs. for maint., 21.5 hrs. (total)	% Stuttered words (pre 7; post 1; 1yr. post 90% subjects at 1%)
14	Weiner (1984)	Breath control, easy voice onset, optimum oral resonance, desensitization	66/37 children and adults	1 hr. 40 mins./wk, 14–156 sessions (range)	[5.7%] 'Stuttering events' (pre, none reported; post, none reported; 1 to 6 yrs. post (95%) fluent, 10 subjects)

ADULTS

15	[2]**Andrews and Tanner (1982b)**	Regulated breathing	/6 26 yrs. (mean)	6 hrs./day, 1 day/wk. for 2 wks.	4.7% Stuttered syllables (pre 15.6; post 5.9; 2 wks. post; 12 wks. post 9.1)
16	[2]**Andrews and Tanner (1982a)**	Passive airflow technique	/6 adult	8 hrs./day on days 1, 2, 3, 8 and 30, 40 hrs. (total)	4.7%Stuttered syllables (pre 12.5; post 2.7; 6 mos. post; 12 mos. post 9.9)
17	**Boberg et al. (1983)**	Prolonged speech, easy voice onset and articulation, continuous airflow	11/11 29.2 yrs. (mean)	7 hrs./day, 5 days/wk. for 3 wks.	7% Stuttered syllables (pre 12.5; post .7)
18	**Evesham and Huddleston (1983)** [1]**Evesham and Fransella (1985)**	Prolonged speech, token economy, personal construct therapy	48/46 adult 18–65 yr. (range)	5 days/wk. for 2 wks. then weekly, fortnightly and monthly sessions	7% Stuttered syllables pre: 29 subjects ≥ 10% pre: 18 subjects 2–10% post: 43 subjects 0–1% post: 4 subjects 1–5% 9 mos. post 18 mos. post, 24 subjects 16 subjects 0–1% 5 subjects 1–5% 3 subjects ≥ 10%
19	**Franck (1980)**	Prolonged speech	441/103 20.2 yrs. (mean)	weekly for 6 mos., then 5 days/wk. for 1 wk., then monthly 128.5 hrs. (maximum)	percentage of increase in fluent syllables 20% subjects — 80–100% 39% subjects — 50–79% 21% subjects — 1–49% 20% subjects — no improvement

Table 1. Recent stuttering treatment studies. (continued)

	Clinicians	Methods	Total Clients/ No. for Study and Client Ages	Therapy Schedule and Duration	Measures of Effectiveness and Averaged Results
			ADULTS		
20	Howie et al. (1981)	Slow onset of phonation, continuous airflow and movement of articulators, extension of vowel and consonant durations	/40 adult	12 hrs./day for 3 wks.	[4.7]% Stuttered syllables (pre 12.1; post .5; 6 mos. post; 2 yrs. post 4.1)
21	Kuhr and Rustin (1985)	Relaxation, regulated-breathing exercises, counseling	8/7 33.75 yrs. (mean)	5 days/wk. for 3 wks., outpatient for 6 mos., phase out for 6–9 mos.	[4]% Stuttered syllables (pre 14.3; post 2.4; 6 mos. post; post 5.9)
22	Ladouceur et al. (1982)	Regulated breathing, relaxation	/12 17–74 yrs. (range)	90 min./session for 2 sessions	[4]% Stuttered words (pre 11.5; post 5.6; 2 mos. post 8.4)
23	[3]Maxwell (1982)	Verbal setting and information giving, cognitive appraisal, thought reversal, vicarious observation, description, identification, termination, anticipation, regulation, cognitive restructuring, coping skills, self-management and self-monitoring	/23 24 yrs. (mean)	1 hr./wk., 1.5 yrs. (mean)	[5,7]Stuttering Severity Instrument scores and severity equivalent ratings (pre 11% stuttered words, moderate; post 4% stuttered words, mild)

	Treatment techniques	N / age	Duration	Measures / results
24 [1,3]**Peins et al. (1984)**	Rate control, modification of phonatory patterns and self-monitoring	/31 13–43 yrs. (range)	12 home lessons, and 30 min. sessions every 2 wks. 6 mos. (total)	Average ratings (1 to 7) of stuttering severity (pre 4.90; post 3.77; 6–12–18–24 mos. post; 30 mos. post 2.85, 7 subjects)
25 **Perkins (1984)**	Rate control, phrasing, modification of vocal, articulatory and prosodic factors	/300 teens to adults	50 hrs. (approx.) for establishment	Clinician's rating of post fluency (95% fluent at slow to normal rate, 80% with normally expressive speech)
26 **Ramig (1984)**	Prolonged speech (on initial syllable of sentences only)	/9 18–37 yrs. (range)	3–5 hrs./wk., 10.5 mos. (mean)	[4]Average disfluencies/reading 200-word passage (pre 32.66; post 9.44)
27 **Sacco (1986)**	(For severe clients) implosion therapy, proprioceptive awareness, breath and rate control	/135 teens and adults	5 days/wk. for 5 wks. 200 hrs. (total)	[7]% Stuttered words (pre 25.91; post .44)
28 **Stromsta (1986)**	Education about stuttering, voluntary coarticulation, counseling	/30 young adult	2 hrs/wk. 12 weeks (total)	[5,7]% Stuttered words (pre 24; post approx. 2.5)
29 **Webster (1980)**	Rate and breath control, easy voice onset and articulation	/200 adult	5 days/wk. for 3 wks.	% Stuttered words (pre 15.2; post 1.3; avg. 10 mos. post 3.2)
30 **Wingate (1984)**	Education about stuttering, modification of voice onset, articulatory pressure and prosody	/14 college-age adults (avg.)	1.5 hrs./week	Clinician's 'qualitative' judgment of fluency (pre, short-term effect, long-term effect)

[1] Incorporated comparison of therapies.
[2] Involved replication of therapy techniques.
[3] Used control groups.
[4] Also measured speaking rate.
[5] Also measured stuttering severity.
[6] Also measured social maturity.
[7] Also measured general anxiety or attitude.

As in the description of methods, an attempt has been made to explain measures of effectiveness and averaged results in the terms used by the individual authors. Empirical evidence of progress is given when this was provided by the author. Time periods between post-therapy and final follow-up assessments are listed for only the final follow-up. Twelve of the thirty studies reported no information on effectiveness past the post-therapy assessment. Eight studies reported follow-up data during the first year following therapy. Seven studies reported assessment for 1 to 2 years following therapy. Three studies followed clients for 4 to 6 years after therapy. When the information was provided, the number of subjects remaining in the final post-therapy assessment was included in the table. Although several studies replicated or compared therapies, only two studies provided information from control groups.

Twenty-one studies measured frequency of stuttering; four studies used severity ratings to measure effectiveness. Other measures included were percentage of increase in fluency, speaking rate, measures of social maturity, general anxiety, and attitude. One study (Wakaba, 1983) allowed parents to join in judging therapy effectiveness, and one study (Maxwell, 1982) reported data on client's judgments of stuttering, speech-related stress, and effective use of controls. Most follow-up data revealed some degree of relapse, but none of the level of pre-treatment measures. This was true even for the three studies with 4- to 6-year follow-up data (Riley and Riley, 1984; Shine, 1984a,b; Weiner, 1984). A tendency was noted amongst adult patients for higher final follow-up levels of dysfluency than was seen in children, indicating that relapse, when it occurs, is more pronounced in adults.

Enhancing Clinical Effectiveness

The preceding review suggests that stutterers can be treated effectively. It is also clear that accepting all clinical and research reports at face value will undoubtedly result in overly optimistic expectations. This point is dramatically true to many practitioners who regularly treat stutterers outside the main stuttering research and treatment centers. We have consulted with practitioners, mostly in public school settings, who, like others surveyed, openly admit that they are pessimistic about the results of stuttering therapy (Cooper, 1986b; Cooper and Cooper, 1985a; Cooper and Rustin, 1985; St. Louis and Lass, 1981; Wingate, 1971). Among the common complaints we hear are: 'I don't know what to do with stutterers'; 'I tried X treatment, and it didn't work'; 'He was completely fluent, but now he is stuttering as much as ever'; 'I'm discouraged'. These are legitimate concerns which must be addressed if stutterers who are not fortunate enough to attend the best programs are to be effectively treated. The remainder of this chapter is devoted to suggestions, drawn as much from our own clinical experience as the research data and 'expert opinion' which may enhance and facilitate better short-term and long-term success with stutterers.

Clinicians' concerns about stuttering therapy seem to center on two simple questions: 'How do you get stutterers fluent?' and 'How do you keep them fluent?' Perhaps these are so obvious as to be trite, like the boxer who is told he has only two things to worry about, his opponent's 'right' and his 'left'. Nevertheless, they do place clinician concerns into a useful perspective. Clinicians are unlikely to be concerned about issues concerning the definition of stuttering, reducing total treatment time, or atypical influences if they have been unable to eliminate stuttering even temporarily in the majority of their clients. Likewise, clinicians who cannot get clients to transfer their fluency from the therapy room to the classroom are unlikely to be concerned about long-term maintenance strategies. We suggest that the clinician must arrive first at a satisfactory method to get stutterers fluent, and then address the issue of how to keep them fluent.

Getting Stutterers Fluent

Therapeutic techniques

The most comprehensive attempt to compare therapeutic techniques used in the treatment of stuttering was the meta-analysis conducted by Andrews, *et al.* (1980). They concluded that therapies which taught 'prolonged speech' or gentle vocal onset were the most effective, followed by the rhythm, airflow, attitude, desensitization, and all other therapies. We find that there is no reason to change that conclusion, although it is possible that popularity may be confused with success (Ingham, 1984b). Recent research reviewed in Table 1 does not suggest the superiority of any one technique but has reaffirmed that stuttering in most stutterers can be effectively reduced with such techniques as precision fluency shaping, delayed auditory feedback, and teaching a slow, prolonged form of speech. There is also reason to believe that operant techniques such as reinforcing progressively longer and more complex fluent utterances while simultaneously punishing occasions of stuttering are usually effective.

We hasten to point out that the efficacy of the above techniques has been shown with groups of 'typical' stutterers which we can assume has mild to moderate dysfluency (Ryan, 1986; Soderberg, 1962) without complicating psychological, neurological, or cultural factors (Bloodstein, 1981). As stuttering symptoms can be compounded by other problems such as extreme anxiety, psychological or social problems, articulation and language disabilities, or other atypical influences, further individually-tailored therapy techniques are likely to be useful (Gregory, 1984a; Riley and Riley, 1983, 1984; St. Louis, 1986b, Van Riper, 1973).

Nevertheless, although unproven, it is important to keep in mind that a few stutterers probably cannot be effectively treated with any program currently available (Cooper, 1986b; Martin, 1981). Adult stutterers reach this conclusion quite frequently on their own.

Therapy model

As noted previously, the delivery model is assumed to play an important role in determining the success of stuttering therapy. Based on our own experience and discussions with clinicians we would suggest that this factor makes the greatest difference between the outcome of stuttering therapy at the well-known stuttering centers and the remaining treatment locations, including public schools and out-patient clinics.

It is beyond the scope of this chapter to review the historical development of delivery models for stuttering therapy. It seems plausible that the typical delivery models for stuttering therapy evolved as much to suit clinicians' tastes, administrators' desires, school, university, or hospital schedules, or physicians' prescriptions as they did to provide the maximum benefit to stutterers. Regardless of why stuttering therapy is carried out as it is, most clients are treated in either intensive or non-intensive settings. Moreover, it appears that intensive therapy is characteristic of most successful research reports (Ingham, 1984b; Shames and Florance, 1980; Van Riper, 1973; Webster, 1986), although there are advocates for non-intensive schedules (Cooper, 1986b). Our interaction with public school personnel leads us to be pessimistic about the advisability of attempting to make stutterers fluent through brief sessions a few times a week (e.g., 20 minutes twice a week). Frequently, there is neither the amount nor duration of training necessary to establish the skills required for improved fluency with these schedules. Clients often do not learn the skills well, forget or fail to practise them between sessions, and end up losing interest in therapy.

A careful look at the most successful therapy programs suggests that a mix of the two models may be better than either alone (e.g., Cooper, 1979a). Intensive therapy seems to be highly effective in helping stutterers become fluent early in the therapy process (Ingham, 1975; 1984b; Prins, 1976; Shames and Florance, 1980; Van Riper, 1973; Webster, 1986). Problems with relapse arise when stutterers are dismissed after intensive therapy with no long-term, non-intensive maintenance program (Kuhr and Rustin, 1985; Prins, 1970).

For adults, intensive residential programs are typically run for a few (e.g., three to five) weeks (Andrews, Craig, and Feyer, 1983; Hasbrouck and Lowry-Romero, 1983; Rustin and Kuhr, 1983; Sacco, 1986; Webster, 1980). Less information is available for children, but intensive therapy durations have been reported from two to six weeks (St. Louis, 1986a; Williams, 1971). Other variants of intensive programs have been developed, such as referral to the stuttering expert in a school district (Mallard and Westbrook, 1983; Van Riper, 1977) or intensive weekend workshops (Boberg, 1983).

Criteria for success

It is axiomatic that when individuals are trained in a new skill, they perform that skill better under the controlled conditions of training than in other situations. Therefore, it is not surprising that stutterers, like other speech or language clients, do better while in therapy than in extra-therapy settings.

For this reason a number of clinicians have argued that stutterers in direct therapy should be expected to achieve speech entirely free of stuttering before being permitted to advance in therapy (Andrews *et al.* 1983; Ingham, 1980; Ryan, 1986). This reduces the occurrence of stuttering in later therapy steps or in untrained settings (Webster, 1986). Clinical supervisory experience also suggests that clinicians who expect fluent speech from their clients are more likely to get it than those who are more 'flexible'. For all but the youngest stutterers, we therefore suggest that whenever possible, clinicians set strenuous criteria of 'no stuttering' or other abnormalities for their stutterers in the early stages of theory in order to enhance their later progress, transfer, and maintenance. For pre-school stutterers such strict criteria are not necessary (Gregory and Hill, 1984) and may not even be desirable.

Recent evidence suggests that speech which is free of stuttering is not perceived by listeners to be normal (e.g., Runyan, Hames and Prosek, 1982). We recommend that clinicians insist that their stutterers learn to vary prosodic elements in their speech (i.e., intonation, syllable stress, and pauses), such that their non-stuttered speech appears more spontaneous or natural to the listener. A recent study done in the USA and Australia demonstrated that stutterers *could* improve their listener-perceived 'speech naturalness' ratings (Ingham *et al.* 1985).

Atypical influences

In spite of our best efforts to achieve complete fluency from our clients some will not respond like most stutterers in therapy due to atypical characteristics relating to etiology, severity, or other factors (St. Louis, 1986b). In such cases the clinician should consider altering the usual therapeutic regimen so that the individual needs of the client may be met. Ordinarily, the client's prognosis for improvement is adjusted downward as well. There is some disagreement about the desirability of such changes (e.g., Webster, 1986) and certainly we do not mean that clinicians should look for reasons to fail in their attempts to instill fluent speech, or to give up after the first evidence of difficulty encountered by the client. Instead, clinicians simply need to be aware that it is acceptable not to succeed with every client. In this regard we might recall the closing words in Bloodstein's (1981) book:

the basic therapeutic problem posed by stuttering may represent about the same kind and degree of difficulty as is involved in the problem of rooting out a superstition, dogma, or prejudice. Perhaps the ultimate advances in our ability to cope with stuttering must await more adequate scientific theories of learning and cognition that will enable us to deal better with the common-place irrationalities of everyday living (p. 394).

Keeping Stutterers Fluent

Therapeutic techniques

As noted previously, stutterers should be free of stuttering before being dismissed from training. Nevertheless, this is not enough; relapse is a ubiquitous and familiar problem in stuttering therapy (e.g., Bloodstein, 1981; Kuhr and Rustin, 1985; Perkins, 1981; Shames, 1981; Silverman, 1981; Van Riper, 1973). The evidence is fairly clear that transfer and maintenance activities are helpful in preventing relapse among treated stutterers (Boberg, 1981; Ryan, 1974, 1981) although research in this area is limited and difficult to do (Ingham, 1981, 1984a).

Transfer activities

Transfer of fluency refers to the generalization of gains made in the original therapy setting to extra-therapy situations. It could logically be argued that transfer is a part of getting stutterers fluent in the first place (Van Riper, 1973; Webster, 1986). Neverthe-less, it is also true that most programs do not attempt to generalize fluency to other settings until the stutterer has been able to speak fluently in the original clinical setting (Ryan, 1974; Shames and Florance, 1980).

Carrying out transfer activities is often one of the most difficult aspects of stutter-ing therapy. Transfer is often resisted by stutterers because it frequently involves con-fronting the stuttering in real social situations where anxiety is at its greatest (Van Riper, 1973). Nevertheless, numerous reports document the necessity of these transfer activities (Ryan, 1974; Sacco, 1986; Shames and Florance, 1980; Van Riper, 1958, 1973).

We take the position that the therapeutic effort devoted to transfer will increase the time in therapy but will also increase the likelihood that fluency will be maintained. Obviously, it will be easier for most clients to remain fluent while describing a tele-vision program for 30 minutes to a familiar clinician than to carry out an assignment to schedule and go through a job interview without stuttering.

Table 2   A sampling of transfer of fluency activities for stutterers. [1]

Varying the audience

    Number of listeners
    Status of listeners
    Age of listeners

Varying listeners reactions

    Degree of listener sensitivity (i.e., positive to negative)

Varying speaking situations

    Perceived ease or difficulty of situation
    Length of situations
    Degree of rehearsal

Varying location

    Similarity or dissimilarity to usual clinical setting
    Familiarity or nonfamiliarity of setting

Varying the time of day

Varying speaking tasks

    Type of speech task (e.g., oral reading, monologue, or conversation)
    Pragmatic function (e.g., informing, persuading, requesting, warning or joking)
    Hierarchy of difficulty (e.g., conversations with friends, conversations with strangers,
        opinion surveys, or job interviews)
    Perceived ease or difficulty of words within the speaking task
    Using the telephone
    Client's conversational role (i.e., initiating or receiving calls)
    Practice of other transfer activities on the telephone
    Role-playing speaking situations
    Rehearsal of assigned situations
    'Psychodramas' to explore new feelings and attitudes
    Practising at home
    Talking to other family members
    Talking or reading alone

Practising in outside situations

    Presence or absence of clinician
    Presence or absence of clinician planning
    Evaluation carried out simultaneously or later
    Collection of large 'quotas' of stuttering (i.e., 'stuttering bath')

Table 2   Continued

Practising in the classroom

Class participation which is prearranged and rehearsed or spontaneous
Discussion of client's therapy with the rest of the class
Oral reading while volunteer(s) count stutterings

Negotiating behavioral contracts

Practice in specified situations
Practice during specified time periods

Enlisting the aid of, and training, volunteers to assist in monitoring

Parents or family members
Other stutterers
Friends

Monitoring speech in outside situations

Counting stutterings
Concentrating on fluency enhancing targets

Pseudostuttering in communicative situations

Training in self-responsibility

Self-instruction
Self-monitoring
Self-evaluation
Self-consequation

Beginning to gradually reduce clinic contacts

[1]This list is not exhaustive and contains activities which overlap with others. Clinicians are advised to select those techniques which are pertinent to their clients' needs. Sources for this list of transfer activities include: Van Riper (1958, 1973), Ryan (1974), Dell (1980), Shames and Florance (1980), Howie, Tanner and Andrews (1981), St. Louis (1982), Boberg (1983), Williams (1983), Boberg and Kully (1984), and the authors' clinical experience.

St. Louis (1982) recommended that clinicians consider a number of transfer activities to solidify their stutterers' fluency and, thereby, reduce the likelihood of future relapse. Table 2 provides a list of such activities, extracted from clinical and research reports, which could be utilized by clinicians interested in bolstering the transfer components of their therapy programs.

Maintenance activities

As noted earlier, the issue of maintenance has become critically important in evaluating

Table 3   A sampling of maintenance of fluency activities for stutterers.[1]

Completing all establishment, transfer, and maintenance activities

Reducing clinic contacts gradually

Not contingent on maintaining fluency
Contingent on maintaining fluency

Self-monitoring and/or practicing regularly

Assessing stuttering

Overt and covert checks by clinician and others
Analysis of self-recorded tapes
Periodic questionnaires
Randomly-spaced telephone calls

Improving fluency

Continuous reading or free association
Shadowing other speakers
Repeating sequences (e.g., jokes) over and over until fluent
Scanning for fluency instead of stuttering
Making new techniques and strategies automatic
Continuing monitoring of speech
Practicing 'hard' words over and over until perfect
Overlearning motor responses
Increasing speech rate with new strategies
Verbalizing and planning for potentially difficult strategies
Reinforcing monitored speech with unmonitored speech until they sound alike
Practising overcorrection for errors or nonperformance

Guiding stutterers into self-help groups with clear purposes and time limits

Utilizing consequences during establishment which enhance maintenance

Using variable schedules
Using delayed reinforcement
Fading out contingencies

Assisting stutterers in changing their self-concepts toward those of fluent speakers

Reassurance and support by a trusted, respected clinician
Group sessions among stutterers to discuss problems
Psychological counseling by trained counselors
Following and assisting clients for at least two years (possibly as long as five years)

Table 3   Continued

Improving or regenerating stutter–reducing or fluency–enhancing skills

> Refresher sessions at clinic
> Booster sessions
> Specific days or weekends
> Reunions
> Recycling through the therapy program

Teaching skills of self-control, problem solving, and self-management

> Improve self-observation and self-monitoring
> Improve skills in modifying one's own environment
> Slowing down during periods of anticipated difficulty

Providing clinician models which are consistent and disciplined

Utilizing different maintenance strategies for high versus low self reinforcers

Preventing relapse

> Discussing reasons for relapse
> Planning imaginary relapses and vicarious courses of action
> Training clients to become their own clinicians
> Encouraging activities or jobs which require considerable talking
> Striving for healthy acceptance of necessary daily monitoring or practice for continued
> fluency
> Discussing new life style changes

[1]This list is not exhaustive and contains activities which overlap with others. Clinicians are advised to select those techniques which are pertinent to their clients' needs. Sources for this list of maintenance activities include: Van Riper (1958, 1973), Ryan (1974, 1981), Ingham and Packman (1977), Ingham (1980a, 1982). Shames and Florance (1980), Boberg (1981, 1983, 1986), Howie, Tanner and Andrews (1981), Perkins (1981, 1983), Andrews and Craig (1982), St. Louis (1982), Craig, Franklin and Andrews (1984), Webster (1986), Sacco (1986), and the authors' clinical experience.

therapeutic effectiveness. In spite of this, there is an 'empirical lag' in the stuttering literature pertaining to documented effectiveness of maintenance activities compared to stutter-reducing establishment activities (St. Louis, 1982). Many maintenance activities are drawn from other areas, such as weight loss, physical fitness, or smoking cessation programs (Owen, 1981) and are derived from a wide variety of theoretical rationales (Ingham, 1984a). Yet, as noted above, consensus is growing that therapy programs which include maintenance activities are more likely to result in the long-term stability of fluency than programs which do not (Boberg, 1981; Boberg, Howie, and Woods, 1979; Ryan, 1974).

Table 3 provides another list of techniques which clinicians might consider employing in the construction or strengthening of the maintenance component of their therapy program (St. Louis, 1982). It will be clear from this list that the therapy delivery model is important since a gradually reducing schedule of clinical contacts appears useful. Client motivation is also important and may, in fact, be the most important variable in whether or not maintenance activities are necessary. Attitudes and role concepts of the stutterer are important too, as these change more slowly than the stutterer's speech fluency (Perkins, 1979, 1981; Shames, 1986; Van Riper, 1973).

Conclusion

Our purposes in writing this chapter were to raise issues, present recent data, and make therapeutic suggestions relative to the effectiveness of treatment of stutterers. If we have succeeded it should be abundantly clear to the reader that clinical effectiveness with stutterers is not a simple unitary phenomenon.

Investigators frequently disagree on the definition of success in stuttering therapy, and success is influenced by the factors covered in the chapter. Moreover, clinical investigators strive for different goals, and assess different variables in different ways. Given this state of affairs, our energy is perhaps best expended in learning from each other. We can be encouraged by the fact that even with increasingly vigorous long-term analyses we are able to conclude that our efforts do benefit people who stutter. It is not advisable, however, to accept simplistic evaluations of clinical effectiveness. Varying degrees of relapse after therapy serve to remind us of the complexity of stuttering, and complex problems rarely yield to simple solutions. Our self-examinations must continue to be thorough and relentless so that the therapy we provide will meet the challenge of serving those who seek our help.

14 The Psychology of Treatment Evaluation Studies

Harry Purser

Introduction

Advances in the understanding of human problems occur in a variety of ways. Some gradually yield their secrets over the years as painstaking coordinated research leads to steady increments in our knowledge. Others are solved more rapidly, either because of some dramatic new technological innovation or a chance discovery. One further avenue of rapid progress opens up when investigators begin to tackle the problem in a completely new way. The latter case would be an example of what the philosopher of science Kuhn (1962) terms a 'paradigm shift' in investigative method. After many years of thinking about the problem in some established way a new conception emerges which quickly integrates previously disparate findings and welds them into a unified theory.

The history of the study of stuttering reveals that paradigm shifts have occurred on a few occasions (see Rosenfield and Sussman, this volume) but these have been confined to the earliest conceptions of the problem. The more recent history of stuttering depicts a cyclical movement of theoretical ideas alternating between hypotheses about the constitutional and neurological basis of speech dysfluency on the one hand to social psychological explanations on the other. Many contemporary students of the causation of stuttering now argue that the only way to integrate the research evidence is in terms of an interactional model. Davison and Neale (1974, 1986) have proposed a similar position in their study of abnormal psychology. There is strong evidence that many forms of psychopathology have some genetic or constitutional basis and that environmental factors such as life events play an important role in precipitating (and conversely in preventing) the emergence of disturbed behaviour. In what Davison and Neale term the *diathesis–stress* model of psychopathology it is assumed that people who develop particular psychological problems have a general *predisposition* towards psychopathology (diathesis). If there are sufficient environmental forces impinging on that individual the *interaction* between the diathesis and the psychological stress results in dysphoria and disturbed overt behaviour.

Whether or not an interactionist model of speech dysfluency will eventually be looked back upon as a true paradigm shift remains to be seen. However, the immediate benefit of such interactionist models of stuttering lies in the hope they offer to both therapists and their clients. There may be little therapists can do to address the diathesis of stuttering, but clearly speech dysfluency *can* be modified under the right environmental circumstances. The focus of the next generation of fluency researchers is likely to be upon the effects of particular forms of treatment for stuttering rather than speculating about the diathesis that underlies the condition.

If this shift in emphasis progresses it is possible that in addition to being able to offer stutterers more effective treatments we will also learn a great deal about the mechanisms involved in stuttering. If we are to achieve these advances the next generation of research workers will need a thorough grounding in the design and evaluation of treatment outcome studies. This chapter emphasises the need for more treatment evaluation studies in stuttering conducted in service contexts and outlines the basic principles that guide the design of modern treatment evaluation studies.

Evaluating the Effects of Therapy

Careful studies of psychological and rehabilitative treatments have only arisen in the past three decades. Prior to this period the transactions that took place between clients and their therapists were shrouded in mystique. It was the Rogerian movement in counselling (Rogers, 1951) that first opened up the therapy room to sympathetic study and gave birth to two distinct traditions in treatment evaluation. The first is *therapy process research* which derives its name from its focus on the methods, techniques and interpersonal dynamics that arise in the process of conducting therapy. The other tradition is *therapy outcome research* where the effects of therapeutic treatments are studied and compared between different schools of therapy. There are formidable technical and conceptual difficulties in both these traditions and in order to appreciate the problems that confront treatment research we need to explore some very basic issues in scientific methodology.

Theory and therapy

Research during the past three decades into the fundamental basis of stuttering reveals a healthy partnership between theory and practice. It seems that for every new theoretical idea about the nature of stuttering that has been advanced a corresponding therapeutic technique has been introduced. In general, if the therapy has shown promise then this has tended to strengthen the credibility of the theory that inspired it.

At first glance this process of theory construction leading to experimental test (therapy), and the therapy outcome informing further theoretical development, looks for all the world like the classic model of applied science. On closer inspection however the arrangement is not always as elegant as it may seem. Whilst well conducted treatment outcome research may be able to *disprove* some theoretical proposition or other it is never the case that theory can be *proven* experimentally (Popper, 1959, 1963). There are always competing explanations of *why* particular treatment effects have been obtained, and many of these explanations have little or nothing to do with the theoretical ideas that inspired the therapy in the first place.

Fundamental ideas about the theoretical nature of stuttering may well serve as a source of inspiration to therapists, but there is rarely any unequivocal relationship between theory and therapy. In modern clinical science therapy has moved away from its role as the test of theory. Therapy has now become a topic in its own right for theoretical development, but the path is rocky, and there are innumerable pitfalls for the unwary. The prime goal of therapy is *to achieve a successful treatment outcome*. Of course the question of what constitutes a 'successful' treatment outcome in stuttering begs a number of further questions. Suffice it to say at this stage that there can be many valid definitions of 'success' for different treatment approaches but determining whether or not success has been achieved is certainly the most salient reason for evaluating the effects of therapy.

Therapy is also essentially an experimental process. The purpose of any experiment is to test some prior hypothesis. The main hypothesis that every therapist tries to test is: *this treatment will lead to a significant improvement in this client's problem*. But further possibilities exist. Regardless of the treatment outcome that is actually obtained (i.e., whether it be positive or negative) the scientific therapist will want to go further and ask the next logical question: *how has this particular treatment outcome come about?* By seeking answers here therapists move away from emotional interpretations of the observed effects and towards being able to *maximise* the impact of their treatments. Therapists can try to distinguish between the various components of a therapy programme in terms of their individual contribution to outcome. Further, the interaction of therapy with various levels of problem severity, therapist experience and client characteristics can then be studied. In the course of this kind of enquiry it is likely that a very great deal will be learned about the nature of stuttering. If treatment evaluation studies are to answer questions about 'success' *and* fundamental questions about the nature of stuttering then special care needs to be taken in their design and execution.

Therapy and methodology

Ever since the searing critique by Eysenck (1952) of the apparent ineffectiveness of analytic psychotherapy in the treatment of neurotic disorders a substantial effort has been made in clinical psychology to evaluate the effects of various forms of psychological treatment. In the past thirty years the clinical psychology literature has been peppered with treatment evaluation studies. Many eminent scholars have tried their best to review these studies and reach reliable conclusions about the efficacy of various treatment approaches (e.g., Bergin, 1971; Bergin and Lambert, 1978; Luborsky *et al.* 1975; Meltzoff and Kornreich, 1970; Rachman and Wilson, 1980; Shapiro and Shapiro, 1982; Smith and Glass, 1977; Smith *et al.* 1980). Whilst their methods have differed considerably, and their conclusions even more, a general consensus has emerged to the effect that most forms of psychological treatment are effective for the range of disorders they address. However, there is also general agreement on the fact that many interesting and promising studies are fatally flawed by serious 'methodological inadequacies'. St. Louis and Westbrook (this volume) highlight a number of methodological problems which continue to confound many dysfluency treatment studies. The presence of such inadequacies in the majority of treatment evaluation studies makes the task of advocating some forms of treatment over others highly problematic.

The newcomer to treatment evaluation research may wonder if there is really any agreement at all between research workers on what constitutes an adequate treatment evaluation study. After all, most of the reported methodological inadequacies feature in studies which have been published in eminent scientific journals employing careful peer review procedures. It seems that on the one hand we are eager to see the publication of studies which have direct implications for practicing clinicians. We want to demonstrate that treatment successes are possible in stuttering and to promote those methods of treatment that achieve positive results. On the other hand we also want to establish higher standards for scientific rigour in the process of treatment evaluation. Competing demands such as these may go some way to explaining the diversity of opinion found in the treatment evaluation literature.

Many see this tension between practical research into the benefits of treatment and the need to attain a high degree of experimental rigour in the process as leading to a state of affairs where treatment evaluation studies become little more than esoteric exercises in experimental design. There is the danger that we may become 'too scientific' in our approach with the result that we lose sight of the basic purpose of therapy. It is important to remind ourselves whenever difficult decisions have to made in both process and outcome research that the first goal of therapy is to achieve a successful treatment outcome and not simply to provide a vehicle for the illustration of advanced treatment evaluation methodology.

The context of therapy evaluation

Given the methodological minefield that treatment evaluation has become in recent years it is hardly surprising that the majority of such studies are undertaken by trained research staff in clinical research centres rather than by practising clinicians in service contexts. To the outside observer it might seem incredible that despite the volume of clinical treatment undertaken in service contexts so few published evaluation studies actually emerge from these settings. Instead the literature is replete with studies which have been undertaken by established research workers specifically to highlight the effects of particular treatment programmes.

There are of course reasons in addition to this lack of methodological expertise why so little service-based research into treatment efficacy is carried out. It may be hard for therapists to appreciate that it is the procedures and techniques that are on trial in a treatment evaluation study rather than the professionals who administer them. Next comes the 'pressure of work' argument. Many clinicians express the view that they simply do not have the time to undertake research into the effectiveness of their treatments. This argument is increasingly difficult to sustain in the face of mounting pressure from a variety of agencies for therapists to provide unambiguous evidence of the benefits of their treatments. In future it seems as if the advancement of many professions will depend on their ability to provide objective rather than emotional evidence of their value to society. Further, the 'applied clinical science' model of professional practice emphasises the evaluation of treatment effects as an integral part of the treatment process. Unless evidence is collected about the impact of treatment there will be no data on which to base decisions about the next stages of treatment.

To press the case for an increase in service-based outcome research we need look no further than one of the most common 'methodological flaws' identified by comtemporary critics of outcome research. It concerns the lack of what is termed 'ecological validity' in the majority of treatment evaluation studies. The point being made here is that studies conducted in research settings may generate results that are highly specific to these settings. For example, a study may be carried out on the premises of a prestigious teaching hospital. The therapists may be highly motivated clinical research workers with a relatively light clinical caseload. The treatments being offered may be novel, attractive, systematic and powerful, but they may also be quite impractical to administer in regular service contexts. The results that are obtained from this form of therapy practised in these settings may have relatively few implications for professional clinicians and their clients in traditional service settings. The results may of course inform us about the fundamental nature of stuttering, and may well highlight what can be achieved under such well resourced circumstances, but the study would not be considered 'ecologically valid'.

If treatment evaluation studies are to make real contributions to speech therapy practice then the focus must be shifted from research to service contexts. Further, studies need to assess methods of therapy that can be accommodated within the resource constraints of service settings. If well-conducted outcome research were to become a regular feature of clinical practice then our understanding of both treatment dynamics and the nature of stuttering might grow at an unprecedented rate.

Traditional Methodology

We need to be clear from the outset about the aims of treatment evaluation studies. Is the purpose to discover whether a particular treatment 'works' or is it to compare the relative efficacy (power) of two or more different forms of treatment? Unless the aims of the study can be unambiguously stated at the outset there is a high probability that a variety of 'methodological flaws' will gradually creep into the design of the study and subsequently undermine a great deal of time and clinical effort. Rachman and Wilson (1980) in their classic critique of the state of treatment outcome research make the point that many studies are initiated primarily to demonstrate that a specific form of therapy can 'master' the problem in question. Relatively few studies start from what in contrast they call the 'mystery' point of view. In the former 'mastery' model the re-searchers may have some personal investment in the treatment under scrutiny and any-thing less than positive findings is hardly likely to be satisfactory. In contrast the 'mystery' approach is characteristic of clinical scientists who genuinely want to learn more about the process and outcome of different treatments. Here positive *and* negative findings are welcome because both sets of results fuel the continuing search for more effective therapeutic methods.

In order to clarify some of the traditional features of evaluation methodology a practical example will be helpful. Suppose a revolutionary new therapy for alleviating stuttering behaviour has burst onto the scene. The first task for any responsible clinician would be to *validate* the new treatment by demonstrating that it does indeed lead to significant reductions in problem severity. There are at least three ways of going about this validation process with the choice of methodology depending on whether the therapy is seen as a panacea for *all* stuttering, whether its effectiveness is likely to be limited to only *some* forms of stuttering, or whether it is claimed the therapy helps some stutterers to achieve higher levels of fluency than could ever be achieved using other established forms of treatment.

Treatment benefits all stutterers: The single case study design

If it is felt the new therapy will help *every* stutterer then a series of single case studies may be all that is required to test this claim (Hersen and Barlow, 1976; Kazdin, 1981,

1982; Kratchowill, 1978). Whilst single case methodology can never be used to *generalise* about the likely effects of a particular treatment it can be used to *disprove* a general claim of the type above. If even *one* client in the series of case studies failed to achieve fluency with this new therapeutic approach it could be safely concluded that the therapy is no panacea for stuttering. One of the major limitations in employing single case study methodology to test the efficacy of therapy lies in the paucity of appropriate statistical techniques with which to evaluate the null hypothesis (that treatment has no effect). Only by using a series of measurements during the process of therapy can suitable statistical techniques be brought to bear (e.g., time series analysis, see Kratchowill *et al.* 1984 for further discussion of this topic).

However, it is rare to come across the claim that a new therapy will help *all* stutterers. Most therapists introducing a new form of treatment adopt more conservative estimates of the likely effects and would therefore begin the validation process with the hypothesis that the therapy will be beneficial to at least some stutterers. Rather than engage in a series of single case studies the most efficient methodology here would be to adopt a group study.

Treatment benefits some stutterers: The single group design

The basic logic of the single group design involves assembling an adequate and representative sample of stutterers and measuring the severity of each individual's dysfluency prior to the application of treatment and again at the conclusion of treatment. Here an 'adequate' sample means a sufficient number of problem sufferers to bring either parametric or non-parametric statistical procedures to bear on the pre- and post-treatment severity measurements. The 'representativeness' of the sample would hinge upon having the right male to female ratio (reflecting the typical ratios found in the population of problem sufferers), a good mix of age ranges, and a good spread of initial problem severity. If the sample was biased on any one of these factors it might seriously limit the kinds of conclusions that could be drawn from the study.

Next, a number of therapists would be trained in the methods and techniques of the new therapy and proceed to treat the dysfluent client for a specified number of sessions. At the end of the treatment period each client would be reassessed on the same measures that were employed at the outset of the study. The therapists would now have two sets of data to compare: the pre-treatment problem definition measures and the post-treatment outcome measures. Typically these two sets of scores would be summarised using descriptive statistics to highlight group mean scores and variance estimates. The pre-treatment and post-treatment means and variances would then be compared using a related samples analysis of variance (Meddis, 1973) and an F ratio obtained which would indicate the amount of variance in the outcome that was due to the therapy process. This F value would then be checked for statistical rarity to ensure that it is unlikely that such a value could have arisen in the study purely by chance. This is known as the *statistical significance* of the outcome.

If the analysis of variance did yield a significant F ratio (say at the .05 level of probability) then the therapists can assume that the differences in scores are not simply due to chance fluctuations in their clients' performance on the two assessment occasions. Further, if it is apparent that the mean severity score has reduced substantially between the pre- and post-treatment assessments it may be claimed that the treatment has also produced a *clinically significant* effect. The clients have become substantially more fluent in their speech.

Treatment benefits some stutterers and achieves better outcomes than established treatments: The two group design

Even if the second claim (that the treatment is better than anything else currently available) was not made it would be a logical extension of the above methodology to look at the *power* of the new therapy in relation to some other established form of treatment for stuttering. There may currently be a treatment of choice for stuttering that is generally acknowledged to have a powerful and reliable impact on the problem. By comparing the treatment effects obtained using the established therapy with those obtainable with the new therapy we can say something about the relative power of the two treatments. This would be a comparative outcome design employing two groups and would effectively replicate the earlier study (i.e., test whether the new therapy continues to demonstrate clinical promise when used with a different sample of stutterers) whilst providing evidence of its impact relative to a second form of treatment of known efficacy. A larger sample of dysfluent clients would be assembled and individuals would be randomly assigned to either the new therapy group or the established therapy group. Therapists would be trained in both methods of treatment and would administer both treatments. Again pre-treatment scores would be compared with post-treatment scores to determine whether statistically and clinically significant results have been obtained. Next, the average magnitude of improvement would be compared.

Suppose it now emerges from this second study that once again the new therapy has produced an outcome which is both statistically and clinically significant, but these gains have fallen short of the results achieved by the established treatment. Should the new therapy now be abandoned in favour of the established procedure? Not quite. There is more to establishing the effectiveness of a therapy than simply gauging its immediate post-treatment impact. If judgement were suspended for six months and the two samples of clients were then recalled for follow-up assessments we would have new data on which to perform a further analysis to establish the relative *duration* of the treatment effects. By comparing the immediate post-treatment scores with the six month follow-up scores for both groups it might emerge that those treated with the new therapy retained their relatively modest post-treatment gains at the follow-up whereas those treated with the established therapy had suffered some deterioration. If this were found to be the case then we would have adequate grounds for continuing the new therapy. It may not be as immediately powerful as the established therapy, but its effects on stuttering have been shown to persist for longer.

There is one further area in which the new therapy might be legitimately superior to the established treatment. Most treatment evaluation studies have to specify a fairly arbitrary treatment period. If resources are scarce this may be in the region of eight consecutive one hour treatment sessions over an eight week period. Suppose instead a criterion-referenced treatment period is employed. Here it would be stated in advance that treatment will continue until each client in the study has achieved some clinically significant level of improvement, say a 25 per cent reduction in their stuttering behaviour. Treatment would be discontinued only when this criterion of improvement had been achieved by each client. It would now be possible to compare the two treatments in terms of their relative *cost effectiveness*. By finding the mean treatment duration and the variance in the number of treatment hours it took for each group to achieve the target criterion it would be possible to say something about the relative *efficiency* of the two forms of treatment.

Summary

By employing the most basic experimental designs we would now have evidence about a. the effectiveness and relative power of the new therapy, b. the duration of the treatment effects, and c. the cost-effectiveness of the therapy in clinical practice. The question now becomes how good is this 'evidence'? Traditional experimental methodology makes a number of assumptions about both the nature of the problem under investigation (in this case stuttering) and the nature of treatment. For example, in the two group comparative design above it is assumed first that the problem being treated is stable over time. Second, it is assumed that the samples of problem sufferers are fairly homogeneous as far as personality and other individual characteristics are concerned. Obviously people differ in age, sex and problem severity, but as long as these characteristics are equally distributed between the two groups then all is well. Third, the assumption is made that 'therapy' is comparable to a drug. It can be administered in standard 'doses' of known 'strength' over a period of time. Finally, the methodology of traditional treatment evaluation assumes that the therapy alone is responsible for any observed changes in the levels of problem severity at the conclusion of the study.

Modern Methodology

The limitations of traditional treatment evaluation studies have been exhaustively catalogued elsewhere (Rachman and Wilson, 1980). Briefly the heart of the problem lies in treating the phenomena under study as if they are akin to some 'quasi-illness'. The best model on which to base the treatment evaluation process then becomes the classic medical drug trial with all the assumptions inherent in this model being brought into play. But therapy for stuttering is not at all like a drug and stuttering is certainly quite unlike an organic disease. Even the more adventurous experimental designs that are found in drug trials such as the treatment crossover strategy (where half the group receive drug A for a period of time whilst the other half receive drug B, then the two drugs are switched between the groups to gauge any improvement or deterioration) are quite meaningless when applied to therapy. Drugs have a finite lifespan in the body but we know little about the lifespan of different therapies.

By treating complex problems and complex treatments as if they were much simpler processes the traditional treatment evaluation model may be doing a great disservice to both therapists and their clients. Although the vocabulary of the traditional treatment evaluation study may sound scientific the acid test of good science is how comprehensively it addresses the phenomena under study. Many clinicians now feel that traditional treatment evaluation strategies only scratch the surface of the treatment process and are in desperate need of new ideas. A new perspective on the methodological issues of treatment evaluation studies has now emerged based on a *realist* philosophy of science (Bhaskar, 1975).

In traditional empirical science the purpose of experimentation is to isolate hypothetical causal mechanisms by manipulating the independent variable(s) and observing the outcome on the dependent variable. In this process there is also a need to control other extraneous variables that may interfere with the dependent variable. In human experimentation this degree of experimental control is seldom possible. The traditional empirical approach to handling this problem is to treat any contamination from uncontrolled variables as 'error'. It is assumed the 'error' is inherent in all experimental conditions and therefore it can be safely ignored. From a realist perspective this is a very dangerous assumption. Below, a number of issues in outcome research are raised which might improve the scientific credibility of treatment outcome studies in stuttering.

Internal validity

In treatment evaluation research the 'internal validity' of a study refers to the extent to which we can be sure that the effects observed at the end of treatment are the direct and sole consequence of the treatment methods. Questions about the internal validity of any evaluation study are really questions about the degree of experimental control that has been achieved over a range of variables with the potential to influence the individual's response to treatment.

For example, many types of problems improve simply with the passage of time. We know that stuttering is a variable phenomenon and it is just possible that the speech of some clients may improve significantly over a period of weeks without any formal therapeutic intervention. Similarly, we know that many stutterers seek help at times when their dysfluency is particularly acute (Andrews and Harvey, 1981). Therefore there is the possibility that some clients may well 'improve' during the course of treatment through simple regression to the mean (i.e., stabilising at their usual level of stuttering severity). Clients such as these represent a real threat to the internal validity of treatment evaluation studies for their 'improvement' during treatment may be quite independent of the therapy being administered.

The traditional way of controlling for these so-called 'spontaneous recovery' effects is to employ a 'no treatment' control group. Here a proportion of the subjects in the study are assessed and randomly assigned to either the treatment group(s) or the 'no treatment' control group. Those in the treatment group(s) proceed to therapy whilst those in the 'no treatment' group are assigned to a 'waiting list' and scheduled for treatment at the end of a defined period of time. All the subjects (including the 'no treatment' group) are then reassessed at the conclusion of the study and any changes in problem severity in the control group can be attributed to the base rate of spontaneous recovery. If the treated groups evidence greater improvement than the control group then it is assumed this difference is due to the treatments they received. But the issue of internal validity does not end here. Although the treatment groups may indeed have improved more than the control group how can we be sure this difference was *exclusively* due to the treatment(s) they received? A variety of other factors could conceivably account for this improvement. In the past several years there has been an upsurge of interest in the role of so-called 'non-specific' factors in therapy. These are factors which are common to all forms of therapy and which may, independently of the specific techniques and methods employed in treatment, account for much of the improvement that clients achieve. Amongst these so-called 'non-specific' factors are variables like the prestige of the settings in which treatment takes place, the personal charisma of the therapists, the novelty of the treatment, the social contact that all therapies inevitably involve and the levels of expectancy for change that clients generate when they enter a therapy programme (Frank, 1961; Kazdin and Wilcoxon, 1976; Shapiro, 1981; Strupp and Hadley, 1979; Wilkins, 1979a, 1979b).

The role of non-specific factors in treatment outcome has become a topic of study in its own right in clinical psychology under the general (and rather misleading) heading of the *placebo effect* (Shapiro, 1971; Shapiro and Morris, 1978). The main lesson for those engaged in treatments evaluation is to ensure that the presence of such non-specific factors are at least equally represented in the treatments under study. This strategy ensures that the potential effects of non-specific factors are held steady between the different treatment programmes under scrutiny. It will not however enable the researcher to discriminate between the effects of the specific treatment and these non-specific influences.

It seems the only way to address the latter issue is to employ special types of control groups (attention-placebo control groups) where the vast majority of the identifiable sources of non-specific effects are represented (e.g., Jacobson and Baucom, 1977; O'Leary and Borkovec, 1978). If these control groups are to work at all they need to generate the same levels of expectancy for change and credibility in the 'treatment' process that the main treatments under study induce in their subjects (Kazdin and Wilcoxon, 1976). Yet the 'treatments' that are offered in these groups must, on all theoretical grounds, be therapeutically inert. Of course this type of strategy naturally raises serious ethical objections as well as some formidable practical and conceptual difficulties (Parloff, 1986).

Nevertheless, the problem of non-specific influences is very pertinent in the treatment of stuttering. There are many anecdotal reports of minimal and often quite bizarre treatments leading to a substantial improvement in the problem. Clearly this is an issue that awaits further development in the evaluation of treatment for stuttering.

External validity

External validity refers to the extent to which it is possible to *generalise* from the findings of a particular treatment study to other populations and settings. Where a study reports positive findings in respect of particular treatment(s) there is the implication that the same outcomes could be obtained in other settings by different therapists treating different clients. But this may not always be the case. As mentioned earlier much depends on the ecological validity of the original study.

In addition to considering the characteristics of the setting, the clients and the therapists who administered the treatment, we need to decide on whether the form of treatment used is replicable. Too often in published studies there is insufficient detail on the specifics of particular treatments. Instead a label is used to convey the likely orientation of the treatment. This lack of treatment process specificity is now considered a very serious obstacle to evaluating the external validity of a study. In psychotherapy research the problem is considered serious enough to warrant the publication of detailed treatment manuals which operationally define *all* aspects of the various treatment processes under investigation. It can only be a matter of time before similar strategies are adopted in the field of stuttering.

One final point needs to be made about the external validity of outcome studies. It concerns the use of a very narrow range of treatment outcome measures. It is obvious that the choice of suitable treatment outcome measures is dictated by the treatment(s) under scrutiny. Inevitably in stuttering research the target of treatment is overt motor speech dysfluency. Unless significant reductions in problem severity are seen here it is hardly likely that a treatment will receive more than passing interest from other clinicians. Yet many modern cognitive–behavioural treatments for stuttering predict changes both in the level of speech dysfluency and the stutterer's attitudes and beliefs. This raises the issue of how far the outcome net should be cast to detect change as a consequence of treatment. Also, there is very little in the literature about the possible *iatrogenic* (adverse) effects of different therapies. It seems we always assume that the only possible treatment outcomes are positive change or no change in target symptoms. But clinicians need to be able to make informed decisions about whether to put some new treatment into practice. If it emerged that a particular treatment had very good outcomes for the majority of clients, but also resulted in catastrophic outcomes in others, then this information would allow a decision to be made on the likely risks associated with some forms of treatment.

Recommendations

The questions that surround the external validity of treatment evaluation studies beg the same action from researchers that the issues of internal validity pose. The hallmark of modern clinical research must be a greater emphasis on *specificity*. We need to become more specific in formulating the aims of the study, in the operational definition of the problem, in the sample definition, in the treatment process definition and in selecting the outcome measures to gauge efficacy. In a thoughtful review of the treatment evaluation literature Strupp (1978) concluded that the burning question for therapists was not whether therapy 'works', but rather:

> What specific therapeutic interventions produce specific changes in specific individuals under specific conditions?

Only by posing this question at the outset of any treatment evaluation study is there a chance that the design will meet the methodological standards that are rapidly moving into place in clinical research. We need to see greater specificity and operational precision in the following areas of treatment evaluation.

Problem definition and pre-treatment measures

Although there is general agreement about the definition of 'stuttering', a precise operational definition of the problem is a good starting point for any research initiative. If we accept that stuttering is a context–sensitive problem then we need to assess it in a representative sample of everyday situations. We need to ensure that the measurement of the severity of the problem is not confined to artificial environments such as the therapy room and arbitrary speech acts such as reading aloud. Although a naturalistic assessment of the problem may be difficult it is not beyond the resources that are available in most clinical contexts, for example through the use of unobtrusive measures via modern technology.

Further, as Lang (1969) and Rachman and Hodgson (1980) have demonstrated, most problems can be defined at three distinct levels of analysis: cognitive, behavioural and physiological. These authors remark on the fact that the three systems are not always synchronised. There are problem sufferers who manifest clear behavioural difficulties but who are not cognitively concerned about the problem nor are they physiologically labile when their problem is at its worst. Similarly it has been discovered that treatment may have a differential impact on one or other of the three systems. One treatment may result in a significant decrease in the physiological activation of the problem sufferer; the same treatment may have a major impact on the behavioural responses of another sufferer but little or no effect at either the cognitive or physiological levels. Such examples of *desynchrony* in the three response systems may have profound implications for the evaluation of treatment for stuttering.

It is also worthwhile considering the secondary problems that might be troubling a chronic or acute stutterer. For example, Seligman's (1975) theory of *learned helplessness* would predict that clinical depression and anxiety are likely byproducts of such chronic handicapping conditions. These secondary components of the problem might usefully be addressed in the problem definition phase of a treatment project. By employing a much broader operational definition of the problem there is a greater chance of detecting subtypes of stutterers and correlating these factors with response to treatment.

Adequate sample definition

There are two principal reasons for taking great care in defining the sample of problem sufferers used in a treatment evaluation study. First, by highlighting individual differences within the sample it becomes possible to examine a variety of person by treatment interactions. With the addition of a higher resolution on the individual's stuttering problem even more sophisticated problem by person by treatment interactions can be studied. This kind of analysis is long overdue in the stuttering literature (e.g., St. Louis and Westbrook, this volume). What is required is a broad range of individual assessments encompassing age, sex, personality variables, psychological adjustment, previous treatment history, I.Q., social circumstances, social networks, and so on. There may be a great difference in the response to treatment we observe in someone who has received treatment on many occasions, is rather lonely, has an uninspiring occupation and is moderately depressed and someone who is sociable, outgoing, well adjusted and happy in his employment. Multivariate statistical techniques allow these kinds of interactions to be highlighted.

The second reason for undertaking an adequate sample definition is simply to allow colleagues to determine the external validity of the study. It will also help future research workers to assemble comparable samples of problem sufferers for replication purposes.

Adequate treatment process specificity

Over twenty years ago Kiesler (1966) warned of the dangers of the 'therapy uniformity assumption' in outcome research. If we simply assume that when different therapists are trained to practice the same treatment we have achieved uniformity in that treatment process we run a serious risk (e.g., Sundland, 1977). It is important to ensure that therapist characteristics are carefully measured and that there is adequate homogeneity amongst therapists in terms of level of experience, therapeutic style and training in the treatment approach under scrutiny. There are two ways in which treatment process uniformity can be enhanced. First it may be advisable to draw up manuals which guide the treatment processes under study. Second it is possible to 'sample' a range of treatment sessions using video or audio recording equipment in order to check whether the treatment guidelines are being observed by the therapists. This strategy was employed in what is generally considered to be one of the best treatment evaluation studies undertaken to date (Sloane *et al.* 1975).

Get specific about 'non-specifics'

There are many obvious sources of 'non-specific' influences in all treatments for stuttering. In comparative outcome research it is vital that sources of these effects should at least be equated between the treatment groups. Perhaps the clearest way to conceive of non-specific influences in therapy is to consider what Greenwood (1981) (after Frank, 1961) calls the *natural negotiation hypothesis* of therapeutic change which states:

> Therapeutic improvement is the result of an interaction between a client and
> a trusted and respected person (or persons) in activities that *both* believe may
> effect a change in attitude and behaviour.

The challenge for all forms of psychosocial or psychoeducational therapy is to demonstrate that their techniques and methods result in consistently superior outcomes to 'natural negotiation' treatments or control groups.

Adequate treatment outcome measures

Although the choice of treatment outcome measures is largely determined by the kinds of pre-treatment measures that were adopted at the outset of the study it is worth emphasising again the need to employ broad assessments of the impact of treatment. There is as much to be gained from pinpointing the failures in the therapy process as there is from demonstrating areas of positive change. Narrow outcome measures such as frequency and rate of behavioural stuttering tell us nothing about the cognitive and physiological sequelae of treatment. Another relatively new avenue in outcome measurement concerns the use of individualised treatment outcome measures (Beutler and Hamblin, 1986) where each client in the study has a series of highly individualised outcome measures which focus on specific target symptoms and difficulties. By using a common metric for these measures it is possible to compare progress between individual clients in terms of standard 'effect sizes'.

If in doubt it may be helpful to bear in mind the distinction between the technical and ethical goals of treatment. Many therapists offer help to individuals who suffer from chronic and intractable problems which simply do not respond to treatment. Here therapists are adopting a moral goal for treatment: to help the individual adjust and come to terms with their handicap. Whilst some treatments may do little to alleviate the overt problem they may have a very great impact on the sufferer's view of himself and his problem.

The final point here concerns the technical aspects of outcome measurement. A variety of measurement devices are available to therapists ranging from formal standardised assessment procedures to ad hoc clinical rating scales of observable behaviour. When choosing a battery of outcome measures it is always best to employ a mixed measurement methodology. A happy mixture of clinical observation, peer ratings, informant opinions, self-assessments, standard tests, objective measures and self-report questionnaires diffuses the many technical objections that are raised about outcome measurements and ultimately increases the reliability of the study.

Conclusion

Stuttering therapies warrant a new emphasis on specificity if further progress is to be made in both the understanding and the treatment of this fascinating problem. We need an increase in the amount of well-conducted comparative outcome research. There is an urgent need to stimulate new projects in service contexts. In the short term this may mean moving the research worker out of his research centre and into the community. In the longer term this need will have to be addressed by training and professional bodies. In the meantime I hope some of the issues raised in this chapter might stimulate a new treatment outcome effort which will be capable of addressing both practical and theoretical problems in stuttering.

References

ABBS, J. H. and ROSENFIELD, D. B. (1986) Motor impairments of speech: Nonaphasic disorders of communication. In S. H. Appel (Ed.), *Current Neurology. Vol 6*. Chicago: Yearbook Medical Publishers.

ABBS, J. H., GRACCO, V. L. and COLE, K. J. (1984) Control of multimovement coordination: sensorimotor mechanisms in speech motor programming. *Journal of Motor Behavior*, **16**, 195–232.

ADAMCZYK, B., SADOWSKA, E. and KUNISZYK-JOZKOWIAK, E. (1975) Influence of reverberation on stuttering. *Folia Phoniatrica*, **27**, 1–6.

ADAMS, M. R. (1977) A clinical strategy for differentiating the normally nonfluent child and the incipient stutterer. *Journal of Fluency Disorders*, **2**, 141–148.

ADAMS, M R. (1978) Stuttering theory, research, and therapy: The present and future. *Journal of Fluency Disorders*, **3**, 139–147.

ADAMS, M. R. (1980) The young stutterer: diagnosis, treatment and assessment of progress. In W. H. Perkins (Ed.), *Seminars in Speech, Language and Hearing*. New York: Thieme-Stratton Inc.

ADAMS, M. R., (1981) The speech production abilities of stutterers: Recent, ongoing and future research. *Journal of Fluency Disorders*, **6**, 311–326.

ADAMS, M. R. (1982) Fluency, non-fluency and stuttering in children. *Journal of Fluency Disorders*, **7**, 171–185.

ADAMS, M. R. (1984a) Laryngeal dynamics of stutterers: Laryngeal onset and reaction time of stutterers. In R. F. Curlee and W. H. Perkins (Eds.), *Nature and Treatment of Stuttering: New Directions*. San Diego, CA: College-Hill Press.

ADAMS, M. R., (1984b) The young stutterer: Diagnosis, treatment, and assessment of progress. In W. H. Perkins (Ed.), *Stuttering Disorders*. New York: Thieme-Stratton.

ADAMS, M. R. (1984c) Laryngeal onset and reaction time of stutterers. In R. F. Curlee and W. H. Perkins (Eds.) *Nature and Treatment of Stuttering: New Directions*. San Diego: College-Hill Press.

ADAMS, M. R. (1984d) Stuttering theory, research and therapy: A five-year retrospective and look ahead. *Journal of Fluency Disorders* **9**, 103–113.

ADAMS, M. R. (1985) The speech physiology of stutterers: present status. In E. Boberg (Ed.), *Seminars in Speech and Language, Stuttering: Part Two*, **6**, 2. New York: Thieme-Stratton Inc.

ADAMS, M. R. and RUNYAN, C. (1981) Stuttering and fluency: exclusive events or points on a continuum? *Journal of Fluency Disorders*, **6**, 197–218.

ADAMS, M. R. and REIS, R. (1971) The influence of the onset of phonation on the frequency of stuttering. *Journal of Speech and Hearing Research*, **14**, 639–44.

ADAMS, M. R. and REIS, R. (1974) The influence of the onset of phonation in the frequency of stuttering: A replication and re-evaluation. *Journal of Speech and Hearing Research*, **17**, 752–54.

ADAMS, M. R. and RAMIG, P. (1980) Vocal characteristics of stutterers and normal speakers during choral reading. *Journal of Speech and Hearing Research*, **3**, 457–465.

ADAMS, M. R. and HAYDEN, P. (1976) The ability of stutterers and nonstutterers to initiate and terminate phonation during production of an isolated vowel. *Journal of Speech and Hearing Research*, **19**, 290–296.

ADLER, A. (1914) *Verdrängung und männlicher Protest; ihre Rolle und Bedeutung für die neurotische Dynamik.* Heilen und Bilden.

AINSWORTH, S. (1957) Method for integrating theories of stuttering. In L. Travis (Ed.), *Handbook of Speech Pathology*. New York: Appleton-Century-Crofts.

AINSWORTH, S. (Ed.) (1981) *If Your Child Stutters: A Guide for Parents*. Memphis, TN: Speech Foundation of America.

AMMONS, R. and AMMONS, R. (1962) The Quick Test (QT): Provisional manual. *Psychological Reports*, **11**, 111–161.

AMSTER, B. (1984) *The Rate of Speech in Normal Preschool Children*. Doctoral Dissertation, Temple University, USA.

AMSTER, B. and STARKWEATHER, C. (1986) Unpublished manuscript.

ANAND, B. K. (1974) *Introduction to Control Systems*. Oxford: Pergamon.

ANDOLFI, M. (1974) Paradox and psychotherapy. *American Journal of Psychoanalysis*, **34**, 221–228.

ANDREWS, G. (1984a) Evaluation of the benefits of treatment. In W. H. Perkins (Ed.), *Current Therapy of Communication Disorders: Stuttering Disorders*. New York: Thieme-Stratton.

ANDREWS, G. (1984b) The epidemiology of stuttering. In R. F. Curlee and W. H. Perkins (Eds.), *Nature and Treatment of Stuttering: New Directions*. San Diego: College-Hill Press.

ANDREWS, G. and CRAIG, A. (1982) Stuttering: Overt and covert measurement of the speech of treated subjects. *Journal of Speech and Hearing Disorders*, **47**, 96–99.

ANDREWS, G. and CUTLER, J. (1974) Stuttering therapy: The relation between changes in symptom level and attitudes. *Journal of Speech and Hearing Disorders*, **37**, 312–319.

ANDREWS, G. and FEYER, A. M. (1985) Does behavior therapy still work when the experimenters depart: An analysis of a behavioral treatment program for stuttering. *Behavior Modification*, **9**, 443–547.

ANDREWS, G. and HARRIS, M. (1964) *The Syndrome of Stuttering*. Levenham, London: Spastics Society Medical Education and Information Unit.

ANDREWS, G. and HARVEY, R. (1981) Regression to the mean in pretreatment measures of stuttering severity. *Journal of Speech and Hearing Disorders*, **46**, 204–207.

ANDREWS, G. and INGHAM, R. (1971) Stuttering: Considerations in the evaluation of treatment. *British Journal of Disorders of Communication*, **6**, 129–38.

ANDREWS, G. and TANNER, S. (1982a) Stuttering: The result of 5 days treatment with an airflow technique. *Journal of Speech of Hearing Disorders*, **47**, 427–429.

ANDREWS, G. and TANNER, S. (1982b) Stuttering treatment: An attempt to replicate the regulated-breathing method. *Journal of Speech and Hearing Disorders*, **47**, 138–140.

ANDREWS, G., CRAIG, A., FEYER, A.-M., HODDINOTT, S., HOWIE, P. and NEILSON, M. (1983) Stuttering: A review of reserach findings and theories circa 1982. *Journal of Speech and Hearing Disorders*, **48**, 226–246.

ANDREWS, G., CRAIG, A. and FEYER, A.-M. (1983) *Therapist's manual for the stuttering treatment programme*. Sydney: Division of Communication Disorders, The Prince Henry Hospital.

ANDREWS, G., GUITAR, B. and HOWIE, P. (1980) Meta-analysis of the effects of stuttering treatment. *Journal of Speech and Hearing Disorders*, **45**, 287–307.

ANDREWS, G., QUINN, P. T. and SORBY, W. A. (1972) Stuttering: An investigation into cerebral dominance of speech. *Journal of Neurology, Neurosurgery, and Psychiatry*, **25**, 414–418.

ARDILA, A. and LOPEZ, M. D. (1986) Severe stuttering associated with right hemisphere lesion. *Brain and Language,* **27**, 239–246.

ARMSON, J. (1986) Stuttering considered from a motor control perspective. Unpublished manuscript.

ARON, M. (1965) The effects of the combination of trifluoperazine and amylobarbitone on adult stutterers. *Medical Proceedings* (South Africa), **11**, 227–33.

ASCHER, L. M. (1979) Paradoxical intention in the treatment of urinary retention. *Behavioral Research and Therapy,* **17**, 267–270.

ASCHER, L. M. (1981) Employing paradoxical intention in the treatment of agoraphobia. *Behaviour Research and Therapy,* **19**, 533–542.

ASCHER, L. M. and TURNER, R. M. (1980) A comparison of two methods for the administration of paradoxical intention. *Behaviour Research and Therapy,* **18**, 121–126.

ASCHER, L.M., SCHOTTE, D.E. and GRAYSON, J.B. (1986) Enhancing effectiveness of paradoxical intention in treating travel restriction in agoraphobia. *Behaviour Therapy,* **17**, 124–130.

AYLLON, T. (1963) Intensive treatment of psychotic behavior by stimulus satiation and food reinforcement. *Behaviour Research and Therapy,* **1**, 53–62.

BAILEY, A. and BAILEY, W. (1982) Managing the environment of the stutterer. In H. Luper (Ed.), Intervention with the Young Stutterer, *Journal of Childhood Communication Disorders,* **6**, 15–25.

BANNISTER, D. and FRANSELLA, F. (1986) *Inquiring Man* (3rd Ed) London: Croom-Helm.

BARBARA, D. A. (1965) *New Directions in Stuttering.* Springfield, IL: Charles C. Thomas.

BARBER, J. (1981) *The Development and Evaluation of an Instrument Assessing Stutterers' Communication Attitudes* (Doctoral dissertation), Northwestern University, Evanston, IL.

BARRETT, R. S. and STOECKEL, C. M. (1979) Unilateral eyelid movement control in stutterers and non-stutterers. Convention Address, *ASHA.*

BEECH, H. R. and FRANSELLA, F. (1968) *Research and Experiment in Stuttering.* Oxford: Pergamon.

BENSON, D. F. and GESCHWIND, N. (1985) The aphasias and related disturbances. In A. B. Baker and R. J. Joynt (Eds.), *Clinical Neurology.* Philadelphia: Harper and Row.

BENTON, A. L. (1968) Differential behavioral effects in frontal lobe disease. *Neuropsychologia,* **6**, 53–60.

BERGIN, A. E. (1971) The evaluation of therapeutic outcome. In: A. E. Bergin and S. L. Garfield (Eds.), *Handbook of Psychotherapy and Behavior Change.* New York: Wiley.

BERGIN, A. E. and LAMBERT, M. J. (1978) The evaluation of therapeutic outcomes. In S. L. Garfield and A. E. Bergin (Eds.), *Handbook of Psychotherapy and Behavior Change.* (2nd Ed.). New York: Wiley.

BERLIN, A. (1954) *An Exploratory Attempt to Isolate Types of Stuttering.* (Doctoral dissertation), Northwestern University, Evanston, IL.

BERRY, (1938) Developmental history of stuttering children. *Journal of Pediatrics,* **12**, 209–217.

BEUTLER, L. E. and HAMBLIN, D. L. (1986) Individualized outcome measures of internal change: Methodological considerations. *Journal of Consulting and Clinical Psychology,* **54**, 48–53.

BHASKAR, R. (1975) *A Realist Theory of Science.* Brighton: Harvester.

BJERKAN, B. (1980) Word fragmentations and repetitions in the spontaneous speech of 2–6 year old children. *Journal of Fluency Disorders,* **5**, 137–148.

BLACK, J. (1951) The effect of delayed sidetone upon vocal rate and intensity. *Journal of Speech and Hearing Disorders,* **16**, 56–60.

BLACKBURN, B. (1931) A study of the diaphragm, tongue, lips and jaw in stutterers and normal speakers. *Psychological Monographs,* **41**, 1–13.

BLODGETT, E. G. (1985) *The Metalinguistic Abilities Checklist: A Developmental Study.* Unpublished doctoral dissertation. The University of Alabama, Tuscaloosa.

BLOOD, G. and SEIDER, R. (1981). The concomitant problems of young stutterers. *Journal of Speech and Hearing Disorders,* **46**, 31–33.

BLOOD, G.W. (1985) Laterality differences in child stutterers: Heterogeneity, severity levels, and statistical treatments. *Journal of Speech and Hearing Disorders,* **50,** 66–72.

BLOODSTEIN, O. (1958) Stuttering as an anticipatory struggle reaction. In J. Eisenson (Ed.), *Stuttering: a Symposium.* New York: Harper and Row.

BLOODSTEIN, O. (1975) Stuttering as tension and fragmentation. In J. Eisenson (Ed.), *Stuttering: A Second Symposium.* New York: Harper and Row.

BLOODSTEIN, O. (1981) *A Handbook on Stuttering* (3rd Ed.). Chicago: National Easter Seal Society.

BLOODSTEIN, O. and GANTWERK, B. F. (1967) Grammatical function in relation to stuttering in young children. *Journal of Speech and Hearing Research,* **10,** 786–789.

BLUEMEL, C. (1930) *Mental Aspects of Stuttering.* Baltimore: Williams and Wilkins.

BLUMSTEIN, S., GOODGLASS, H. and TARTER, B. (1975) The reliability of ear advantage in dichotic listening. *Brain and Language,* **2,** 226–236.

BOBERG, E. (1981) Maintenance of fluency: An experimental program. In E. Boberg (Ed.), *Maintenance of Fluency.* New York: Elsevier.

BOBERG, E. (1983) Behavioral transfer and maintenance programs for adolescent and adult stutterers. In J. Fraser Gruss (Ed.). *Stuttering Therapy: Transfer and Maintenance.* Memphis: Speech Foundation of America.

BOBERG, E. (1986) Postscript: Relapse and outcome. In G. H. Shames and H. Rubin (Eds.), *Stuttering Then and Now.* Columbus, OH: Merrill.

BOBERG, E., and KULLY, D. (1984) Techniques for transferring fluency. In W. H. Perkins (Ed.), *Current Therapy of Communication Disorders: Stuttering Disorders.* New York: Thieme-Stratton.

BOBERG, E. and YEUDALL, L. (1984) Some clinical successes and failures: possible relationships to CNS functions. Paper presented at the *Annual Convention of the American Speech Language Hearing Association,* San Francisco.

BOBERG, E., HOWIE, P. and WOODS, L. (1979) Maintenance of fluency: A review. *Journal of Fluency Disorders,* **4,** 93–116.

BOBERG, E., YEUDALL, L., SCHOPFLOCHER, D. and BO-LASSEN, P. (1983) The effects of an intensive behavioral program on the distribution of EEG alpha power in stutterers during the processing of verbal and visuospatial information. *Journal of Fluency Disorders,* **8,** 245–263.

BOEHMLER, R. M. (1958) Listener responses to non-fluencies. *Journal of Speech and Hearing Research,* **1,** 132–141.

BOGEN, J. and GORDON, H. (1971) Musical tests for functional lateralization with intracarotid amobarbital. *Nature,* **230,** 524.

BORDEN, G. J. and ARMSON, J. (1985) Lip/jaw coordination with larynx in the speech of stutterers. Convention paper, *Acoustical Society of America.*

BOTTERILL, W. and RUSTIN, L. (1987) Teaching parents to manage their stuttering child. *Proceedings of the XX Congress of the IALP,* Tokyo, Japan.

BRADSHAW, J. L. (1980) Right-hemisphere language: familial and nonfamilial sinistrals, cognitive defects and writing hand position in sinistrals and concrete-abstract, imageable-nonimageable dimensions in word recognition. A review of interrelated issues. *Brain and Language,* **10,** 172–188.

BRADY, J. (1969) Studies on the metronome effect on stuttering. *Behaviour Research and Therapy,* **7,** 197–204.

BRADY, J. P. and BERSON, J. (1975) Stuttering, dichotic listening and cerebral dominance. *Archives of General Psychiatry,* **32,** 1449–1459.

BRANSCOM, M., HUGHES, J. and OXTOBY, E. (1955). Studies of nonfluency in the speech of preschool children. In W. Johnson and R. Leutenegger (Eds.), *Stuttering in Children and Adults.* Minneapolis, MN: University of Minnesota Press.

BRONFENBRENNER, U. (1976) Is early intervention effective? In A. Clarke and A. Clarke (Eds.), *Early Experience: Myth and Evidence.* London: Open Books.

BROWN, J. W. (1972) *Aphasia, Apraxia and Agnosia: Clinical and Theoretical Aspects.* Springfield, IL: Thomas.

BROWN, J. W. (1975) On the neural organization of language: thalamic and cortical relationships. *Brain and Language,* **2,** 18–30.

BROWN, S. F. (1938) Stuttering with relation toward accent and word position. *Journal of Abnormal and Social Psychology,* **33,** 112–120.

BROWN, S. F. (1945) The loci of stuttering in the speech sequence. *Journal of Speech Disorders,* **10,** 181–192.

BROWN, W. S., MARSH, J. T. and SMITH, J. C. (1973) Contextual meaning effects on speech evoked potentials. *Behavioral Biology,* **9,** 755–761.

BROWN, W. S., MARSH, J. T. and SMITH, J. C. (1976) Evoked potential waveform differences produced by the perception of different meanings of an ambiguous phrase. *Electroencephalography and Clinical Neurophysiology,* **41,** 113–123.

BROWNELL, W. (1973) *The Relationship of Sex, Social Class, and Verbal Planning to the Disfluences Produced by Non-stuttering Preschool Children* (Doctoral Dissertation), State University of New York at Buffalo.

BRUTTEN, E. and SHOEMAKER, D. (1967) *The Modification of Stuttering.* Englewood Cliffs, NJ: Prentice-Hall.

BRUTTEN, G. (1982) Speech situation checklist for children: A discriminant analysis. Paper presented to the annual meeting of the *American Speech Language Hearing Association,* Toronto, Ontario.

BRUTTEN, G. J. and TROTTER, A. C. (1985) Hemispheric interference: A dual-task investigation of youngsters who stutter. *Journal of Fluency Disorders,* **10,** 77–85.

BRYDEN, M. P. and MURRAY, J. E. (1985) Toward a model of dichotic listening performance. *Brain and Cognition,* **4,** 241–257.

BRYNGELSON, B. (1943) Stuttering and personality development. *The Nervous Child,* **2,** 162–166.

BRYNGELSON, B. (1950) *Know Yourself: A Workbook for Those who Stutter.* Minneapolis: Burgess.

BURNS, D. and BRADY, J. P. (1980) The treatment of stuttering. In A. Goldstein and E. B. Foa (Eds.), *Handbook of Behavioral Interventions.* New York: Wiley.

BUTLER, R. J. (1985) Towards an understanding of childhood difficulties. In N. Beail (Ed.), *Repertory Grid Technique and Personal Constructs.* London: Croom Helm.

CARROLL, J. and TANEHAUS, M. (1978) Functional clauses and sentence segmentation. *Journal of Speech and Hearing Research,* **21,** 793–808.

CARTLEDGE, G. and FELLOWES-MILBURN, J. (Eds.) (1980) *Teaching Social Skills to Children: Innovative approaches.* Oxford: Pergamon.

CARUSO, A.J., CONTURE, E. and COLTON, R. (in press) Selected temporal parameters of coordination associated with stuttering in children. *Journal of Fluency Disorders.*

CARUSO, A. J., GRACCO, V., and ABBS, J. (in press). A speech motor control perspective on stuttering: Preliminary observations. In H. Peters and W. Hulstijn (Eds.), *Speech Motor Dynamics in Stuttering.* New York: Springer Press.

CASE, H. W. (1960) Therapeutic methods in stuttering and speech blocking. In H. J. Eysenck (Ed.), *Behavior Therapy and the Neuroses.* Oxford: Pergamon.

CERF, A. and PRINS, D. (1974) Stutterers' ear preference for dichotic syllables. Paper presented to the *Annual Convention of the American Speech and Hearing Association,* Las Vegas.

CHEASMAN, C. (1983) Therapy for adults: An evaluation of current techniques for establishing fluencey. In P. Dalton (Ed.), *Approaches to the Treatment of Stuttering.* London: Croom Helm.

CHERRY, B. and SAYERS, B. (1956) Experiments upon the total inhibition of stammering by external control and some clinical results. *Journal of Psychosomatic Research,* **1,** 233–246.

CIMORELL-STRONG, J. M., GILBERT, H. R. and FRICK, J. V. (1983) Dichotic speech perception: A comparison between stuttering and nonstuttering children. *Journal of Fluency Disorders,* **8,** 77–91.

CLARK, E. F. (1978) Awareness of language: Some evidence from what children say and do. In A. Sinclair, R. J. Jarvell and W. J. M. Levelt (Eds.), *The Child's Conception of Language.* New York: Springer-Verlag.

COLBURN, N. and MYSAK, E. (1982a) Developmental disfluency and emerging grammar I: Disfluency characteristics in early syntactic utterances. *Journal of Speech and Hearing Research,* 25, 414–420.

COLBURN, N. and MYSAK, E. (1982b) Developmental disfluency and emerging grammar II: Co-occurrence of disfluency with specified semantic–syntactic structures. *Journal of Speech Hearing Research,* 25, 421–427.

CONTURE, E. G. (1982a) *Stuttering.* Englewood Cliffs, NJ: Prentice-Hall.

CONTURE, E. G. (1982b) Youngsters who stutter: Diagnosis, parent counseling, and referral. *Journal of Developmental Behavioral Pediatrics,* 3, 163–169.

CONTURE, E. G. (1984) Observing laryngeal movements of stutterers. In R. F. Curlee and W. H. Perkins (Eds.), *Natur and Treatment of Stuttering,* San Diego: College-Hill Press.

CONTURE, E. G. and CARUSO, A. (1978) A review of the Stocker Probe Technique for diagnosis and treatment of stuttering in young children. *Journal of Fluency Disorders,* 3, 297–298.

CONTURE, E. G. and SCHWARTZ, H. (1984) Children who stutter: Diagnosis and remediation. *Communicative Disorders,* 9, 1–18.

CONTURE, E. G. and VAN NAERSSEN, E. (1977) Reading abilities of school-age stutterers. *Journal of Fluency Disorders,* 2, 295–300.

CONTURE, E. G., ROTHENBERG, M. and MOLITOR, R. (1986) Electroglottographic observations of young stutterers' fluency. *Journal of Speech and Hearing Research,* 29, 384–393.

COOPER, E. B. (1965) An inquiry into the use of inter-personal communications as a source for therapy with stutterers. In D. Barbara (Ed.), *New Directions in Stuttering.* Springfield, IL: Charles C. Thomas.

COOPER, E. B. (1968) A therapy process for the adult stutterer. *Journal of Speech and Hearing Disorders,* 33, 246–260.

COOPER, E. B. (1969) An integration of behaviour therapy and traditional therapy procedures for stutterers. *Association for the Advancement of Behaviour Therapy Newsletter,* 2 (2) 10–11.

COOPER, E. B. (1971) Integrating behaviour therapy and traditional insight therapy procedures with stutterers. *Journal of Communication Disorders,* 4, 40–43.

COOPER, E. B. (1972) Recovery from stuttering in a junior and senior high school population. *Journal of Speech and Hearing Research,* 15, 632–638.

COOPER, E. B. (1973a) Integrating relationship and behaviour therapy procedures for adult stutterers. In L. Emmerick and S. Hood (Eds.), *The Client Clinician Relationship.* Springfield, IL: Charles C. Thomas.

COOPER, E. B. (1973b) The development of a stuttering chronicity prediction checklist for school aged stutterers: A research inventory for clinicians, *Journal of Speech and Hearing Research,* 38, 215–223.

COOPER, E. B. (1976) *Personalised Fluency Control Therapy: An Integrated Behavior and Relationship Therapy for Stutterers.* Austin, Texas: Learning Concepts Press.

COOPER, E. B. (1979a) Intervention procedures for the young stutterer. In H. H. Gregory (Ed.), *Controversies about Stuttering Therapy.* Baltimore: University Park Press.

COOPER, E. B. (1979b) *Understanding Stuttering: Information for Parents.* Chicago, IL: National Easter Seal Society.

COOPER, E. B. (1980) Etiology and treatment of stuttering. *Ear Nose and Throat Journal,* 59, 60–76.

COOPER, E. B. (1984) Personalized fluency control therapy: A status report. In M. Peins (Ed.), *Contemporary Approaches in Stuttering Therapy.* Boston: Little, Brown and Co.

COOPER, E. B. (1986a) The mentally retarded stutterer. In K. O. St. Louis (Ed.), *The Atypical Stutterer: Principles and Practices of Rehabilitation.* New York: Academic Press.

COOPER, E. B. (1986b) Treatment of dysfluency: Future trends. *Journal of Fluency Disorders,* 11, 317–327.

COOPER, E. B. and COOPER, C. S. (1976) *Personalized Fluency Control Therapy.* Hingham, MA: Teaching Resources.

COOPER, E. B. and COOPER, C. S. (1980) *Personalized Fluency Control Therapy Individualized Education Program Forms.* Hingham, MA: Teaching Resources.

COOPER, E. B. and COOPER, C. S. (1985a) Clinician attitudes toward stuttering: A decade of change (1973-1983). *Journal of Fluency Disorders,* 10, 19–33.

COOPER, E.B. and COOPER, C.S. (1985b) *Cooper Personalized Fluency Control Therapy Revised.* Allen, TX: DLM Teaching Resources.

COOPER, E. B. and RUSTIN, L. (1985) Clinician attitudes toward stuttering in the United States and Great Britain: A cross-cultural study. *Journal of Fluency Disorders,* 10, 1–17.

CORIAT, I. H. (1943) In E. Hahn (Ed.), *Stuttering: Significant Theories and Therapies.* Stanford, CA: Stanford University Press.

COSTELLO, J. M. (1984a) Treatment of the young chronic stutterer: Managing fluency. In R. G. Curlee and W. H. Perkins (Eds.), *The Nature and Treatment of Stuttering: New Directions.* San Diego: College-Hill Press.

COSTELLO, J. M. (1984b) Operant conditioning and the treatment of stuttering. In W. H. Perkins (Ed.), *Stuttering Disorders.* New York: Thieme-Stratton.

COSTELLO, J. M. and INGHAM, R. J. (1984) Assessment Strategies for stuttering. In R. F. Curlee and W. H. Perkins (Eds.), *Nature and Treatment of Stuttering: New Directions.* San Diego: College-Hill Press.

COX, M. D. (1986) The psychologically maladjusted stutterer. In K. St. Louis (Ed.), *The Atypical Stutterer: Principles and Practices of Rehabilitation.* New York: Academic Press.

CRAIG, A. R. and CLEARY, P. J. (1982) Reduction of stuttering by young male stutterers using EMG feedback. *Biofeedback and Self Regulation,* 7, 241–245.

CRAIG, A. R., FRANKLIN, J. A. and ANDREWS, G. (1984) A scale to measure locus of control of behaviour. *British Journal of Medical Psychology,* 57, 173–180.

CROSS, D. and LUPER, H. (1979) Voice reaction time of stuttering and nonstuttering children and adults. *Journal of Fluency Disorders,* 4, 59–77.

CRYSTAL, D., FLETCHER, P. and GARMAN, M. (1976) *The Grammatical Analysis of Language Disability.* London: Edward Arnold.

CULLINAN, W. and SPRINGER, M. (1980) Voice initiation and termination times in stuttering and non-stuttering children. *Journal of Speech and Hearing Research,* 23, 344–361.

CULP, M. (1984) The preschool fluency development program: Assessment and treatment: In M. Peins (Ed.), *Contemporary Approaches in Stuttering Therapy.* Boston: Little, Brown and Co.

CURLEE, R. F. (1980) A case selection strategy for young disfluent children. In W. H. Perkins (Ed.), *Seminars in Speech Language and Hearing, Vol. 1.* New York: Thieme-Stratton.

CURLEE, R. F. (1984) Stuttering disorders: An overview. In J. M. Costello (Ed.), *Speech Disorders in Children: Recent Advances.* San Diego: College-Hill Press.

CURLEE, R. F. and PERKINS, W. H. (Eds.) (1984) *The Nature and Treatment of Stuttering. New Directions.* San Diego, CA: College-Hill Press.

CURLEE, R. F. and PERKINS, W. H. (1969) Conversational rate control therapy for stuttering. *Journal of Speech and Hearing Disorders,* 34, 245–250.

CURRY, F. and GREGORY, H. (1969) The performance of stutterers on dichotic listening tasks thought to reflect cerebral dominance. *Journal of Speech and Hearing Research,* 12, 73–82.

DALTON, P. (1983a) Maintenance of change: Towards the integration of behavioural and psychological procedures. In P. Dalton (Ed.), *Approaches to the Treatment of Stuttering.* London: Croom Helm.

DALTON, P. (1983b) Psychological approaches to the treatment of stuttering. In P. Dalton (Ed.), *Approaches to the Treatment of Stuttering.* London: Croom Helm.

DALTON, P. and HARDCASTLE, W. (1977) *Disorders of Fluency and their Effects on Communication.* London: Arnold.

DALY, D. A. (1981a) Differentiation of stuttering subgroups with Van Riper's developmental tracks: a preliminary study. *Journal of the National Student Speech and Hearing Association,* 9, 89–101.

DALY, D. A. (1981b) An investigation of immediate auditory memory skills in 'functional' stutterers. Paper presented at the Annual Meeting of the *International Neuropsychological Society,* Atlanta.

DALY, D. A. (1985) Intensive versus conventional treatment for stutterers. Unpublished paper presented at Speech Foundation of America sponsored conference, Champaign, Illinois.

DALY, D. A. (1986) The clutterer. In K. St. Louis (Ed.), *The Atypical Stutterer: Principles and Practices of Rehabilitation.* New York: Academic Press.

DALY, D. A., KIMBARROW, M. L. and SMITH, A. (1977) Further definitions of neuropsychological deficits in 'functional stutterers'. Paper presented at the Annual Convention of the *American Speech Language Hearing Association,* Chicago.

DARLEY, F., ARONSON, A. and BROWN, J. (1975) *Motor Speech Disorders.* Philadelphia, PA: W. B. Saunders Company.

DAVENPORT, R. W. (1979) Dichotic listening in four severity levels of stuttering. Paper presented at the Annual Convention of the *American Speech and Hearing Association,* Atlanta.

DAVIS, D. M. (1939) The relation of repetitions in the speech of young children to certain measures of language maturity and situational factors: Part I. *Journal of Speech Disorders,* 4, 303–318.

DAVIS, D. M. (1940) The relation of repetitions in the speech of young children to certain measures of language maturity and situational factors. Parts II and III. *Journal of Speech Disorders,* 5, 235–246.

DAVISON, G. C. and NEALE, J. M. (1974) *Abnormal Psychology: An Experimental Clinical Approach.* New York: Wiley.

DAVISON, G. C. and NEALE, J. M. (1986) *Abnormal Psychology: An Experimental Clinical Approach.* (4th Ed.) New York: Wiley.

DAY, J. (1977) Right-hemisphere language processing in normal right-handers. *Journal of Experimental Psychology: Human Perception and Performance,* 13, 518–528.

DAY, J. (1979) Visual half-field word recognition as a function of syntactic class and imageability. *Neuropsychologia,* 17, 515–519.

DEJOY, D. (1975) *An Investigation of the Frequency of Nine Individual Types of Disfluency and Total Disfluency in Relation to Age and Syntactic Maturity in Nonstuttering Males, Three and One Half Years of Age and Five Years of Age.* (Doctoral dissertation) Evanston, IL: Northwestern University.

DEJOY, D. and GREGORY, H. H. (1985) The relationship between age and frequency of disfluency in preschool children. *Journal of Fluency Disorders,* 10, 107–123.

DELANEY, C. M. (1979) The function of the middle ear muscles in stuttering. *South African Journal of Communication Disorders,* 26, 20–34.

DELL, C. W. (1980) *Treating the School Age Stutterer: A Guide for Clinicians.* Memphis: Speech Foundation of America.

DELL, P. F. (1981a) Paradox redux. *Journal of Marital and Family Therapy,* 7, 127–134.

DELL, P. F. (1981b) Some irreverent thoughts on paradox. *Family Process,* 20, 37–42.

DENNIS, M. (1980a) Capacity and strategy for syntactic comprehension after left or right hemidecortication. *Brain and Language,* 10, 287–317.

DENNIS, M. (1980b) Language acquisition in a single hemisphere: semantic organization. In D. Caplan (Ed.), *Biological Studies of Developmental Processes.* Cambridge: MIT Press.

DENNIS, M. and WHITAKER, H. A. (1976) Language acquisition following hemidecortication: linguistic superiority of the left over the right hemisphere. *Brain and Language,* **3,** 404–433.

DENNIS, M. and KOHN, B. (1975) Comprehension of syntax in infantile hemiplegics after cerebral hemidecortication: left-hemispheric superiority. *Brain and Language,* **2,** 472–482.

DEVILLIERS, P. A. and DEVILLIERS, J. G. (1972) Early judgements of semantic and syntactic acceptability by children. *Journal of Psycholinguistic Research,* **1,** 229–310.

DORMAN, M. F. and PORTER, R. J., Jr. (1975) Hemispheric lateralization for speech perception in stutterers. *Cortex,* **11,** 181–185.

DOUGLASS, L. C. (1943) A study of bilaterally recorded electroencephalograms of adult stutterers. *Journal of Experimental Psychology,* **32,** 247–265.

DUNLAP, K. (1928) A revision of the fundamental law of habit formation. *Science,* **67,** 360–362.

DUNLAP, K. (1942) The technique of negative practice. *American Journal of Psychology,* **55,** 270–273.

DUNLAP, K. (1946) *Personal Adjustment.* New York: McGraw Hill.

DUNLAP, K. (1972) *Habits Their Making and Unmaking.* New York: Liveright.

DUNN, L. and DUNN, L. (1981) *The Peabody Picture Vocabulary Test – Revised.* Circle Pines, MN: American Guidance Service.

ECKEL, F. and BOONE, D. (1981). The s/z ratio as an indicator of laryngeal pathology. *Journal of Speech Hearing Disorders,* **46,** 147–149.

EDWARDS, M. L. and SHRIBERG, L. D. (1983) *Phonology: Applications in Communicative Disorders,* San Diego, CA: College Hill Press.

ELLIS, A. (1977) *Die Rational-emotive Therapie.* Munchen: Pfeiffer.

ENTUS, A., (1977) Hemispheric asymmetry in processing of dichotically presented speech and nonspeech stimuli by infants. In S. J. Segalowitz and F. A. Gruber (Eds.), *Language Development and Neurological Theory.* New York: Academic Press.

ERICKSON, R. L. (1969) Assessing communication attitudes among stutterers. *Journal of Speech and Hearing Research,* **12,** 711–724.

EVESHAM, M. and FRANSELLA, F. (1985) Stuttering relapse: the effect of a combined speech and psychological reconstruction programme. *British Journal of Disorders of Communication,* **20,** 237–248.

EVESHAM, M. and HUDDLESTON, A. (1983) Teaching stutterers the skill of fluent speech as a preliminary to the study of relapse. *British Journal of Disorders of Communication,* **18,** 31–38.

EYSENCK, H. J. (1952) The effects of psychotherapy: An evaluation. *Journal of Consulting and Clinical Psychology,* **16,** 319–324.

FABER-CLARK, M. and MOORE, W. H., Jr. (1983) Sex, task, and strategy effects in hemispheric alpha asymmetries for the recall and recognition of arousal words: results from perceptual and motor tasks. *Brain and Cognition,* **2,** 233–250.

FAHMY, M. (1950) The theory of habit control and negative practice as a corrective for stammering. *Speech,* **14,** 24–30.

FAIRBANKS, G. (1954) Systematic research in experimental phonetics: I. A theory of the speech mechanism as a servosystem. *Journal of Speech and Hearing Disorders,* **19,** 133–139.

FAIRBANKS, G. (1955) Selected vocal effects of delayed auditory feedback. *Journal of Speech and Hearing Disorders,* **20,** 336–346.

FAIRBANKS, G. (1960) *Voice and Articulation Drillbook.* Second Edition. New York: Harper and Row.

FEDIO, P. and VAN BUREN, J. M. (1975) Memory and perceptual deficits during electrical stimulation in the left and right thalamus and parietal subcortex. *Brain and Language,* **2,** 78–100.

FIEDLER, P. and STANDOP, R. (1983) *Stuttering: Integrating Theory and Practice* (Translated by S. Silverman) Rockville, MD: Aspen Publications.

FISHMAN, H. C. (1937) A study of the efficacy of negative practice as a corrective for stammering. *Journal of Speech Disorders,* **2,** 67–72.

FLEET, W. S. and HEILMAN, K. M. (1985) Acquired stuttering from a right hemisphere lesion in a right-hander. *Neurology, 35,* 1345–1346.

FLETCHER, J. (1928) *The problem of stuttering.* New York: Longmans, Green and Co.

FLETCHER, S. (1972) Time-by-count measurement of diadochokinetic syllable rate. *Journal of Speech and Hearing Research, 15,* 763–770.

FLOYD, S. and PERKINS, W. H. (1974) Early syllable dysfluency in stutterers and non-stutterers: A preliminary report. *Journal of Communication Disorders, 7,* 279–282.

FOPPA, K. (1968) *Lernen, Gedachtnis, Verhalten.* Koln: Kiepenheuer and Witsch.

FOX, B. and ROUTH, D. K. (1975) Analyzing spoken language into words, syllables, and phonemes: A developmental study. *Journal of Psycholinguistic Research, 4,* 331–342.

FRANCK, R. (1980) Integration of an intensive program for stutterers within the normal activities of a major acute hospital. *Australian Journal Human Communication Disorders, 20,* 237–248.

FRANK, J. D. (1961) *Persuasion and Healing.* Baltimore: John Hopkins.

FRANKL, V. E. (1959) *Man's Search for Meaning: An Introduction to Logotherapy.* Boston: Beacon Press.

FRANKL, V. E. (1961) *Die Psychotherapie in der Praxis.* Wien: Deuticke.

FRANSELLA, F. (1967) Rhythm as a distractor in the modification of stuttering. *Behaviour Reserach and Therapy, 5,* 253–55.

FRANSELLA, F. (1972) *Personal Change and Reconstruction: Research on a Treatment for Stuttering.* London: Academic Press.

FRANSELLA, F. (1983) Mistaken assumptions. *Changes, 1,* 4, 104.

FRANSELLA, F. and BANNISTER, D. (1977) *A Manual for the Repertory Grid Technique.* London: Academic Press.

FREEMAN, F. and USHIJIMA, T. (1978) Laryngeal muscle activity during stuttering. *Journal of Speech and Hearing Research, 21,* 538–562.

FREEMAN, F. J. (1979) Phonation and stuttering. A review of current research. *Journal of Fluency Disorders, 4,* 78–89.

FREEMAN, F. J. (1982) Stuttering. In J. Lass, L. V., McReynolds, J. L. Northern and D. E. Yoder (Eds.), *Speech, Language and Hearing. Vol 2.* Philadelphia: W. B. Saunders.

FREEMAN, F. J. (1984) Laryngeal muscle activity of stutterers. In R. F. Curlee and W. H. Perkins (Eds.), *Nature and Treatment of Stuttering: New Directions.* San Diego: College-Hill Press.

FREEMAN, F. J. and ROSENFIELD, D. B. (1982) 'Source' in disfluency. *Journal of Fluency Disorders, 7,* 295–296.

FREUND, H. (1952) Studies in the interrelationship between stuttering and cluttering. *Folia Phoniatrica, 4,* 146–168.

FRICK, J. (1952) An exploratory study of the effect of punishment (electric shock) upon stuttering behavior. *Speech Monographs, 19,* 146–147.

FRIEDMAN, A. and POLSON, M. D. (1981) Hemispheres as independent resource systems: limited-capacity processing and cerebral specialization. *Journal of Experimental Psychology: Human Perception and Performance, 7,* 1031–1058.

FROMKIN, V. A., KRASHEN, S., CURTISS, S., RIGLER, D. and RIGLER, M. (1974) The development of language in Genie: A case of language acquisition beyond the 'Critical Period'. *Brain and Language, 1,* 81–107.

GALIN, D. and ORNSTEIN, R. (1972) Lateral specialization of cognitive mode: An EEG study. *Psychophysiology, 9,* 412–418.

GAZZANIGA, M. S. (1970) *The Bisected Brain.* New York: Appleton-Century-Crofts.

GERMAN, D. (1986) *Test of Word Finding.* Allen, Texas: DLM Teaching Resources.

GESCHWIND, N. (1984) The biology of cerebral dominance: Implications for cognition. *Cognition, 17,* 192–208.

GESCHWIND, N. and BEHAN, P. (1982) Left-handedness: Association with immune disease, migraine, and developmental learning disorder. *Proceedings of the National Academy of Science,* **79**, 5097–5100.

GESCHWIND, N. and GALABURDA, A. N. (1985a) Cerebral lateralization: Biological mechanisms, associations, and pathology: I. A hypothesis and a program for research. *Archives of Neurology,* **42**, 428–459.

GESCHWIND, N. and GALABURDA, A. N. (1985b) Cerebral lateralization: Biological mechanisms, associations, and pathology: II. A hypothesis and a program for research. *Archives of Neurology,* **42**, 521–552.

GESCHWIND, N. and GALABURDA, A. N. (1985c) Cerebral lateralization: Biological mechanisms, associations and pathology: III. A hypothesis and a program for research. *Archives of Neurology,* **42**, 634–654.

GIFFORD, M. (1943) In E. Hahn (Ed.), *Stuttering: Significant theories and therapy.* Stanford, CA: Stanford University Press.

GLASNER, P. (1970) Developmental view. In J. Sheehan (Ed.), *Stuttering Research and Therapy.* New York: Harper and Row.

GLAUBER, I. (1958) The psychoanalysis of stuttering. In J. Eisenson (Ed.), *Stuttering: A Symposium.* New York: Harper and Row.

GLEITMAN, L. R., GLEITMAN, H. and SHIPLEY, E. F. (1972) The emergence of the child as grammarian. *Cognition: International Journal of Cognitive Psychology,* **1**, 137–164.

GOLDFRIED, M. R. (1980) (Ed.) Special issue: Psychotherapy process. *Cognitive Therapy and Research,* **4**.

GOLDIAMOND, I. (1965) Stuttering and fluency as manipulatable operant response classes. In L. Krasner and L. Ullman (Eds.), *Research in Behavior Modification.* New York: Holt, Rinehart and Winston.

GOLDMAN, R. and FRISTOE, M. (1969) *Goldman-Fristoe Test of Articulation.* Circle Pines, Minn: American Guidance Service Inc.

GOODGLASS, H. and QUADFASEL, F. A. (1954) Language laterality and left-handed aphasics. *Brain,* **77**, 521–548.

GORDON, P. (1982) The effects of syntactic complexity on the occurrence of dysfluencies in five-year-old children. Poster session, ASHA.

GORDON, W. H. (1979) Left hemisphere dominance of rhythmic elements in dichotically-presented melodies. *Cortex,* **15**, 58–58.

GRACCO, V. L. and ABBS, J. H. (1985) Dynamic control of the perioral system during speech; kinematic analyses of autogenic and nonautogenic sensorimotor processes. *Journal of Neurophysiology,* **54**, 418–432.

GREENWOOD, J. D. (1981) *Explanatory Structures in Natural and Human Science.* Unpublished DPhil thesis. University of Oxford, UK.

GREGORY, H. H. (1959) *A Study of the Neurophysiological Integrity of the Auditory Feedback System in Stutterers and Nonstutterers* (Doctoral Dissertation). Evanston, IL: Northwestern University.

GREGORY, H. H. (1968) (Ed.), *Learning Theory and Stuttering Therapy.* Evanston, IL: Northwestern University Press.

GREGORY, H. H. (1973) *Stuttering: Differential Evaluation and Therapy.* Indianapolis, IN: Bobbs-Merrill.

GREGORY, H. H. (1979a) Controversial issues: Statement and review of literature. In: H. H. Gregory (Ed.), *Controversies about Stuttering Therapy.* Baltimore, MD: University Park Press.

GREGORY, H. H. (1979b) The controversies: Analysis and current status. In H. H. Gregory (Ed.), *Controversies about Stuttering Therapy.* Baltimore, MD: University Park Press.

GREGORY, H. H. (1980) The clinicians' attitudes. In J. Fraser-Gruss (Ed.), *Counselling stutterers.* Memphis, TN: Speech Foundation of America.

GREGORY, H. H. (1983) Commentary. In J. Fraser Gruss (Ed.), *Stuttering Therapy: Transfer and Maintenance.* Memphis: Speech Foundation of America.

GREGORY, H. H. (1984a) Prevention of stuttering: Management of the early stages. In: R. F. Curlee and W. H. Perkins (Eds.), *Nature and Treatment of Stuttering:* New Directions. San Diego: College-Hill Press.

GREGORY, H. H. (1984b) *Stuttering Therapy: Prevention and Intervention with Children.* Memphis, TN: Speech Foundation of America.

GREGORY, H. H. (1985a) Environmental manipulation and family counselling. In G. Shames and H. Rubin (Eds.), *Stuttering: Then and Now.* Columbus, Ohio: Charles Merrill.

GREGORY, H. H. (1985b) *The problem of stuttering: Where are we?* Paper presented at The Oxford Dysfluency Conference, England.

GREGORY, H. H. (1986a) *Stuttering: Differential Evaluation and Therapy.* Austin, TX: PRO-ED.

GREGORY, H. H. (1986b) *Stuttering: A contemporary perspective.* Paper presented at XX Congress of the International Association of Logopedics and Phoniatrics, Tokyo.

GREGORY, H. H. (1986c) Stuttering: A contemporary perspective. *Folia Phoniatrica,* **38,** 89–120.

GREGORY, H. H. and GREGORY, C. (1984) *Combining the stutter-more-fluently and speak-more-fluently approaches in stuttering therapy.* Workshop, ASHA convention, San Francisco.

GREGORY, H. H. and HILL, D. (1980) Stuttering therapy for children. In W. H. Perkins (Ed.), *Strategies in Stuttering Therapy.* New York: Thieme-Stratton.

GREGORY, H. H. and HILL, D. (1984) Stuttering therapy for children. In W. H. Perkins (Ed.), *Current Therapy of Communication Disorders: Stuttering Disorders.* New York: Thieme-Stratton.

GREGORY, H. H. and MANGAN, J. (1982) Auditory processes in stutterers. In J. Lass (Ed.), *Speech and Language: Advances in Basic Research and Practice* (Vol. 7). New York: Academic Press.

GRUBER, F. and SEGALOWITZ, S. (1977) Some issues and methods in the neuropsychology of language. In S. Segalowitz and F. Gruber (Eds.) 6, *Language Development and Neurological Theory.* New York: Academic Press.

GRUSS, J. (Ed.) (1983) *Stuttering Therapy: Transfer and Maintenance.* Memphis, TN: Speech Foundation of America.

GUITAR, B. (1975) Reduction of stuttering frequency using analog electro-myographic feedback. *Journal of Speech and Hearing Research,* **18,** 672–685.

GUITAR, B. (1976) Pretreatment factors associated with the outcome of stuttering therapy. *Journal of Speech and Hearing Research,* **19,** 590–600.

GUITAR, B. and BASS, C. (1978) Stuttering therapy: The relation between attitude change and long-term outcome. *Journal of Speech and Hearing Disorders,* **43,** 392–400.

GUITAR, B. and PETERS, T. J. (1980) *Stuttering: An integration of contemporary theories.* Memphis: Speech Foundation of America.

GUR, R. C. and REIVICH, M. (1980) Cognitive task effects on hemispheric blood flow in humans: evidence for individual differences in hemispheric activation. *Brain and Language,* **9,** 78–92.

HAGGARD, M. P. and PARKINSON, A. M. (1971) Stimulus and task factors as determinants of ear advantages. *Quarterly Journal of Experimental Psychology,* **23,** 168–177.

HAKES, D. (1980) *The Emergence of Metalinguistic Abilities in Children.* New York: Springer-Verlag.

HALEY, J. (1963) *Strategies of Psychotherapy.* New York: Grune and Stratton.

HALEY, J. (1976) *Problem-Solving Therapy.* San Francisco: Jossey Bass.

HALL, J. W. and JERGER, J. (1978) Central auditory function in stutterers. *Journal of Speech and Hearing Research,* **21,** 324–337.

HAM, R. (1985). *Techniques of Stuttering Therapy.* Englewood Cliffs, NJ: Prentice-Hall.

HAND, C. R. and HAYNES, W. O. (1983) Linguistic processing and reaction time differences in stutterers and nonstutterers. *Journal of Speech and Hearing Research,* **26,** 181–185.

HANNAH, E. P. and GARDNER, J. G. (1968) A note on syntactic relationships in nonfluency. *Journal of Speech Hearing Disorders,* **11,** 853–860.

HANSON, D., GRONHOYD, K. and RICE, P. (1981). A shortened version of the Southern Illinois University speech situation checklist for the identification of speech-related anxiety. *Journal of Fluency Disorders,* **6,** 351–360.

HASBROUCK, J. M. and LOWRY-ROMERO, F. (1983) *An intensive therapy approach to eliminating stuttering and maintaining fluency.* Videotape forum presented at the American Speech-Language-Hearing Association Convention, Cincinnati, OH.

HAYHOW, R. (1983) The assessment of stuttering and the evaluation of treatment. In P. Dalton (Ed.), *Approaches to the Treatment of Stuttering.* London: Croom Helm.

HAYNES, W. and HOOD, S. (1978) Dysfluency changes in children as a function of the systematic modification of linguistic complexity. *Journal of Communication Disorders,* **11,** 79–93.

HAYNES, W. O. and MOORE, W. H., Jr. (1981a) Sentence imagery and recall: an electroencephalographic evaluation of hemispheric processing in males and females. *Cortex,* **17,** 49–62.

HAYNES, W. O. and MOORE, W. H., Jr., (1981b) Recognition and recall: an electroencephalographic investigation of hemispheric alpha asymmetries for males and females on perceptual and retrieval tasks. *Perceptual and Motor Skills,* **53,** 283–290.

HEESCHEN, C. and JURGENS, R. (1978) Pragmatic-semantic and syntactic factors influencing ear differences in dichotic listening. *Cortex,* **14,** 17–24.

HELM, N. A., BUTLER, R. B. and BENSON, D. F. (1978) Acquired stuttering. *Neurology,* **28,** 1159–1165.

HELM-ESTABROOKS, N. (1986) Diagnosis and management of neurogenic stuttering in adults. In, K. St. Louis (Ed.), *The Atypical Stutterer: Principles and Practices of Rehabilitation.* New York: Academic Press.

HELM-ESTABROOKS, M., YEO, R., GESCHWIND, N., FREEDMAN, M. and WEINSTEIN, C. (1986) Stuttering: Disappearance and reappearance with acquired brain lesions. *Neurology,* **36,** 1109–1112.

HELTMAN, H. (1938) Psychosocial phenomena of stuttering and their etiological and therapeutic implications. *Journal of Social Psychology,* **9,** 79–96.

HENKE, W. L. (1966) *Dynamic Articulatory Model of Speech Production Using Computer Simulation.* Doctoral dissertation, Massachusetts Institute of Technology.

HERSEN, M. and BARLOW, D. H. (1976) *Single Case Experimental Designs: Strategies for Studying Behavior Change.* New York: Pergamon.

HIGGINBOTHAM, P. and BANNISTER, D. (1983) *The GAB computer program for the analysis of repertory grid data.* Department of Psychology, University of Leeds, UK.

HINKLE, D. E. (1965) *The Change in Personal Constructs from the Viewpoint of a Theory of Implications.* Unpub PhD thesis, Ohio State University, USA.

HINZMAN, A. R. and ST. LOUIS, K. O. (1983) *Success vs. failure in alleviating stuttering: A retrospective study.* Paper presented at the American Speech-Language-Hearing Association Convention, Cincinnati, OH., USA.

HOMZIE, M. J. and LINDSAY, J. S. (1984) Language and the young stutterer: a new look at old theories and findings. *Brain and Language,* **22,** 232–252.

HORNER, J. and MASSEY, E. W. (1983) Progressive dysfluency associated with right hemisphere disease. *Brain and Language,* **18,** 71–85.

HOWIE, P. and ANDREWS, G. (1984) Treatment of adults: Managing fluency. In R. F. Curlee and W. H. Perkins (Eds.), *Nature and Treatment of Stuttering: New Directions:* San Diego: College-Hill Press.

HOWIE, P. M., TANNER, S., and ANDREWS, G. (1981) Short- and long-term outcome in an intensive treatment program for adult stutterers. *Journal of Speech and Hearing Disorders,* **46,** 104–109.

HOWIE, P. WOODS, C. and ANDREWS, J. (1982) Relationship between covert and overt speech measures immediately before and immediately after stuttering treatment. *Journal of Speech and Hearing Disorders,* **47,** 419–422.

HRESKO, W. D., REID, D. and HAMMILL, D. (1982) *Test of Early Language Development.* Austin, Texas: PRO-ED.

HUDSON, P. (1980) Different strokes different folks: A comparative examination of behavioural, structural and paradoxical method in family therapy. *Journal of Family Therapy,* **2**, 181–197.

HUGGINS, A. W. F. (1978) Speech timing and intelligibility. In J. Requin (Ed.), *Attention and performance VII.* Hillsdale, N.J.: Lawrence Erlbaum.

HUNNICUTT, S. (1985) Intelligibility versus redundancy: conditions of dependency. *Language and Speech,* **28**, 47–56.

HUTT, D. (1986) *Parent-child Speech Rate Differences: Boys v. Girls.* M.A. Thesis, Temple University.

INGHAM, R. J. (1975) Operant methodology in stuttering therapy. In J. Eisenson (Ed.), *Stuttering: A Second Symposium.* New York: Harper and Row.

IINGHAM, R. J. (1980a) Modification of maintenance and generalization during stuttering treatment. *Journal of Speech and Hearing Research,* **23**, 732–745.

INGHAM, R. J. (1980b) *Stuttering therapy manual: Hierarchy control schedule. A clinician's guide.* Sydney: School of Communication Disorders, Cumberland College of Health Sciences.

INGHAM, R. J. (1981) Evaluation and maintenance in stuttering treatment: A search for ecstacy with nothing but agony. In E. Boberg (Ed.), *Maintenance of Fluency.* New York: Elsevier.

INGHAM, R. J. (1982) The effects of self-evaluation training on maintenance and generalisation during stuttering treatment. *Journal of Speech and Hearing Disorders,* **47**, 271–280.

INGHAM, R. J. (1983) Spontaneous remission of stuttering. In D. Prins and R. J. Ingham (Eds.), *Treatment of Stuttering in Early Childhood: Methods and Issues.* San Diego: College-Hill Press.

INGHAM, R. J. (1984a) Generalization and maintenance of treatment. In R. F. Curlee and W. H. Perkins (Eds.), *Nature and Treatment of Stuttering: New Directions.* San Diego: College-Hill Press.

INGHAM, R. J. (1984b) *Stuttering and Behavior Therapy: Current Status and Experimental Foundations.* San Diego: College-Hill Press.

INGHAM, R. J. (1984c) Toward a therapy assessment procedure for treating stuttering in children. In H. H. Gregory (Ed.), *Stuttering Therapy: Prevention and Intervention with Children.* Memphis, TN: Speech Foundation of America.

IINGHAM, R. J. and COSTELLO, J. M. (1985) Stuttering treatment outcome evaluation. In J. M. Costello (Ed.), *Stuttering Disorders in Adults: Recent Advances.* San Diego, CA: College-Hill Press.

INGHAM, R. J. and PACKMAN, A. (1977) Treatment and generalization effects in an experimental treatment for a stutterer using contingency management and speech rate control. *Journal of Speech and Hearing Disorders,* **42**, 394–407.

INGHAM, R. J. and ONSLOW, M. (1985) Measurement and modification of speech naturalness during stuttering therapy. *Journal of Speech and Hearing Disorders,* **50**, 261–281.

INGHAM, R. J., ANDREWS, G. and WINKLER, R. (1972) Stuttering: A comparative evluation of the short-term effectiveness of four treatment techniques. *Journal of Communication Disorders,* **5**, 91–117.

INGHAM, R. J., GOW, M. and COSTELLO, J. M. (1985) Stuttering and speech naturalness: Some additional date. *Journal of Speech and Hearing Disorders,* **50**, 217–219.

INGHAM, R. J., MARTIN, R. R., HAROLDSON, S. K., ONSLOW, M. and LENEY, M. (1985) Modification of listener-judged naturalness in the speech of stutterers. *Journal of Speech and Hearing Research,* **28**, 495–504.

JACOBSON, E. (1938) *Progressive Relaxation.* Chicago: University of Chicago Press.

JACOBSON, N. S. and BAUCOM, D. H. (1977) Design and assessment of nonspecific control groups in behavior modification research. *Behavior Therapy,* **8**, 709–719.

JAYARAM, M. (1984) Distribution of stuttering in sentences: relationships to sentence length and clause position, *Journal of Speech and Hearing Research,* **27**, 338–341.

JOHNSON, J., SOMMERS, R. K. and WEIDNER, W. E. (1977) Dichotic ear preference in aphasia. *Journal of Speech and Hearing Research,* **20**, 116–129.

JOHNSON, W. (1934) *Stuttering in the preschool child.* University of Iowa Welfare Pamphlet No. 37.

JOHNSON, W. (1944) The Indians have no name for it. *Quarterly Journal of Speech,* **30,** 330–337.

JOHNSON, W. (1946) *People in Quandries.* New York. Harper and Row.

JOHNSON, W. (1948) Stuttering. In W. Johnson, S. F. Brown, J. F. Curtis, C. W. Edney and J. Keester (Eds.), *Speech and Handicapped School Children.* New York: Harper and Row.

JOHNSON, W. (1955) A study of the onset and development of stuttering. In W. Johnson and R. R. Leutenegger (Eds.), *Stuttering in Children and Adults.* Minneapolis: University of Minnesota Press.

JOHNSON, W. (1955) *Stuttering in Children and Adults.* Minneapolis, MN: University of Minnesota Press.

JOHNSON, W. (1959) *The Onset of Stuttering.* Minneapolis, MN: University of Minnesota Press.

JOHNSON, W. (1961a) *Stuttering and What You Can Do About It.* Danville, IL: Interstate Printers and Publishers.

JOHNSON, W. (1961b) Measurements of oral reading and speaking rate and disfluency of adult male and female stutterers and nonstutterers. *Journal of Speech and Hearing Disorders, Monograph Supplement,* **7,** 1–20.

JOHNSON, W. (1967) Stuttering. In W. Johnson and E. Moeller (Eds.), *Speech Handicapped School Children.* New York: Harper and Row.

JOHNSON, L. (1984) Facilitating parental involvement in therapy of the preschool disfluent child. In W. H. Perkins (Ed.), *Current Therapy of Communication Disorders: Stuttering Disorders.* New York: Thieme-Stratton.

JOHNSON, W. and BROWN, S. F. (1935) Stuttering in relation to various speech sounds. *Quarterly Journal of Speech,* **21,** 481–496.

JOHNSON, W., BOEHMLER, R., DAHLSTROM, W., DARLEY, F., GOODSTEIN, L., KOOLS, S., NEELEY, J., PRATHER, W., SHERMAN, D., THURMAN, C., TROTTER, W. and WILLIAMS, D. (1959) *The Onset of Stuttering.* Minneapolis, MN: University of Minnesota Press.

JOHNSON, W., DARLEY, F. and SPRIESTERSBACH, D. (1963). *Diagnostic Methods in Speech Pathology.* New York: Harper and Row.

JONES, D. (1944) Chronemes and tonemes. *Acta Linguistica,* **4,** 1–10.

JONES, R. K. (1966) Observations on stammering after localized cerebral injury. *Journal of Neurology, Neurosurgery and Psychiatry,* **29,** 192–195.

JURGENS, U. and PLOOG, D. (1981) On the neural control of mammalian vocalization. *Trends in Neurosciences,* **4,** 135–137.

KAIL, R. and LEONARD, L. (1986) Word-finding abilities in language impaired children. *ASHA Monograph 25.*

KASPRISIN-BURRELLI, A., EGOLF, D., and SHAMES, G. (1972) A comparison of parental verbal behavior with stuttering and nonstuttering children. *Journal of Communicative Disorders,* **5,** 335–346.

KATZ, A. H. and BENDER, E. (1976) *The Strength in Us: Self-help Groups in the Modern World.* New York: Franklin Watts.

KAZDIN, A. E. (1981) Drawing valid inferences from case studies. *Journal of Consulting and Clinical Psychology,* **49,** 183–192.

KAZDIN, A. E. (1982) *Single Case Research Designs: Methods for Clinical and Applied Settings.* New York: Oxford Press.

KAZDIN, A. E. and WILCOXON, L. A. (1976) Systematic desensitisation and nonspecific treatment effects: A methodological evaluation. *Psychological Bulletin,* **83,** 729–758.

KELLY, G. A. (1955a) *The Psychology of Personal Constructs. Vol 1* New York: Norton.

KELLY, G. A. (1955b) *The Psychology of Personal Constructs. Vol 2* New York: Norton.

KELSO, J. A. S., and TULLER, B. (1984) Converging evidence in support of common dynamical principles for speech and movement coordination. *American Journal of Physiology,* **246,** R928–R935.

KELSO, J. A. S., TULLER, B. and FOWLER, C. A. (1982) The functional specificity of articulatory control and coordination (abstract). *Journal of the Acoustical Society of America,* **72,** Supplement 1, S103.

KENT, R. D. (1983) Facts about stuttering: Neuropsychological perspectives. *Journal of Speech and Hearing Disorders,* **48,** 249–255.

KENT, R. D. (1984) Stuttering as a temporal programming disorder. In R. F. Curlee and W. H. Perkins (Eds.), *Nature and Treatment of Stuttering: New Directions.* San Diego: College-Hill Press.

KICKBUSCH, I. and HATCH, S. (1983) A Re-orientation of Health Care? In S. Hatch and I. Kickbusch (Eds.), *Self-help and Health in Europe: New Approaches in Health Care.* Copenhagen: WHO.

KIDD, K. (1980) Genetic models of stuttering. *Journal of Fluency Disorders,* **5,** 187–201.

KIDD, K. (1983) Recent progress on the genetics of stuttering. In C. Ludlow and E. Cooper (Eds.), *Genetic Aspects of Speech and Language.* New York: Academic Press.

KIDD, K. K. (1984) Stuttering as a genetic disorder. In R. F. Curlee and W. H. Perkins (Eds.), *Nature and Treatment of Stuttering: New Directions.* San Diego: College-Hill Press.

KIESLER, D. J. (1966) Some myths of psychotherapy research and the search for a paradigm. *Psychological Bulletin,* **65,** 110–136.

KIMURA, D. (1961a) Some effects of temporal-lobe damage on auditory perception. *Canadian Journal of Psychology,* **15,** 156–165.

KIMURA, D. (1961b) Cerebral dominance and the perception of verbal stimuli. *Canadian Journal of Psychology,* **15,** 166–175.

KIMURA, D. (1964) Left-right differences in the perception of melodies. *Quarterly Journal of Experimental Psychology,* **16,** 355–358.

KIMURA, D. (1967) Functional asymmetry of the brain in dichotic listening. *Cortex,* **13,** 163–178.

KINSBOURNE, M. (1971) The minor cerebral hemisphere as a source of aphasic speech. *Archives of Neurology,* **25,** 302–306.

KLATT, D. (1976) Linguistic uses of segmental duration in English: acoustic and perceptual evidence. *Jurnal of the Acoustical Society of America,* **59,** 1208–1221.

KNOTT, J. R. and TJOSSEN, T. D. (1943) Bilaterial encephalograms from normal speakers and stutterers. *Journal of Experimental Psychology,* **32,** 357–362.

KOHN, B. and DENNIS, M. (1974) Selective impairments of visuo-spatial abilities in infantile hemiplegics after right cerebral hemidecortication. *Neuropsychologica,* **12,** 505–512.

KOLB, B. and WHISHAW, I. Q. (1980) *Fundamentals of Human Neuropsychology.* New York: W. H. Freeman and Company.

KOZHEVNIKOV, V. A. and CHISTOVICH, L. A. (1965) *Speech: Articulation and Perception.* Washington, D.C.: Joint Publication Research Service.

KRATCHOWILL, T. R. (1978) (Ed.), *Single Subject Research: Strategies for Evaluating Change.* New York: Academic Press.

KRATCHOWILL, T. R., MOTT, S. E. and DODSON, C. L. (1984) Case study and single case research in clinical and applied psychology. In A. S. Bellack and M. Hersen (Eds.), *Research methods in Clinical Psychology.* New York: Pergamon.

KUHN, T. S. (1962) *The Structure of Scientific Revolutions.* Chicago: University of Chicago Press.

KUHR, A. and RUSTIN, L. (1985) The maintenance of fluency after intensive in-patient therapy: Long-term follow-up. *Journal of Fluency Disorders,* **10,** 229–236.

LADOUCEUR, R., COTE, C. LEBLOND, G. and BONCHARD, L. (1982) Evaluation of regulated-breathing method and awareness training in the treatment of stuttering. *Journal of Speech and Hearing Disorders,* **47,** 422–426.

LANG, P. E. (1969) The mechanics of desensitiation and the laboratory study of fear. In C. Franks (Ed.), *Behavior Therapy: Appraisa and Status.* New York: McGraw-Hill.

LANKFORD, S. D. and COOPER, E. B. (1974) Recovery from stuttering as viewed by parents of self-diagnosed recovered stutterers. *Journal of Communication Disorders,* **7,** 171–180.

LANYON, R. (1977) Effect of biofeedback-based relaxation on stuttering during reading and spontaneous speech. *Journal of Consulting Clinical Psychology,* **45**, 860–866.

LASHLEY, K. A. (1951) The problem of serial order in behaviour. In L. A. Jeffress (Ed.), *Cerebral Mechanisms in Behaviour.* New York: Wiley.

LASSEN, N. A., INGVAR, D. H. and SKINHOJ, E. (1978) Brain Function and Blood Flow. *Scientific American,* **239**, 62–71.

LAZARUS, A. A. (1971) *Behavior Therapy and Beyond.* New York: McGraw-Hill.

LEE, B. (1951) Artificial stutter. *Journal of Speech and Hearing Disorders,* **16**, 53–55.

LEES, R. (1983) Adjuncts to speech therapy. In P. Dalton (Ed.), *Approaches to the Treatment of Stuttering.* London: Croom Helm.

LEHISTE, I. (1972) Syllable nucleus as a unit of timing, *Journal of the Acoustical Society of America,* **52**, 182.

LEITH, W. (1971) Clinical training in stuttering therapy: A survey. *ASHA,* **13**, 6–8.

LEITH, W. (1986) Treating the stutterer with atypical culture influences. In K. St. Louis (Ed.), *The Atypical Stutterer: Principles and Practices of Rehabilitation.* Nw York: Academic Press.

LENNEBERG, E. (1967) *Biological Foundations of Language.* New York: Wiley.

LIBERMAN, I. Y., SHANKWEILER, D., FISCHER, F. W. and CARTER, B. (1974) Explicit syllable and phoneme segmentation in the young child. *Journal of Experimental Child Psychology,* **18**, 201–212.

LIEBETRAU, R. M. and DALY, D. A. (1981) Auditory processing and perceptual abilities of 'organic' and 'functional' stutterers. *Journal of Fluency Disorders,* **6**, 219–231.

LINDBLOM, B. (1968) Temporal organization of syllable production. *Speech Transmission Laboratory Quarterly Progress and Status Report,* Stockholm, October.

LINGWALL, J. B. and BERGSTRAND, G. G. (1979). Perceptual boundaries for judgments of 'normal', 'abnormal' and 'stuttered' prolongations. *ASHA,* **21**, 733.

LOMAS, J. (1980) Competition within the left hemisphere between speaking and unimanual tasks performed without visual guidance. *Neuropsychologia,* **18**, 141–149.

LOMAS, J. and KIMURA, D. (1976) Intrahemispheric interaction between speaking and sequential manual activity. *Neuropsychologia,* **14**, 23–33.

LUBORSKY, L., SINGER, B. and LUBORSKY, L. (1975) Comparative studies of psychotherapies: Is it true that everyone has won and all must have prizes? *Archives of General Psychiatry,* **32**, 995–1008.

LUESSENHOP, A. J., BOGGS, J. S., LABORWIT, L. J. and WALLE, E. L. (1973) Cerebral dominance in stutterers determined by Wada testing. *Neurology,* **23**, 1190–1192.

LUPER, H. and CROSS, D. (1978) *Finger reaction time of stuttering and nonstuttering children and adults.* Annual ASHA Convention, San Francisco.

MALECOT, A., JOHNSTON, R. and KIZZIAR, P. A. (1972) Syllabic rate and utterance length in French. *Phonetica,* **26**, 235–251.

MALLARD, A. R. and WESTBROOK, J. B. (1983) *The public school specialist in stuttering therapy.* Paper presented at the XIX Congress of the International Association of Logopaedics and Phoniatrics, Edinburgh, Scotland.

MANN, M. B. (1955) Nonfluencies in the oral reading of stutterers and nonstutterers of elementary school age. In W. Johnson and R. R. Leutenegger (Eds.), *Stuttering in Children and Adults.* Minneapolis: University of Minnesota Press.

MARTIN, F. (1926) *Manual of Speech Training.* Ithaca, NY: Frederick and Louise Martin.

MARTIN, R. R. (1981) Introduction and perspective: Review of published research. In E. Boberg (Ed.), *Maintenance of Fluency.* New York: Elsevier.

MARTIN, R. R., HAROLDSON, S. K. and TRIDEN, K. A. (1984) Stuttering and speech naturalness. *Journal of Speech and Hearing Disorders,* **49**, 53–58.

MATEER, C. A. (1983) Motor and perceptual functions of the left hemisphere and their interaction. In S. J. Segalowitz (Ed.), *Language Functions and Brain Organization.* New York: Academic Press.

MAVISSAKALIAN, M., MICHELSON, L., GREENWALD, D., KORNBLITH, S. and GREENWALD, M. (1983) Cognitive behavioral treatment of agoraphobia: Paradoxical intention vs self-treatment training. *Behavior Research and Therapy,* **21**, 75–86.

MAXWELL, D. L. (1982) Cognitive and behavioral self-control strategies: Applications for the clinical management of adult stutterers. *Journal of Fluency Disorders,* **7**, 403–432.

McFARLANE, S. and PRINS, D. (1978) Neural response time of stutterers in selected oral instruction tasks. *Journal of Speech and Hearing Research,* **21**, 768–778.

McKEE, G., HUMPHREY, B. and McADAM, D. (1973) Scaled lateralizations of alpha activity during linguistic and musical tasks. *Psychophysiology,* **10**, 441–443.

McKEEVER, W. F. and HULING, M. D. (1971) Lateral dominance in tachistoscopic word recognition as a function of hemisphere stimulation and interhemispheric transfer time. *Neuropsychologia,* **9**, 291–299.

McLEAN, T. (1985) *Metal Jam – the Story of a Diabetic.* London: Hodder and Stoughton.

McLELLAND, J. K. and COOPER, E. B. (1978) Fluency-related behaviours and attitudes of 178 young stutterers. *Journal of Fluency Disorders,* **8**, 253–263.

MEDDIS, R. (1973) *Elementary Analysis of Variance for the Behavioural Sciences.* London: McGraw-Hill.

MELTZOFF, J. and KORNREICH, M. (1970) *Research in Psychotherapy.* New York: Atherton.

MEYERS, S. and FREEMAN, F. (1985) Mother and child speech rate as a variable in stuttering and dysfluency. *Journal of Speech and Hearing Research,* **28**, 436–444.

MILLER, G. A. (1951) Speech and Language. In S. S. Stevens (Ed.), *Handbook of Experimental Psychology.* New York: Wiley.

MILLER, N. (1944) Experimental studies of conflict. In J. Hunt (Ed.), *Personality and the Behavior Disordered 1.* New York: Ronald Press.

MILNER, B. (1975) Psychological effects of focal epilepsy and its neurological management. *Advances in Neurology,* **8**, 299–321.

MILNER, B. (1982) Some cognitive effects of frontal-lobe lesions in man. In D. E. Broadbent and L. Weiskrantz (Eds.), *The Neuropsychology of Cognitive Function.* London: The Royal Society.

MILNER, B., BRANCH, C. and RASMUSSEN, T. (1966) Evidence for bilateral speech representation in some non-right-handers. *Transactions of the American Neurological Association,* **91**, 306–308.

MILSUM, J. H. (1966) *Biological Control Systems Analysis.* New York: McGraw Hill.

MITCHELL, L. (1977) *Simple Relaxation: The Physiological Method for Easing Tension.* London: John Murray.

MITCHELL, K. M., BOZARTH, J. D. and KRAUFT, C. C. (1977) A reappraisal of the therapeutic effectiveness of accurate empathy, non-possessive warmth, and genuiness. In A. S. Gurman and A. M. Razin (Eds.), *Effective Psychotherapy: A Handbook of Research.* Oxford: Pergamon.

MOLFESE, D. L. (1977) Infant cerebral asymmetry. In S. J. Segalowitz and F. A. Gruber (Eds.), *Language Development and Neurological Theory.* New York: Academic Press.

MOLFESE, D. L. (1978a) Electrophysiological correlates of categorical speech perception in adults. *Brain and Language,* **5**, 25–35.

MOLFESE, D. L. (1978b) Left and right hemisphere involvement in speech perception. Electrophysiological correlates. *Perception and Psychophysics,* **23**, 237–243.

MOLFESE, D. L. (1980) Hemispheric specialization for temporal information: Implications for the perception of voicing cues during speech perception. *Brain and Language,* **11**, 285–299.

MOLFESE, D. L. (1983) Event related potentials and language processes. In A. Gillard and W. Ritter (Eds.), *Tutorials in ERP: Endogenous Components.* Amsterdam: North-Holland Publishing Company.

MOLFESE, D. L. (1984) Left hemispheric sensitivity to consonant sounds not displayed by the right hemisphere: electrophysiological correlates. *Brain and language,* **22**, 109–127.

MOLFESE, D. L., FREEMAN, R. B., Jr. and PALERMO, D. S. (1975) The ontogeny of brain lateralization for speech and nonspeech stimuli. *Brain and Language,* **2**, 356–368.

MOORE, W. H., Jr. (1976) Bilateral tachistoscopic word perception of stutterers and normal subjects. *Brain and Language,* 3, 434–442.

MOORE, W. H., Jr. (1984a) Hemispheric alpha asymmetries during an electromyographic biofeedback procedure for stuttering: A single-subject experimental design. *Journal of Fluency Disorders,* 17, 143–162.

MOORE, W. H., Jr. (1984b) The role of right hemispheric information processing strategies in language recovery in aphasia: An electroencephalographic investigation of hemispheric alpha asymmetries in normal and aphasic subjects. *Cortex,* 20, 193–205.

MOORE, W. H., Jr. (1984c) Central nervous system characteristics of stutterers. In R. F. Curlee and W. H. Perkins (Eds.), *The Nature and Treatment of Stuttering*: New Directions. San Diego, CA: College-Hill Press.

MOORE, W. H., Jr. (1986a) Hemispheric alpha asymmetries of stutters and non-stutterers for the recall and recognition of words and connected reading passages: Some relationships to severity of stuttering. *Journal of Fluency Disorders,* 11, 71–89.

MOORE, W. H., Jr. (1986b) Hemispheric alpha asymmetries and behavorial responses of aphasic and normal subjects for the recall and recognition of active, passive and negative sentences. *Brain and Language* (In Press).

MOORE, W. H., Jr. and HAYNES, W. O. (1980a) Alpha hemispheric asymmetry and stuttering: Some support for a segmentation dysfunction hypothesis. *Journal of Speech and Hearing Research,* 23, 229–247.

MOORE, W. H., Jr. and HAYNES, W. O. (1980b) A study of alpha hemispheric asymmetries and their relationship to verbal and nonverbal abilities in males and females. *Brain and Language,* 9, 338–349.

MOORE, W. H., Jr. and LANG, M. K. (1977) Alpha asymmetry over the right and left hemispheres of stutterers and control subjects preceding massed oral readings: A preliminary investigation. *Perceptual and Motor Skills,* 44, 223–230.

MOORE, W. H., Jr. and LORENDO, L. (1980) Alpha hemispheric asymmetries of stuttering and nonstuttering subjects for words of high and low imagery. *Journal of Fluency Disorders,* 5, 11–26.

MOORE, W. H., Jr. and WEIDNER, W. E. (1974) Bilateral tachistoscopic word perception in aphasic and normal subjects. *Perceptual and Motor Skills,* 39, 1001–1011.

MOORE, W. H., Jr., CRAVEN, D. C. and FABER, M. M. (1982) Hemispheric alpha asymmetries of words with positive, negative and neutral arousal values preceding tasks of recall and recognition: Electrical, physiological and behavioral results from stuttering males and nonstuttering males and females. *Brain and Language,* 17, 211–224.

MORDECAI, D. (1979) *An Investigation of the Communicative Styles of Mothers and Fathers of Stuttering versus Nonstuttering Preschool Children During a Triadic Interaction* (Doctoral dissertation). Evanston, IL: Northwestern University.

MORGAN, S. H., McDONALD, P. J. and MACDONALD, H. (1971) Differences in bilateral alpha activity as a function of experimental task with a note on lateral eye movements and hypnotizability. *Neuropsychologia,* 9, 459–469.

MOSCOVITCH, M. (1977) The development of lateralization of language functions and its relation to cognitive and linguistic development: a review and some theoretical speculations. In S. J. Segalowitz and F. A. Gruber (Eds.), *Language Development and Neurological Theory.* New York: Academic Press.

MOZDZIERZ, G., MACCHITELLI, F. and LISIECKI, J. (1976) The paradox in psychotherapy: An Adlerian perspective. *Journal of Individual Psychology,* 32, 169–184.

MUMA, J. (1971) Syntax of preschool fluent and disfluent speech: A transformational analysis. *Journal of Speech and Hearing Research,* 14, 428–441.

MUNHALL, K. G. (1985) An examination of intra-articulator relative timing. *Journal of the Acoustical Society of America,* 78, 1548–1553.

MURRAY, F. P. (1980) *A Stutterer's Story.* Danville: Interstate.

MUTTI, M., STERLING, H. and SPAULDING, N. (1978) *Quick Neurological Screening Test.* Revised Edition. Novato, California: Academic Therapy Publications.

NEELY, N. and TIMMONS, R. (1967) Adaptation and consistency in the disfluent speech behavior of young stutterers and nonstutterers. *Journal of Speech and Hearing Research,* **10,** 250–256.

NELSON, L. (1984) Language formulation related to disfluency and stuttering. In H. Gregory (Ed.), *Stuttering Therapy: Prevention and Intervention with Children.* Memphis, TN: Speech Foundation of America.

NESSEL, E. (1958) Die venzogerte sprachruckkopplung (Tee effekt) bei stotterern. *Folia Phoniatrica,* **10,** 199–204.

NEVILLE, H. J. (1977) Electroencephalographic testing of cerebral specialization in normal and congenitally deaf children: A preliminary report. In S. J. Segalowitz and F. A. Gruber (Eds.), *Language Development and Neurological Theory.* New York: Academic Press.

NIPPOLD, M. A. and FEY, S. H. (1983) Metaphoric understanding in pre-adolescents having a history of language acquisition difficulties. *Language, Speech and Hearing Services in Schools,* **14,** 171–180.

NUDELMAN, H. B., HERBRICH, K. E., HOYT, B. D. and ROSENFIELD, D. B. (1987 in press) Dynamic characteristics of vocal frequency tracking in stutterers and nonstutterers. In H. Peters and W. Hulstijn (Eds.), *Speech Motor Dynamics in Stuttering.* Wien/New York: Springer.

NYSTUL, M. S. and MUSZYSKA, E. (1976) Adlerian treatment of a classical case of stuttering. *Journal of Individual Psychology,* **32,** 194–202.

O'LEARY, K. D. and BORKOVEC, T. D. (1978) Conceptual, methodological and ethical problems of placebo groups in psychotherapy research. *American Psychologist,* **33,** 821–830.

OJEMANN, G. A. (1975) Language and the thalamus: object naming and recall during and after thalamic stimulation. *Brain and Language,* **2,** 101–120.

OJEMANN, G. A., FEDIO, P. and VAN BUREN, J. M. (1968) Anomia from pulvinar and subcortical parietal stimulation. *Brain,* **91,** 99–116.

ORTON, S. T. (1927) Studies in stuttering. *Archives of Neurology and Psychiatry,* **18,** 671–672.

ORTON, S. T. (1928) A physiological theory of reading disability and stuttering in children. *New England Journal of Medicine,* **199,** 1045–1052.

ORTON, S. T. (1937) *Reading, Writing and Speech Problems in Childhood.* New York: Norton.

OSSER, H. and PENG, F. (1964) A cross-cultural study of speech rate. *Language and Speech,* **7,** 120–125.

OWEN, N. (1981) Facilitating maintenance of behavior change. In E. Boberg (Ed.), *Maintenance of Fluency.* New York: Elsevier.

PAIVIO, A. (1978) On exploring visual knowledge. In B. Randhawa and W. Coffman (Eds.), *Visual Thinking, Learning and Communication.* New York: Academic Press.

PALEN, C. and PETERSON, J. M. (1982) Word frequency and children's stuttering: The relationship to sentence structure. *Journal of Fluency Disorders,* **7,** 55–62.

PALMER, F. R. (1974) *The English Verb.* London: Longman.

PARLOFF, M. B. (1986) Placebo controls in psychotherapy research: A sine qua non or a placebo for research problems? *Journal of Consulting and Clinical Psychology,* **54,** 79–87.

PEARL, S. and BERNTHAL, J. (1980) The effect of grammatical complexity upon disfluency behaviour of nonstuttering preschool children. *Journal of Fluency Disorders,* **5,** 55–68.

PEINS, M., McGOUGH, W. E. and LEE, B. S. (1984) Double tape recorder therapy for stutterers. In M. Peins (Ed.), *Contemporary Approaches in Stuttering Therapy.* Boston: Little, Brown and Co.

PENFIELD, W. and ROBERTS, L. (1959) *Speech and Brain Mechanisms.* Princeton, NJ: Princeton University Press.

PERECMAN, E. and KELLAR, L. (1981) The effect of voice and place among aphasic, nonaphasic right-damaged, and normal subjects on a metalinguistic task. *Brain and Language,* **12,** 213–223.

PERKINS, W. H. (1979) From psychoanalysis to discoordination. In H. H. Gregory (Ed.), *Controversies about Stuttering Therapy*. Baltimore: University Park Press.

PERKINS, W. H. (1981) Measurement and maintenance of fluency. In E. Boberg (Ed.), *Maintenance of Fluency*. New York: Elsevier.

PERKINS, W. H. (1983) The problem of definitions: Commentary on 'stuttering'. *Journal of Speech and Hearing Disorders*, **48**, 246–249.

PERKINS, W. H. (1984) Techniques for establishing fluency. In W. H. Perkins (Ed.), *Current Therapy of Communication Disorders: Stuttering Disorders*. New York: Thieme-Stratton.

PERKINS, W. H., BELL, J., JOHNSON, L. and STOCKS, J. (1979) Phone rate and the effective planning time hypothesis of stuttering. *Journal of Speech and Hearing Research*, **22**, 747–755.

PERKINS, W. H., RUDAS, J., JOHNSON, L. and BELL, J. (1976) Stuttering: Discoordination of phonation with articulation and respiration. *Journal of Speech and Hearing Research*, **19**, 509–522.

PERRIN, K. L. and EISENSON, J. (1970) An examination of ear preference for speech and nonspeech stimuli in a stuttering population. Paper presented at the Annual Convention of the *American Speech and Language Association*, New York.

PETERSON, H. A. and MARQUARDT, T. P. (1981) *Appraisal and Diagnosis of Speech and Language Disorders*. Englewood Cliffs, New Jersey: Prentice-Hall.

PETTIT, J. and NOLL, J. (1979) Cerebral dominance and aphasia recovery. *Brain and Language*, **7**, 191–200.

PINDZOLA, R. (1986) A description of some selected stuttering instruments. *Journal of Childhood Communication Disorders*, **9**, 183–200.

PINSKY, S. D. and McADAM, D. W. (1980) Electroencephalographic and dichotic indices of cerebral laterality in stutterers. *Brain and Language*, **11**, 374–397.

PLAKOSH, P. (1978) *The Functional Asymmetry of the Brain: Hemispheric Specialization in Stutterers for Processing of Visually Presented Linguistic and Spatial Stimuli*. Unpublished doctoral dissertation, the Palo Alto School of Professional Psychology.

PONSFORD, R., BROWN, W., MARSH, J. and TRAVIS, L. (1975) Evoked potential correlates of cerebral dominance for speech perception in stutterers and nonstutters. *Electroencephalography and Clinical Neurophysiology*, **39**, 434.

POPPER, K. R. (1959) *The Logic of Scientific Discovery*. New York: Harper.

POPPER, K. R. (1963) *Conjectures and Refutations*. New York: Harper.

PORFERT, A. R. and ROSENFIELD, D. B. (1978) Prevalence of stuttering. *Journal of Neurology, Neurosurgery and Psychiatry*, **41**, 954–956.

PRATT, J. (1972) *Comparison of Linguistic Perception and Production in Preschool Stutterers and Nonstutterers* (Doctoral dissertation). Champaign: University of Illinois.

PREUS, A. (1981) *Identifying Subgroups of Stutterers*. Oslo, Norway: Universitetsforlaget.

PRIESTLY, P., McGUIRE, J., FLEGG, D., HEMSLEY, V. and WELHAM, D. (1978) *Social Skills and Personal Problem Solving*. London: Tavistock.

PRINS, D. (1970) Improvement and regression in stutterers following short-term intensive therapy. *Journal of Speech and Hearing Disorders*, **35**, 123–135.

PRINS, D. (1976) Stutterers' perceptions of therapy improvement and of post-therapy regression: Effects of certain program modifications. *Journal of Speech and Hearing Disorders*, **41**, 452–463.

PRINS, D. and INGHAM, R. J. (1983) *Treatment of Stuttering in Early Childhood: Methods and Issues*. San Diego, CA: College-Hill Press.

QUINN, P. T. (1972) Stuttering, cerebral dominance and the dichotic word test. *Medical Journal of Australia*, **2**, 639–643.

QUIRK, R., GREENBAUM, S., LEECH, G. and SVARTVIK, J. (1972) *A Grammar of Contemporary English*. London: Longman.

RACHMAN, S. J. and HODGSON, R. (1980) *Obsessions and Compulsions*. Englewood Cliffs, NJ: Prentice-Hall.

RACHMAN, S. J. and WILSON, G. T. (1980) *The Effects of Psychological Therapy* (2nd Ed.). Oxford: Pergamon.

RAMIG, P. R. (1984) Rate changes in the speech of stutterers after therapy. *Journal of Fluency Disorders,* **9,** 285–294.

RASMUSSEN, T. and MILNER, B. (1975) Clinical and surgical studies of the cerebral speech areas in man. In K. J. Zulch, O. Creutzfeldt and G. C. Calbraith (Eds.), *Cerebral Localization.* Berlin and New York: Springer-Verlag.

RAVENETTE, A. T. (1980) The exploration of consciousness: personal construct intervention with children. In A. W. Landfield and L. M. Lietner (Eds.), *Personal Construct Psychology, Psychotherapy and Personality.* Chichester: Wiley.

READ, C. (1978) Children's awareness of language with emphasis on sound systems. In A. Sinclair, R. J. Jarvella, and W. J. M. Levelt (Eds.), *The Child's Conception of Language.* New York: Springer-Verlag.

REICH, A., TILL, J. and GOLDSMITH, H. (1981) Laryngeal and manual reaction times of stuttering and nonstuttering adults. *Journal of Speech and Hearing Research,* **24,** 192–196.

RICHARDSON, A. and GOODMAN, M. (1983) *Self-help and Social Care: Mutual Aid Organisations in Practice.* London: Policy Studies Institute.

RIEBER, R. W. and WOLLOCK, J. (1977a) The historical roots of the theory and therapy of stuttering. *Journal of Communication Disorders,* **10,** 3–24.

RIEBER, R. W. and WOLLOCK, J. (1977b) The history of the theory and therapy of stuttering. In R. W. Rieber (Ed.), *The Problem of Stuttering: Theory and Therapy.* New York: Elsevier.

RILEY, G. (1980). *Stuttering Severity Instrument for Children and Adults.* Revised Edition. Tigard, Oregon: C.C. Publications.

RILEY, G. (1981). *Stuttering Prediction Instrument for Young Children.* Tigard, Oregon: C.C. Publications.

RILEY, G. and RILEY, J. (1979) A component model for diagnosing and treating children who stutter. *Journal of Fluency Disorders,* **4,** 279–293.

RILEY, G. and RILEY, J. (1980) Motoric and linguistic variables among children who stutter: A factor analysis. *Journal of Speech and Hearing Disorders,* **45,** 504–514.

RILEY, G. and RILEY, J. (1982) Evaluating stuttering problems in children. In H. Luper (Ed.), Intervention with the Young Stutterer. *Journal of Childhood Communication Disorders, VI,* **1,** 15–25.

RILEY, G. and RILEY, J. (1983) Evaluation as a basis for intervention. In D. Preins and R. Ingham (Eds.), *Treatment of Stuttering in Early Childhood.* San Diego, CA: College-Hill.

RILEY, G. and RILEY, J. (1984) A component model for treating stuttering in children. In M. Peins (Ed.), *Contemporary Approaches in Stuttering Therapy.* Boston: Little, Brown and Co.

RILEY, G. and RILEY, J. (1985) *Oral Motor Assessment and Treatment: Improving Syllable Production.* Tigard, Oregon: C.C. Publications.

ROBB, M. P., LOYBOLT, J. T. and PRICE, H. A. (1985) Acoustic measures of stutterers' speech following an intensive therapy program. *Journal of Fluency Disorders,* **10,** 269–279.

ROBBINS, K. I. and McADAM, D. W. (1974) Interhemispheric alpha asymmetry and imagery mode. *Brain and Language,* **1,** 189–193.

ROGERS, C. (1951) *Client-centered Therapy.* Boston: Houghton-Mifflin.

ROHRBAUGH, M., TENNEN, H., PRESS, S., WHITE, L., RASKIN, P. and PICKERING, M. (1977) Paradoxical strategies in psychotherapy. Paper presented at the *American Psychological Association,* San Francisco.

ROHRBAUGH, M., TENNEN, H., PRESS, S. and WHITE, L. (1981) Compliance, defiance and therapeutic paradox. *American Journal of Orthopsychiatry,* **51,** 454–467.

RONSON, I. (1976) Word frequency and stuttering: the relationship to sentence structure. *Journal of Speech and Hearing Research,* **19,** 813–819.

ROSENBEK, J., MASSERT, B., COLLINS, M. and WERTZ, R. T. (1978) Stuttering following brain damage. *Brain and Language,* **6,** 82–96.

ROSENBEK, J. C. (1984) Stuttering secondary to nervous system damage. In R. F. Curlee and W. H. Perkins (Eds.), *Nature and Treatment of Stuttering: New Directions.* San Diego: College-Hill Press.

ROSENFIELD, D. B. (1972) Stuttering and cerebral ischemia. *New England Journal of Medicine,* **287,** 991–993.

ROSENFIELD, D. B. (1980) Cerebral dominance and stuttering. *Journal of Fluency Disorders,* **5,** 171–185.

ROSENFIELD, D. B. (1984) Stuttering. *CRC Critical Reviews in Clinical Neurobiology,* **1,** 117–139.

ROSENFIELD, D. B. and GOODGLASS, H. (1980) Dichotic testing of cerebral dominance in stutterers. *Brain and Language,* **11,** 170–180.

ROSENFIELD, D. B. and FREEMAN, F. J. (1983) Stuttering onset after laryngectomy. *Journal of Fluency Disorders,* **8,** 265–268.

ROSENFIELD, D. B. and JERGER, J. (1984) Stuttering and auditory function. in D. F. Curlee and W. H. Perkins (Eds.), *Nature and Treatment of Stuttering:* New Directions. San Diego, CA: College-Hill Press.

ROSENFIELD, D. B., MILLER, S. D. and FELTOVICH, M. (1981) Brain damage causing stuttering. *Transactions of the American Neurological Association,* **105,** 181–183.

RUBIN, H. (1986) Postscript: Cognitive therapy. In G. H. Shames and H. Rubin (Eds.), *Stuttering Then and Now.* Columbus, OH: Merrill.

RUNYAN, C. M. and RUNYAN, S. E. (1986) A fluency rules therapy program for young children in the public schools. *Language, Speech and Hearing Services in Schools,* **17,** 276–284.

RUNYAN, C. M. HAMES, P. E. and PROSEK, R. A. (1982) A perceptual comparison between paired stimulus and single stimulus methods of presentation of the fluent utterances of stutterers. *Journal of Fluency Disorders,* **7,** 71–77.

RUSTIN, L. (1978) An intensive group therapy programme for adolescent stammerers. *British Journal of Disorders of Communication,* **13,** 85–92.

RUSTIN, L. (1982) The management of the primary school stammerer with parental involvement. *Northern Ireland Speech and Language Forum,* **8,** 15–19.

RUSTIN, L. (1984) *Intensive Treatment Models for Adolescent Stuttering: a Comparison of Social Skills Training and Speech Fluency Techniques.* Unpublished M.Phil. Thesis, Leicester Polytechnic, UK.

RUSTIN, L. (1987) *The Management of Childhood Stuttering with Parental Involvement.* Windsor: NFER-Nelson (In press).

RUSTIN, L. and COOK, F. (1983) Intervention procedures for the dysfluent child. In P. Dalton (Ed.), *Approaches to the Treatment of Stuttering.* London: Croom-Helm.

RUSTIN, L. and KUHR, A. (1983) The treatment of stammering: A multi-modal approach in an in-patient setting. *British Journal of Disorders of Communication,* **18,** 90–97.

RUSTIN, L. and PURSER, H. (1984) Intensive treatment models for the adolescent stuttering: Social skills versus speech techniques. *Proceedings of the XIX Congress of the IALP, Brussels:* IALP.

RUTTER, M., SHAFFER, D. and STURGE, C. (1983) *A guide to a multi-axial classification scheme for psychiatric disorders in childhood and adolescence.* London: Department of Child and Adolescent Psychiatry, University of London.

RYAN, B. P. (1974) *Programmed Therapy for Stuttering in Children and Adults.* Springfield, IL: Charles C. Thomas.

RYAN, B. P. (1979) Stuttering therapy in a framework of operant conditioning and programmed learning. In H. Gregory (Ed.), *Controversies about Stuttering Therapy.* Baltimore: University Park.

RYAN, B. P. (1981) Maintenance programs in progress – II. In E. Boberg (Ed.), *Maintenance of Fluency.* New York: Elsevier.

RYAN, B. P. (1984) Treatment of stuttering in school children. In W. H. Perkins (Ed.), *Current Therapy of Communication Disorders: Stuttering Disorders.* New York: Thieme-Stratton.

RYAN, B. P. (1986) Postscript: Operant therapy for children. In G. H. Shames and H. Rubin (Eds.), *Stuttering Then and Now.* Columbus, OH: Merrill.

RYAN, B. P. and VAN KIRK, B. (1978) *The Monterey Fluency Programme.* Palo Alto: Monterey Learning Systems.

SACCO, P. T. (1986) The exceptionally severe stutterer. In K. St. Louis (Ed.), *The Atypical Stutterer: Principles and Practices of Rehabilitation.* New York: Academic Press.

SCHACHTER, S. C., McINTYRE, R. and ROSENFIELD, D. B. (1986) *Handedness among stutterers.* Paper presented at the American Academy of Neurology, New Orleans, Louisiana.

SCHIAVETTI, N. (1975) Judgements of stuttering severity as a function of type and locus of disfluency. *Folia Phoniatrica,* **27,** 26–37.

SCHLESINGER, I. M., MELKMAN, R. and LEVY, R. (1966) Word length and frequency as determinants of stuttering. *Psychonomic Science,* **6,** 255–256.

SCHWARTZ, H. and CONTURE, E. (1987) *Subgrouping young stutterers: Behavioral perspectives.* Unpublished Manuscript, Northern Illinois University.

SEITZ, M. R., WEBER, B., JACOBSON, J. and MOREHOUSE, R. (1980) The use of averaged electro-encephalographic response techniques in the study of auditory processing related to speech and language. *Brain and Language,* **11,** 261–284.

Self-Help and the Patient – A directory of national organisations (1984) London: The Patients' Association.

SELIGMAN, M. E. P. (1975) *Helplessness: On Depression, Development and Death.* San Francisco: Freeman.

SELTZER, L. F. (1986) *Paradoxical Strategies in Psychotherapy. A Comprehensive Overview and Guidebook.* New York: Wiley.

SHAMES, G. H. (1981) Relapse in stuttering. In E. Boberg (Ed.), *Maintenance of Fluency.* New York: Elsevier.

SHAMES, G. H. (1986) Postscript: A current view of stutter-free speech. In G. H. Shames and H. Rubin (Eds.), *Stuttering Then and Now.* Columbus, OH: Merrill.

SHAMES, G. H. and EGOLF, D. B. (1976) *Operant Conditioning and the Management of Stuttering.* Englewood Cliffs, NJ: Prentice-Hall.

SHAMES, G. H. and FLORANCE, C. L. (1980) *Stutter Free Speech: A Goal for Therapy.* Columbus, OH: Merrill.

SHAMES, G. and RUBIN, H. (1986) (Eds.), *Stuttering: Then and Now.* Columbus, Ohio: Charles Merrill.

SHAMES, G. and SHERRICK, C. (1963) A discussion of nonfluency and stuttering as operant behavior. *Journal of Speech and Hearing Disorders,* **28,** 3–18.

SHAPIRO, A. (1980) An electromyographic analysis of the fluent and dysfluent utterance of several types of stutterers. *Journal of Fluency Disorders,* **5,** 203–231.

SHAPIRO, A. K. (1971) Placebo effects in medicine, psychotherapy and psychoanalysis. In A. Bergin and S. Garfield (Eds.), *Handbook of Psychotherapy and Behavior Change.* New York: Wiley.

SHAPIRO, A. K. and MORRIS, L. A. (1978) Placebo effects in medical and psychological therapies. In S. Garfield and A. Bergin (Eds.), *Handbook of Psychotherapy and Behavior Change* (2nd Ed.), New York: Wiley.

SHAPIRO, D. A. (1981) Comparative credibility of treatment rationales: three tests of expectancy. *British Journal of Medical Psychology,* **53,** 1–10.

SHAPIRO, D. A. and SHAPIRO, D. (1982) Meta-analysis of comparative therapy outcome studies: A replication and refinement. *Psychological Bulletin,* **92,** 581–604.

SHEEHAN, J. G. (1953) Theory and treatment of stuttering as an approach-avoidance conflict. *The Journal of Psychology,* **36,** 27–49.

SHEEHAN, J. G. (1970a) Role therapy. In J. G. Sheehan (Ed.), *Stuttering: Research and Therapy.* New York: Harper and Row.

SHEEHAN, J. G. (1970b) *Stuttering: Research and Therapy.* New York: Harper and Row.

SHEEHAN, J. G. (1975) Conflict theory and avoidance-reduction therapy. In J. Eisenson (Ed.), *Stuttering: A Second Symposium*. New York: Harper and Row.

SHEEHAN, J. G. (1979) Current issues on stuttering and recovery. In H. Gregory (Ed.), *Controversies about Stuttering Therapy*. Baltimore: University Park Press.

SHEEHAN, J. G. (1980) Problems in the evaluation of progress and outcome. In W. H. Perkins (Ed.), *Strategies in Stuttering Therapy*. New York: Thieme-Stratton.

SHEEHAN, J. G. (1984) Problems in the evaluation of progress and outcome. In W. H. Perkins (Ed.), *Stuttering Disorders*. New York: Thieme-Stratton.

SHEEHAN, J. G. and SHEEHAN, V. M. (1984) Avoidance-reduction therapy: A response suppression hypothesis. In W. Perkins (Ed.), *Stuttering Disorders*. New York: Thieme-Stratton.

SHEEHAN, V. M. (1986) Postscript: Approach-avoidance and anxiety reduction. In G. H. Shames and H. Rubin (Eds.), *Stuttering Then and Now*. Columbus, OH: Merrill.

SHENKER, R. C., HUS, Y., RUBIN, A. and MENDELSON, B. (1983) A peer-mediated approach to intensive stuttering therapy for older children: Results of a pilot study. *Human Communication in Canada*, 7, 149–159.

SHINE, R. E. (1980a) Direct management of the beginning stutterer. *Seminars in Speech, Language and Hearing*, 1, 339–350.

SHINE, R. E. (1980b) *Systematic Fluency Training for Young Children*. Tigard, OR: C.C. Publications.

SHINE, R. E. (1984a) Assessment and fluency training with the young stutterer. In M. Peins (Ed.), *Contemporary Approaches in Stuttering Therapy*. Boston: Little, Brown and Co.

SHINE, R. E. (1984b) Direct management of the beginning stutterer. In W. H. Perkins (Ed.), *Current Therapy of Communication Disorders: Stuttering Disorders*. New York: Thieme-Stratton.

SHUMAK, I. C. (1955) A speech situation rating sheet for stutterers. In W. Johnson and R. Leutenegger (Eds.), *Stuttering in Children and Adults*. Minneapolis, MN: University of Minnesota Press.

SILVERMAN, E. M. (1986) The female stutterer. In K. St. Louis (Ed.), *The Atypical Stutterer: Principles and Practices of Rehabilitation*. New York: Academic Press.

SILVERMAN, E. M. and ZIMMER, C. H. (1982) Demographic characteristics and treatment experiences of women and men who stutter. *Journal of Fluency Disorders*, 7, 273–285.

SILVERMAN, F. H. (1981) Relapse following stuttering therapy. In N. J. Lass (Ed.), *Speech and Language: Advances in Basic Research and Practice, Vol. 5*. New York: Academic Press.

SKINNER, B. (1953) *The Science of Human Behavior*. New York: Appleton-Century-Crofts.

SLOANE, R. B., STAPLES, F. R., CRISTOL, A. H., YORKSTON, N. J. and WHIPPLE, K. (1975a) *Psychotherapy versus Behavior Therapy*. Cambridge, MA: Harvard University Press.

SLOANE, R. B., STAPLES, F. R., CHRISTOL, A. H., YORKSTON, N. J. and WHIPPLE, K. (1975b) Short-term analytically oriented psychotherapy versus behavior therapy. *American Journal of Psychiatry*, 132, 373–377.

SMITH, A. (1975) Neuropsychological testing in neurological disorders. In W. J. Friedlander (Ed.), *Advances in Neurology Volume 7*, New York: Raven Press.

SMITH, A. and DALY, D. A. (1980) Neuropsychological assessment: Implications for treatment of aphasic and stuttering clients. Paper presented at the Annual Convention of the *American Speech Language Hearing Association*, Detroit.

SMITH, J. W. A. (1976) Children's comprehension of metaphor: A Piagetian interpretation. *Language and Speech*, 19, 263–243.

SMITH, M. L. and GLASS, C. V. (1977) Meta-analysis of psychotherapy outcome studies. *American Psychologist*, 32, 752–760.

SMITH, M. L., GLASS, G. V. and MILLER, T. I. (1980) *The Benefits of Psychotherapy*. Baltimore, MD: John Hopkins Press.

SODERBERG, G. A. (1962) What is 'average stuttering'? *Journal of Speech and Hearing Disorders*, 27, 85–86.

SODERBERG, G. A. (1966) The relation of stuttering to word length and word frequency. *Journal of Speech and Hearing Research,* **9**, 584–589.

SODERBERG, G. A. (1967a) Linguistic factors in stuttering. *Journal of Speech and Hearing Research,* **10**, 801–810.

SODERBERG, G. A. (1967b) Phonetic influences upon stuttering. *Journal of Speech and Hearing Research,* **10**, 801–810.

SOMMERS, R. K., BOBKOFF-LEVENTHAL, K., APPLEGATE, J. A. and SQUARE, D. A. (1979) A critical review of a recent decade of stuttering research. *Journal of Fluency Disorders,* **4**, 223–237.

SOMMERS, R. K., BRADY, W. and MOORE, W. H., Jr. (1975) Dichotic ear preferences of stuttering children and adults. *Perceptual and Motor skills,* **41**, 931–938.

SPELLACY, F. and BLUMSTEIN, S. (1970) The influence of language set on ear preference in phoneme recognition. *Cortex,* **6**, 430–439.

SPIVACK, G. and SHURE, M. (1974) *The Social Adjustment of Young Children: The Cognitive Approach to Solving Real Life Problems.* San Francisco: Jossey Bass.

ST. LOUIS, K. O. (1979) Linguistic and motor aspects of stuttering. In N. J. Lass (Ed.), *Speech and Language: Advances in Basic Research and Practice, Vol. 1.* New York: Academic Press.

ST. LOUIS, K. O. (1982) *Transfer and maintenance of fluency in stuttering clients.* Short course presented at the American Speech-Language-Hearing Association Convention, Toronto, Ontario.

ST. LOUIS, K. O. (1986a) *Comprehensive Stuttering Therapy Program: Program Manual for Elementary School-Aged Stutterers.* Morgantown, WV: Communication Disorders Center.

ST. LOUIS, K. O. (1986b) The problem of the atypical stutterer: An introduction. In K. O. St. Louis (Ed.), *The Atypical Stutterer: Principles and Practices of Rehabilitation.* New York: Academic Press.

ST. LOUIS, K. O. and LASS, N. J. (1980) A survey of university training in stuttering. *Journal of the National Student Speech Language Hearing Association,* **10**, 88–97.

ST. LOUIS, K. O. and LASS, N. J. (1981) A survey of communicative disorders students' attitudes toward stuttering. *Journal of Fluency Disorders,* **6**, 49–79.

ST. ONGE, K. R. (1963) The stuttering syndrome. *Journal of Speech and Hearing Research,* **60**, 159–165.

STAMPFL, T. G. and LEVIYS, D. S. (1967) Essentials of implosive therapy. *Journal of Abnormal Psychology,* **72**, 496–503.

STARKWEATHER, C. W. (1981) Speech fluency and its development in normal children. In N. J. Lass (Ed.), *Speech and Language: Advances in Basic Research and Practice,* vol. 4. New York: Academic Press.

STARKWEATHER, C. W. (1982) Stuttering and laryngeal behavior: A review. *ASHA Monographs,* **21**, 1–45.

STARKWEATHER, C. W. (1983) Talking with the parents of young stutterers. In J. Fraser-Gruss (Ed.), *Counselling Stutterers.* Memphis: Speech Foundation of America.

STARKWEATHER, C. W. (1987) *Fluency and Stuttering.* Englewood Cliffs, N.J.: Prentice-Hall, in press.

STARKWEATHER, C. W. and GOTTWALD, S. R. (1985) The prognosis of stuttering. Mini-seminar, ASHA.

STARKWEATHER, C. W. and GOTTWALD, S. R. (1986) Stuttering. In N. Cole (Ed.) *A Manual for the Prevention of Speech, Language and Hearing Disorders,* Rockville, MD: American Speech-Language Hearing Association.

STARKWEATHER, C. W. and MYERS, M. (1979) The duration of subsegments within the intervocalic interval in stutterers and nonstutterers. *Journal of Fluency Disorders,* **4**, 205–214.

STARKWEATHER, C. W., HIRSCHMAN, P. and TANNENBAUM, R. (1976) Latency of vocalization: Stutterers vs. nonstutterers. *Journal of Speech and Hearing Research,* **19**, 481–492.

STES, R. (1979) A directive therapeutic approach with stuttering children. In F. Stounaras (Ed.), *Proceedings of the International Symposium about the Stuttering Child.* Rotterdam.

STOCKER, B. (1976) *Stocker Probe Technique for the Diagnosis and Treatment of Stuttering in Young Children.* Tulsa, OK: Modern Educational Corp.

STOCKER, B. and GERSTMAN, L. J. (1983) A comparison of the Probe Technique and conversational therapy for young stutterers. *Journal of Fluency Disorders,* **8**, 331–339.

STROMSTA, C. (1986) *Elements of Stuttering.* Oshtemo, MI: Atsmorts Publishing.

STRONG, J. C. (1978) Dichotic speech perception: A comparison between stutterers and nonstutterers. *ASHA,* **20**, 728.

STRUPP, H. H. (1978) Psychotherapy research and practice: An overview. In S. Garfield and A. Bergin (Eds.), *Handbook of Psychotherapy and Behavior Change (2nd Ed.).* New York: Wiley.

STRUPP, H. H. and HADLEY, S. W. (1979) Specific vs. nonspecific factors in psychotherapy. *Archives of General Psychiatry,* **36**, 1125–1136.

STUSS, D. T. and BENSON, D. F. (1984) Neuropsychological studies of the frontal lobes. *Psychological Bulletin,* **95**, 3–28.

SUNDLAND, D. (1977) Theoretical orientations of psychotherapists. In A. Gurman and A. Razin (Eds.), *Effective Psychotherapy: A Handbook of Research.* New York: Pergamon.

SUSSMAN, H. M. (1982) Contrastive patterns of intrahemispheric interference to verbal and spatial concurrent tasks in right-handed, left-handed, and stuttering populations. *Neuropsychologia,* **20**, 675–684.

SUSSMAN, H. M. and MacNEILAGE, P. F. (1975a) Hemispheric specialization for speech production and perception in stutterers. *Neuropsychologia,* **9**, 19–26.

SUSSMAN, H. M. and MacNEILAGE, P. F. (1975b) Studies of hemispheric specialization for speech production. *Brain and Language,* **2**, 131–151.

SWIFT, W. (1915) A psychological analysis of stuttering. *Journal of Abnormal and Social Psychology,* **32**, 3–13.

SYKES, J. B. (1978) (Ed.) The Pocket Oxford Dictionary. Oxford: Clarendon.

TALLAL, P. and NEWCOMB, F. (1978) Impairment of auditory perception and language comprehension in dysphasia. *Brain and Language,* **5**, 13–24.

TANNER, D. and CANNON, N. (1978) *Stuttering: Parental Diagnostic Questionnaire.* Tulsa, OK: Modern Education Corporation.

TEUBER, H. L. (1979) Recovery of function after brain injury in man. In *Outcome of severe damage to the nervous system.* Ciba Foundation Symposium 34. Amsterdam: Elsevier-North Holland Publishing Co.

THATCHER, R. W. (1977) Evoked-potential correlates of hemispheric lateralization during semantic information processing. In S. Harnad, R. Doty, L. Goldstein, J. Jaynes and G. Krauthamer (Eds.), *Lateralization in the Nervous System.* New York: Academic Press.

THATCHER, R. W. (1980) Neurolinguistics: theoretical and evolutionary perspectives. *Brain and Language,* **11**, 235–260.

THOMPSON, J. (1983) *Assessment of Fluency in School-Age Children.* Resource Guide. Danville, IL: Interstate Printers and Publishers.

TILL, J., REICH, A., DICKEY, S. and SEIBER, J. (1983) Phonatory and manual reactions times of stuttering and nonstuttering children. *Journal of Speech and Hearing Research,* **26**, 171–180.

TORNICK, G. B. and BLOODSTEIN, O. (1976) Stuttering and sentence length. *Journal of Speech and Hearing Research,* **19**, 651–654.

TOSCHER, M. and RUPP, R. A. (1978) A study of the central auditory processes in stutterers using the Synthetic Sentence Identification (SSI) test battery. *Journal of Speech and Hearing Research,* **21**, 779–792.

TRAVIS, L. E. (1931) *Speech Pathology.* New York: Appleton-Century-Crofts.

TRAVIS, L. E. (1957) The unspeakable feelings of people with special reference to stuttering. In L. Travis (Ed.), *Handbook of Speech Pathology.* New York: Appleton-Century-Crofts.

TROWER, P., BRYANT, B. and ARGYLE, M. (1978) *Social Skills and Mental Health*. London: Methuen.

TUCK, A. E. (1979) An alaryngeal stutterer: a case history. *Journal of Fluency Disorders*, **4**, 239–243.

TULLER, B., KELSO, J. A. S. and HARRIS, K. J. (1982) Interarticulator phasing as an index of temporal regularity in speech. *Journal of Experimental Psychology*, **8**, 460–472. Presented at a conference of the Acoustical Society of America, 1985.

ULLIANA, L. and INGHAM, R. (1984) Behavioral and nonbehavioral variables in the measurement of stutterers' communication attitudes. *Journal of Speech and Hearing Disorders*, **49**, 83–93.

UMEDA, N. (1975) Vowel duration in American English. *Journal of the Acoustical Society of America*, **58**, 434–445.

UMEDA, N. (1977) Consonant duration in American English. *Journal of Fluency Disorders*, **4**, 846–858.

VALSINER, J. (1983) Hemispheric specialisation and integration in child development. In S. Segalwitz (Ed.), *Language Functions and Brain Organisation*. New York: Academic Press.

VAN KLEECK, A. (1981) Children's development of metalinguistic skills: Implications for assessment and intervention with language-disordered children. *Communicative Disorders: An Audio-Journal for Continuing Education*, **6**.

VAN RIPER, C. (1937) The effect of penalty upon the frequency of stuttering. *Journal of Genetic Psychology*, **50**, 193–195.

VAN RIPER, C. (1947) *Speech Correction: Principles and Methods*. Englewood Cliffs, NJ: Prentice-Hall. (Revised 1954, 1956, 1971).

VAN RIPER, C. (1958) Experiments in stuttering therapy. In J. Eisenson (Ed.), *Stuttering: A Symposium*. New York: Harper and Row.

VAN RIPER, C. (1971) *The Nature of Stuttering*. Englewood Cliffs, NJ: Prentice-Hall.

VAN RIPER, C. (1973) *The Treatment of Stuttering*. Englewood Cliffs, NJ: Prentice-Hall.

VAN RIPER, C. (1975) The stutterer's clinician. In J. Eisenson (Ed.), *Stuttering: A Second Symposium*. New York: Harper and Row.

VAN RIPER, C. (1977) The public school specialist in stuttering. *ASHA*, **19**, 467–469.

VAN RIPER, C. (1982) *The Nature of Stuttering*. (2nd Ed.) Englewood Cliffs, NJ: Prentice-Hall.

VIVIANI, P. and TERZUOLO, V. (1980) Space-time invariance in learned motor skills. In G. E. Stelmach and J. Requin, (Eds.), *Tutorials in Motor Behaviour*. Amsterdam: North-Holland.

WADA, J. A. (1949) A new method for the determination of the side of cerebral speech dominance. *Medical Biology*, **14**, 221–222.

WADA, J. and RASMUSSEN, T. (1960) Intracarotid injection of sodium amytal for the lateralization of cerebral speech dominance: Experimental and clinical observation. *Journal of Neurosurgery*, **17**, 266–282.

WAKABA, Y. Y. (1983) Group play therapy for Japanese children who stutter. *Journal of Fluency Disorders*, **5**, 303–320.

WALKER, C. and BLACK, J. (1950) The intrinsic intensity of oral phrases. Joint Project Report No. 2. Pensacola, FL: Naval Air Station, U.S. Naval School of Aviation Medicine.

WALL, M. (1980) A comparison of syntax in young stutterers and nonstutterers. *Journal of Fluency Disorders*, **5**, 345–352.

WALL, M. J. and MYERS, F. L. (1984) *Clinical Management of Childhood Stuttering*. Baltimore: University Park Press.

WALL, M. J. and MYERS, F. L. (1985) *Stuttering therapy: Review and critique*. Short Course, New York Speech-Hearing-Language Convention.

WALL, M. J., STARKWEATHER, C. W. and CAIRNS, H. S. (1981) Syntactic influences on stuttering in young child stutterers. *Journal of Fluency Disorders*, **6**, 283–298.

WALL, M. J., STARKWEATHER, C. W. and HARRIS, K. S. (1981) The influence of voicing adjustments in the location of stuttering in the spontaneous speech of young child stutterers. *Journal of Fluency Disorders*, **6**, 299–310.

WARREN, L. R., PELTZ, L. and HAUETER, E. S. (1976) Patterns of EEG alpha during word processing and relations to recall. *Brain and Language,* **3,** 283–291.

WATSON, B. C. and ALFONSO, P. J. (1986) Prephonatory respiratory activity in stutterers and nonstutters. Technical Paper, American Speech-Language-Hearing Association.

WATZLAWICK, P., BEAVIN, J. and JACKSON, B. (1967) *Pragmatics of Human Communication.* New York: Norton.

WATZLAWICK, P., WEAKLAND, J. and FISCH, R. (1974) *Change: Principles of Problem Formation and Problem Resolution.* New York: Norton.

WEBSTER, R. L. (1977) Concept and theory in stuttering: An insufficiency of empiricism. In R. W. Rieber (Ed.), *The Problem of Stuttering: Theory and Therapy.* New York: Elsevier.

WEBSTER, R. L. (1979) Empirical considerations regarding stuttering therapy. In H. H. Gregory (Ed.), *Controversies about Stuttering Therapy.* Baltimore: University Park.

WEBSTER, R. L. (1980) Evolution of a target-based behavioral therapy for stuttering. *Journal of Fluency Disorders,* **5,** 303–320.

WEBSTER, R. L. (1986) Postscript: Stuttering therapy from a technological point of view. In G. H. Shames and H. Rubin (Eds.), *Stuttering Then and Now.* Columbus, OH: Merrill.

WEBSTER, W. G. (1985a) Neuropsychological models of stuttering – I. Representation of sequential response mechanisms. *Neuropsychologia,* **23,** 263–267.

WEBSTER, W. G. (1986a) Neuropsychological models of stuttering – II. Interhemispheric interference. *Neuropsychologia,* **24,** 737–741.

WEBSTER, W. G. (1986b) Response sequence organization and reproduction by stutterers. *Neuropsychologia,* **24,** 813–821.

WEINER, A. E. (1984) Vocal control therapy for stutterers. In M. Peins (Ed.), *Contemporary Approaches in Stuttering Therapy.* Boston: Little, Brown and Co.

WEIS, D. (1964) *Stuttering.* Englewood Cliffs, NJ: Prentice-Hall.

WELLS, G. B. (1979) Effect of sentence structure on stuttering. *Journal of Fluency Disorders,* **4,** 123–129.

WEXLER, K. and MYSAK, E. (1982) Disfluency characteristics of 2-, 4- and 6-year old males. *Journal of Fluency Disorders,* **7,** 37–46.

WHITE, B. L. (1984) *The First Three Years of Life.* New York: Avon Books.

WICKELGREN, W. A. (1969) Context-sensitive coding, associative memory, and serial order in (speech) behaviour. *Psychological Review,* **76,** 1–15.

WILKINS, C., WEBSTER, R. L. and MORGAN, B. T. (1984) Cerebral lateralization of visual stimulus recognition in stutterers and fluent speakers. *Journal of Fluency Disorders,* **17,** 131–141.

WILKINS, W. (1979a) Expectancies in therapy research: Discriminating amongst heterogeneous nonspecifics. *Journal of Consulting and Clinical Psychology,* **47,** 837–845.

WILKINS, W. (1979b) Getting specific about nonspecifics. *Cognitive Research and Therapy,* **3,** 319–329.

WILLIAMS, D. E. (1971) Stuttering therapy for children. In L. Travis (Ed.), *Handbook of Speech Pathology.* New York: Appleton-Century-Crofts.

WILLIAMS, D. E. (1978) Differential diagnosis of disorders of fluency. In F. Darley and D. Spriestersbach (Eds.) *Diagnostic Methods in Speech Pathology,* (2nd Ed.) New York: Harper and Row.

WILLIAMS, D. E. (1979) A perspective on approaches to stuttering therapy. In H. H. Gregory (Ed.), *Controversies about Stuttering Therapy.* Baltimore, MD: University Park Press.

WILLIAMS, D. E. (1980) Talking with children who stutter. In J. Fraser Gruss (Ed.), *Counselling Stutterers.* Memphis, TN: Speech Foundation of America.

WILLIAMS, D. E. (1983) Working with children in the school environment. In J. Fraser Gruss (Ed.), *Stuttering Therapy: Transfer and Maintenance.* Memphis: Speech Foundation of America.

WILLIAMS, D. E. and KENT, L. (1958) Listener evaluations of speech interruptions. *Journal of Speech and Hearing Research,* **1,** 124–131.

WILLIAMS, D. E., SILVERMAN, F. and KOOLS, J. (1969) Disfluency behavior of elementary-school stutterers and non-stutterers: The consistency effect. *Journal of Speech and Hearing Research,* 12, 301–307.

WILLIS, S. G., WHEATLEY, G. H. and MITCHELL, O. R. (1979) Cerebral processing of spatial and verbal-analytic tasks: An EEG study. *Neuropsychologia,* 17, 473–484.

WINGATE, M. E. (1964) A standard definition of stuttering. *Journal of Speech and Hearing Disorders,* 29, 484–489.

WINGATE, M. E. (1971) The fear of stuttering. *ASHA,* 13, 3–5.

WINGATE, M. E. (1976) *Stuttering: Theory and Treatment.* New York: Irvington Pub.

WINGATE, M. E. (1984) A rational management of stuttering. In M. Peins (Ed.), *Contemporary Approaches in Stuttering Therapy.* Boston: Little, Brown and Co.

WINGATE, M. E. (1985) Stuttering as a prosodic disorder. In R. F. Curlee and W. H. Perkins (Eds.), *Nature and Treatment of Stuttering: New Directions.* San Diego: College-Hill Press.

WINITZ, H. (1961) Repetitions in the vocalisations of children in the first two years of life. *Journal of Speech and Hearing Disorders Monograph Supplement,* 7, 55–62.

WISCHNER, G. (1950) Stuttering behavior and learning: A preliminary theoretical explanation. *Journal of Speech and Hearing Disorders,* 15, 324–335.

WOOD, F. (1980) Theoretical methodological and statistical implications of the inhalation CBF technique for the study of brain-behavior relationships. *Brain and Language,* 9, 1–8.

WOOD, F., STUMP, D., McKEEHAN, A., SHELDON, S. and PROCTOR, J. (1980) Patterns of regional cerebral blood flow during attempted reading aloud by stutterers both on and off haloperidol medication: Evidence for inadequate left frontal activation during stuttering. *Brain and Language,* 9, 141–144.

WOODCOCK, R. (1973) *Woodcock Reading Mastery Tests (Manual),* Circle Pines, Min: American Guidance Service.

WOODS, C. L. and WILLIAMS, D. E. (1976) Traits attributed to stuttering and normally fluent males. *Journal of Speech and Hearing Research,* 19, 267–278.

WOOLF, G. (1967) The assessment of stuttering as struggle, avoidance and expectancy. *The British Journal of Disorders of Communication,* 2, 158–171.

WYKE, B. (1971) The neurology of stammering. *Journal of Psychosomatic Research,* 15, 423–432.

YAIRI, E. (1981) Disfluencies of normally speaking two-year old children. *Journal of Speech and Hearing Research,* 25, 155–160.

YAIRI, E. (1982) Longitudinal studies of disfluencies in two-year-old children. *Journal of Speech and Hearing Research,* 25, 155–160.

YAIRI, E. and LEWIS, B. (1984) Disfluencies at the onset of stuttering. *Journal of Speech and Hearing Research,* 27, 154–159.

YEUDALL, L. T. (1985) A neuropsychological theory of stuttering. In E. Boberg (Ed.), *Seminars in Speech and Language: Stuttering, Part Two.* New York: Thieme-Stratton, Inc.

YOUNG, M. (1984) Identification of stuttering and stutterers. In R. F. Curlee and W. H. Perkins (Eds.), *Nature and Treatment of Stuttering: New Directions.* San Diego, CA: College-Hill Press.

ZAIDEL, E. (1979) The split and half brains as models of congenital language disability. In C. L. Ludlow and Doran-Quine M. D. (Eds.), *The Neurological Bases of Language Disorders in Children: Methods and Directions for Research.* Bethesda: NIH Publication 79–440, 55–89.

ZIMMERMAN, G. N. (1980a) Articulatory behaviors associated with stuttering: a cinefluorographic analysis. *Journal of Speech and Hearing Research,* 23, 108–121.

ZIMMERMAN, G. N. (1980b) Stuttering: a disorder of movement. *Journal of Speech and Hearing Research,* 23, 122–136.

ZIMMERMAN, G. N. (1980c) Articulatory dynamics of fluent utterances of stutterers and nonstutterers. *Journal of Speech and Hearing Research,* **23**, 95–107.

ZIMMERMAN, G. N. and HANLEY, J. N. (1983) A cinefluorographic investigation of repeated fluent productions of stutterers in an adaptation procedure. *Journal of Speech and Hearing Research,* **26**, 35–42.

ZIMMERMAN, G. N. and KNOTT, J. R. (1974) Slow potentials of the brain relation to speech processing in normal speakers and stutterers. *Electroencephalography and Clinical Neurophysiology,* **37**, 599–607.

ZIMMERMAN, J., STEINER, V. and POND, R. (1979) *Preschool Language Scale Revised Edition.* Columbus, Ohio: Charles E. Merrill Co.

ZWITMAN, D. (1978) *The Disfluent Child.* Baltimore, MD: University Park Press.

Index

Acquired stuttering 5, 8, 9
Affect-sensitivity 6
Alpha suppression 22, 23, 28, 29
Anxiety 6, 43, 55, 108, 109, 125, 164, 175,
    183, 185, 187, 189, 190, 192, 195, 196,
    204, 236, 237, 248, 249, 252, 271
Aphasia 8, 10, 11, 32
Assessment 53–56, 58, 59, 63, 72, 84, 88–93,
    98–101, 104, 120, 124, 126–129, 134,
    139–141, 144, 145, 167, 168, 172–174,
    215, 221, 225–227, 231, 240, 241, 248,
    265, 271, 273
  Assessment of Fluency in School-Age
    Children 90
  blocks 36, 109, 172, 193, 197, 224
  Chronicity Prediction Checklist 127, 139,
    140
  electroencephalography (EEG) 20, 22–24,
    28, 30, 31
  electroglottography 114
  electropalatography 64
  electromyography (EMG) 29, 36, 119
  Erickson Communication Attitude Scale 120
  Goldman-Fristoe Test of Articulation 98
  Iowa Scale of Stuttering 89
  laryngography 64
  Michigan Neuropsychological Test
    Battery 30
  Oral Motor Assessment Scale 98
  Peabody Picture Vocabulary Test 96
  pneumotachography 64
  Preschool Language Scale 96
  prolongations 36, 61, 64, 65, 67, 68, 70–73,
    86, 93, 94, 102, 103, 125, 127, 139, 141,
    172, 174, 175
  Quick Neurological Screening Test 98

  Quick Test 96
  reaction time 5, 12, 45, 53–55, 112, 113,
    115
  repetitions 36, 37, 61, 64–73, 86, 93, 94,
    102, 110, 111, 125, 139–141, 144, 172,
    174, 194
  Speech Situations Checklist 91
  Stocker Probe Technique 90, 95
  Stuttering Prediction Instrument (SPI) 90,
    95, 102, 103
  Stuttering Severity Instrument (SSI) 89, 90,
    95, 102, 103
  Test of Early Language Development 96
  Test of Word Finding 98
  Wada Test 4, 10, 11, 24, 27, 31
  Woodcock Reading Mastery Test 100
Assessment of Fluency in School-Age
    Children 90
Association for Stammerers (AFS) 198,
    200–202, 207, 212
Asymmetry 22, 28, 33, 38, 41
Attitude change 91, 119, 120
Attitudes 55, 58, 91, 92, 117, 119, 120, 125,
    127–131, 134–137, 140, 142, 144, 145,
    149, 154, 159, 170, 171, 207, 209, 211,
    213, 214, 236, 257, 270
Auditory feedback 7, 16, 109, 118, 119, 237,
    241, 249
Auditory tracking 12
Averaged evoked response 22, 23

Basal ganglia 9
Behaviour therapy 60, 181, 186, 187, 189
Behaviourism
  contingency management approaches 237
  contingent negative variation 12, 28

Behaviourism (*continued*)
  desensitisation 240
  negative practice 184, 187, 193, 194
Biofeedback 29, 119
Blocks 36, 109, 172, 193, 197, 224
Brainstem 7, 9, 37, 38, 42, 51
Brainstorm technique 163
Broca's area 28, 30, 33

Cerebral blood flow 30
Cerebral dominance 4, 9–12, 22, 26, 107, 112
Choral speech 46
Chronicity Prediction Checklist 127, 139, 140
Cineradiography 50
Cluttering 3, 5, 9, 111, 116, 238
Coarticulation 48, 49
Communicative stress 114
Constructive alternativism 148–150
Contingency management approaches 237
Contingent negative variation 12, 28
Core role constructs 151, 159
Cortex 8, 9, 22, 38
Cortical blood flow 24

Delayed Auditory Feedback (DAF) 46, 109,
  119
Deep breath 115, 132, 136, 137, 140, 142, 145,
  146
Desensitisation 240
Developmental theory 107
Diagnosogenic theory 109, 130
Dichotic listening 4, 5, 11, 20, 21, 25, 26, 34,
  112, 123
Differential diagnosis 86, 87, 89, 172
Double-bind 183, 189, 191
Drug therapy 119
Dysphonia 5

Easy onset 57, 58, 132, 136, 137
Edinburgh Masker 119
Electroencephalography (EEG) 20, 22–24, 28,
  30, 31
Electroglottography 114
Electropalatography 64
Electromyography (EMG) 29, 36, 119
Environmental factors 33, 34, 113, 169, 258
Easy relaxed approach, smooth movement
  (ERA–SM) 116
Erickson Communication Attitude Scale 120

Feedback 5, 7, 14, 16, 109, 115, 118, 119, 136,
  211, 225, 227, 231, 237, 241, 249

Fluency initiating gestures (FIGs) 115, 131,
  136, 137, 140, 146, 168
Fluency-shaping 57, 58
Frequency fallacy 126

Genetic models 39, 112–114, 258
Goldman–Fristoe Test of Articulation 98
Group therapy 163, 200, 207

Handedness 4, 10–13, 24, 27, 107, 108, 112
Hypnosis 119
Hypoglossal nucleus 7

Imagery 22, 23, 28, 35, 40, 106, 107
Internal locus of control 238
Interpersonal stress 114, 115, 117
Iowa Scale of Stuttering 89
Ischnophonia 3

Laddering 155, 156, 159, 161
Laryngeal activity 7
Laryngography 64
Larynx 4, 36, 52, 111
Laterality 4, 9, 11–14, 17, 30, 172
Learned helplessness 271
Limbic system 8
Loudness control 136, 137

Maintenance 58, 106, 109, 120, 121, 134, 136,
  167, 176, 179, 203, 227, 228, 237, 240,
  249–252, 254, 256, 257
Metalinguistics 131
Michigan Neuropsychological Test Battery 30
Midbrain 7, 8, 38
Modeling 101
Morita Therapy 183
Motor control theory 14, 17
Motor dynamics 3, 13, 15, 18
Motoric perspective 43, 53, 54, 57

Negative practice 184, 187, 193, 194
Negative thoughts 55
Neurological theory 107
Neurotic difficulty 108, 113
Nonsense syllables 20, 21, 26

Oral Motor Assessment Scale 98

Palilalia 5, 9
Paradoxical therapy 60, 181, 187, 197
Parental counselling 173, 174

Personal Construct Theory (PCT) 59, 120, 147–165, 168
  core role constructs 151, 159
  laddering 155, 156, 159, 161
  Repertory Grids 120, 152–154, 156, 157
  personal constructs 120, 148–150, 152–155, 157, 165
Peabody Picture Vocabulary Test 96
Personalized Fluency Control Therapy 124
Phase margin 16
Phoneme 26, 48, 51, 64, 65
Placebo effect 268
Pneumotachography 64
Pons 7, 8
Preschool Language Scale 96
Prolongations 36, 61, 64, 65, 67, 68, 70–73, 86, 93, 94, 102, 103, 125, 127, 139, 141, 172, 174, 175
Prolonged speech 204, 237, 240, 241, 249
Proprioceptive feedback 5, 14
Prosody 58, 116, 118, 137, 213

Quick Neurological Screening Test 98
Quick Test 96

Range corollary 150
Reaction time 5, 12, 45, 53–55, 112, 113, 115
Relaxation training 177
Repertory Grids 120, 152–154, 156, 157
Repetitions 36, 37, 61, 64–73, 86, 93, 94, 102, 110, 111, 125, 139, 140, 141, 144, 172, 174, 194
Right hemispheric processing 19, 32–35, 37, 39, 41
Role play 164, 175–177

Segmentation dysfunction 39–41
Self-help 60, 133, 198–208, 210–212, 231
Sex differences 39
Single group design 264
Situational variability 46
Slow speech 16, 115, 132, 137, 140, 142, 145, 146
Smooth speech 115, 136, 137, 145, 213, 215–223, 225, 227–230
Social skills training 163, 176, 206
Specialist in stuttering 122
Speech Situations Checklist 91
Spinal cord 7, 8
STAR Therapy 133, 138, 144
Stocker Probe Technique 90, 95
Stuttering Prediction Instrument (SPI) 90, 95, 102, 103

Stuttering Severity Instrument (SSI) 89, 90, 95, 102, 103
Syllable stress 136, 137, 143, 251

Tachistoscopic studies 21, 22, 27, 31
Test of Early Language Development 96
Test of Word Finding 98
Therapy
  attitude change 91, 119, 120
  choral speech 46
  DAF 46, 109, 119
  deep breath 115, 132, 136, 137, 140, 142, 145, 146
  drug therapy 119
  easy onset 57, 58, 132, 136, 137
  Edinburgh Masker 119
  fluency shaping 57, 58
  group therapy 163, 200, 207
  hypnosis 119
  Morita Therapy 183
  paradoxical therapy 60, 181, 187, 197
  parental counselling 173, 174
  Personal Construct Therapy (PCT) 147–151, 153, 154, 161–165, 168
  Personalized Fluency Control Therapy 124
  placebo effect 268
  prolonged speech 204, 237, 240, 241, 249
  relaxation training 177
  role play 164, 175–177
  self-help 60, 133, 198–208, 210–212, 231
  slow speech 16, 115, 132, 137, 140, 142, 145, 146
  smooth speech 115, 136, 137, 145, 213, 215–223, 225, 227, 228, 229, 230
  social skills training 163, 176, 206
  STAR Therapy 133, 138, 144
  therapy outcome research 259
  therapy process research 259
  voluntary stuttering 108, 193–195, 197
Therapy outcome research 259
Therapy process research 259
Trigeminal motor nucleus 7

Unilateral damage 8

Variability 46, 48, 93, 109, 110, 126, 170
Ventrolateral thalamus 41
Voice initiation 36, 112
Voice onset 5, 12, 36, 113, 115
Voluntary stuttering 108, 193–195, 197

Wada test 4, 10, 11, 24, 27, 31
Wernicke's area 33
Woodcock Reading Mastery Test 100